Handbook of Hematology

Handbook of Hematology

Editor: Malcolm Porter

FOSTER ACADEMICS

www.fosteracademics.com

www.fosteracademics.com

FOSTER ACADEMICS

Cataloging-in-Publication Data

Handbook of hematology / edited by Malcolm Porter.
p. cm.
Includes bibliographical references and index.
ISBN 978-1-63242-886-8
1. Hematology. 2. Blood--Diseases. 3. Internal medicine. I. Porter, Malcolm.
RC633 .H36 2020
616.15--dc23

Foster Academics,
118-35 Queens Blvd., Suite 400,
Forest Hills, NY 11375, USA

ISBN 978-1-63242-886-8 (Hardback)

Contents

Preface

Hematology is a branch of medicine that studies the cause, treatment, prognosis and prevention of diseases of the blood. There are various diseases that affect the production of blood and blood constituents. Some of these diseases are rare leukemia, lymphoma and multiple myeloma. Depending on the pathologies addressed in this field, specializations exist in this field such as the treatment of hemoglobinopathies, hematological malignancies and bleeding disorders as well as bone marrow and stem cell transplantation. The field of hematology also encompasses the examination of bone marrow slides and blood films, and the interpretation of blood clotting and other hematological test results. This book elucidates new techniques and applications of hematology in a multidisciplinary manner. It covers in detail some major hematological disorders and their clinical diagnosis and management. With state-of-the-art inputs by acclaimed experts of this field, this book targets students and professionals.

All of the data presented henceforth, was collaborated in the wake of recent advancements in the field. The aim of this book is to present the diversified developments from across the globe in a comprehensible manner. The opinions expressed in each chapter belong solely to the contributing authors. Their interpretations of the topics are the integral part of this book, which I have carefully compiled for a better understanding of the readers.

At the end, I would like to thank all those who dedicated their time and efforts for the successful completion of this book. I also wish to convey my gratitude towards my friends and family who supported me at every step.

Editor

Peripheral T-Cell Lymphoma of the Submandibular Salivary Gland as an Unusual Manifestation of Richter's Syndrome

Vadim R. Gorodetskiy,[1] Natalya A. Probatova,[2] and Tatiana T. Kondratieva[2]

[1]*Department of Intensive Methods of Therapy, V.A. Nasonova Research Institute of Rheumatology, Russian Academy of Medical Sciences, Kashirskoye shosse 34A, Moscow 115522, Russia*
[2]*Department of Pathology, N.N. Blokhin Russian Cancer Research Center, Russian Academy of Medical Sciences, Kashirskoye shosse 24, Moscow 115478, Russia*

Correspondence should be addressed to Vadim R. Gorodetskiy; gorodetskiyblood@mail.ru

Academic Editor: Kazunori Nakase

Richter's syndrome is the development of high-grade non-Hodgkin lymphoma (NHL) or Hodgkin lymphoma in patients with chronic lymphocytic leukemia (CLL)/small lymphocytic lymphoma (SLL). In most patients with Richter's syndrome, the high-grade NHL is diffuse large B-cell lymphoma. Only a small minority of CLL/SLL patients develop T-cell malignancies. Herein, we describe a 40-year-old male patient presenting with peripheral T-cell lymphoma not otherwise specified (PTCL-NOS) in the submandibular salivary gland, two years after the diagnosis of CLL/SLL. The PTCL-NOS consisted of small lymphocytes, which complicated diagnosis. Immunohistochemical, cytological, and molecular studies allowed the correct diagnosis of composite lymphoma (SLL/PTCL-NOS) of the submandibular salivary gland. The PTCL-NOS had a cytotoxic phenotype and aberrant expression of CD79a. There was no evidence to suggest that the PTCL-NOS of the submandibular salivary gland developed from an intimately associated submandibular lymph node or by PTCL-NOS dissemination. A review of the literature and presented case suppose that the PTCLs developed following CLL/SLL have the cytotoxic phenotype and can clinically mimic typical Richter's syndrome.

1. Introduction

Richter's syndrome is the development of high-grade non-Hodgkin lymphoma (NHL) or Hodgkin lymphoma in patients with chronic lymphocytic leukemia (CLL)/small lymphocytic lymphoma (SLL) [1]. In most patients with Richter's syndrome, the high-grade NHL is diffuse large B-cell lymphoma. In rare cases, T-cell malignancies develop in patients with CLL/SLL. Single cases have been described of the combination of CLL/SLL and anaplastic large-cell lymphoma (ALCL) [2, 3], T-cell large granular leukemia [4, 5], subcutaneous panniculitis-like T-cell lymphoma [6], cutaneous gamma-delta T-cell lymphoma [7], mycosis fungoides [8], and peripheral T-cell lymphoma, not otherwise specified (PTCL-NOS) [8–12]. As some of the cases have been reported a while back [13–17], not all the peripheral T-cell lymphomas (PTCLs) have been subclassified as per the most recent World Health Organization Classification [18]. Herein, we describe an unusual manifestation of Richter's syndrome in the form of extranodal PTCL-NOS in the submandibular salivary gland.

2. Case Presentation

A previously healthy 38-year-old man presented with enlarged lymph nodes in the left supraclavicular and both axillary and inguinal areas. Computed tomography also revealed an increase of mediastinal, hilar, abdominal, retroperitoneal, retrocrural, and iliac lymph nodes, as well as hepatosplenomegaly. Peripheral blood flow cytometry showed 2095 B cells/mL with a CLL-like immunophenotype: CD19+, CD5+, CD23+, CD38+, CD79b−/CD43+, and

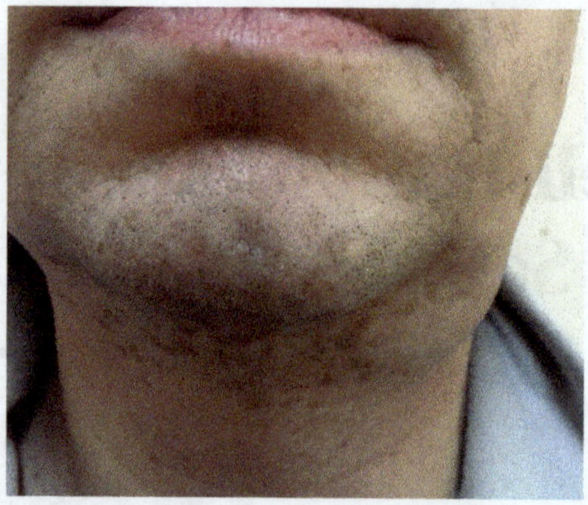

FIGURE 1: A mass in the left submandibular region.

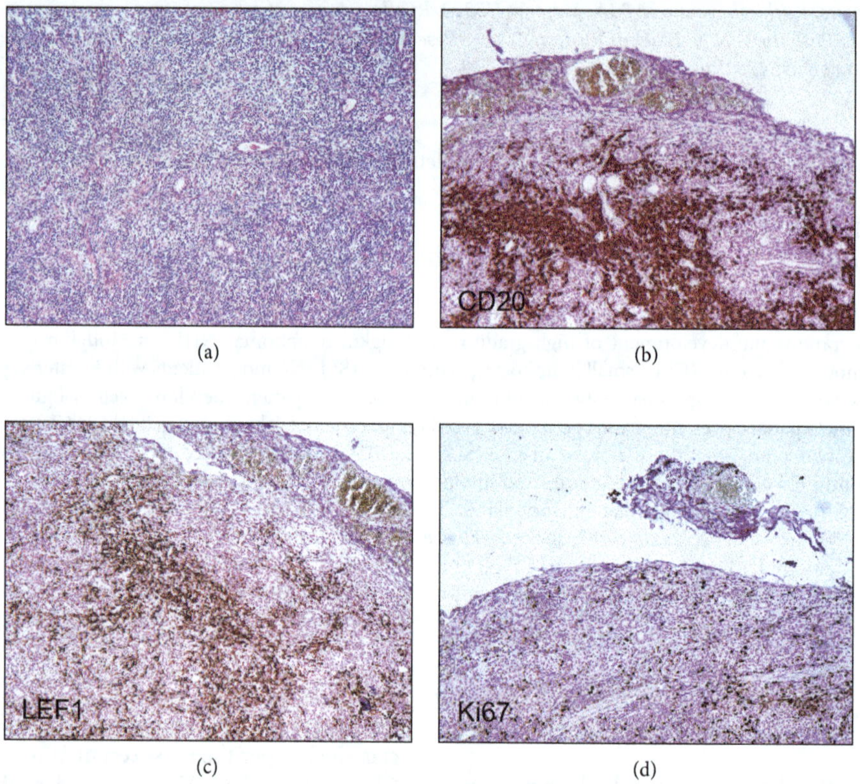

FIGURE 2: Submandibular salivary gland. (a) The architecture of the submandibular salivary gland is replaced by a diffuse small lymphocyte infiltrate H&E staining, ×100. (b) The SLL component strongly expresses CD20, highlighting focal accumulations of CD20+ B cells, ×100. (c) B cells express LEF1, ×100. (d) Proliferative activity marker Ki-67 in the B-cell area is expressed by up to 20% of the cells, ×100.

CD22low/CD81low. Histology of an enlarged right axillary lymph node showed a distortion of the lymph node architecture by small lymphocytes expressing CD20, CD5, CD23, CD43, BCL2, and LEF1, consistent with SLL involvement. Peripheral blood mononuclear cells analyzed by FISH showed ATM (ataxia-telangiectasia mutated) gene deletion (11q23) in 25% of nuclei. A diagnosis of CLL/SLL stage II/B (Rai/Binet) was made. During the next two years, the disease remained stable and did not require any therapy. During a monitoring visit in March 2017, the patient noted the appearance of a dense painless mass in the left submandibular area, which rapidly increased in size within a month (Figure 1). The serum lactate dehydrogenase (LDH) level was elevated to 368 IU/L (normal < 225). Richter's syndrome was suspected. Ultrasound scanning and computed tomography did not allow categorical target organ identification (submandibular lymph node or submandibular salivary gland). Histologic examination revealed diffuse infiltration of the salivary gland tissue with small lymphocytes with atrophy of glandular parenchyma (Figure 2(a)). Immunohistochemical staining showed that only a part of the infiltration, mainly the focal cluster, was composed of lymphocytes expressing CD20 (Figure 2(b)), CD79a, PAX5, CD5, CD23, LEF1 (Figure 2(c)), and CD43. Up to 20% cells

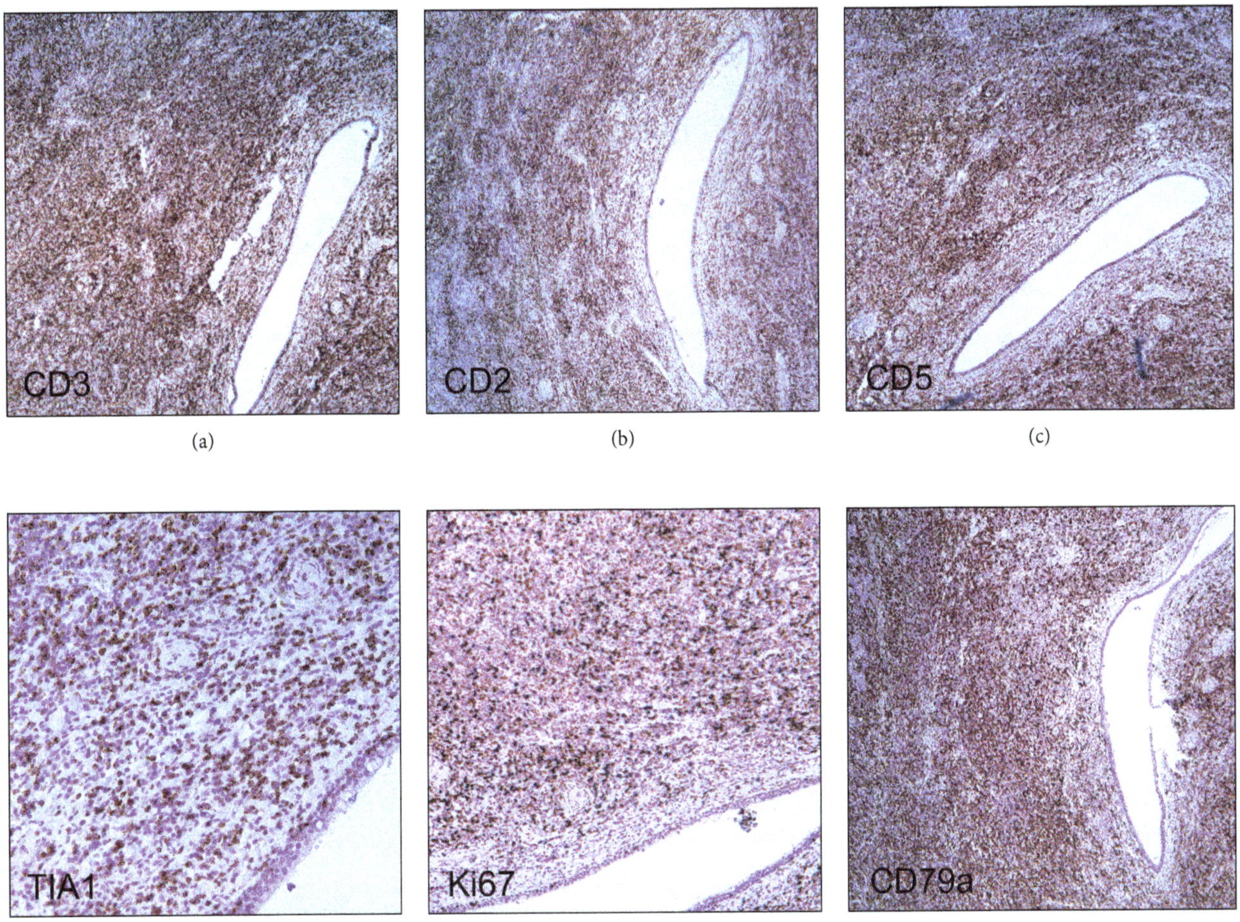

(a) (b) (c) (d) (e) (f)

FIGURE 3: Submandibular salivary gland. (a) Immunohistochemistry for CD3 shows diffuse infiltration by CD3+ T cells, ×50. (b) T cells express CD2, ×50. (c) T cells express CD5, ×50. (d) T cells express TIA1, ×200. (e) Proliferative activity marker Ki-67 in the T-cell area is expressed by up to 70% of the cells, ×100. (f) The neoplastic T cells coexpress CD79a, ×50.

of the focal cluster expressed the proliferative activity marker Ki-67 (Figure 2(d)). The lymphoid infiltration consisted mostly of cells expressing CD2, CD3, CD5, CD7, CD8, CD43, TIA1, and granzyme B and coexpressing CD79a, with 70% Ki-67 positivity (Figure 3). The study of imprints of the submandibular salivary gland showed two types of lymphocytes: one corresponding to CLL/SLL lymphocytes and the other with irregular nuclei and cytoplasmic granules (Figure 4). Study of the DNA extracted from freshly prepared submandibular salivary gland tissue revealed clonal IGH and clonal TCRβ gene rearrangements (Figure 5). A composite SLL/PTCL-NOS lymphoma of the submandibular salivary gland was diagnosed. Positron emission tomography-computed tomography showed an increase in the size of the spleen, right submandibular, bilateral cervical, left supraclavicular and axillary, mediastinal, retrocrural, abdominal, retroperitoneal, and bilateral external iliac lymph nodes, with slightly increased accumulation of fluorine-18 fluorodeoxyglucose (SUV (standard uptake value) max = 3.7) as well as an enlarged pericardial lymph node in the anterior mediastinum (SUVmax = 6.1) (Figure 6). The patient refused a diagnostic biopsy of the pericardial lymph node, bone marrow study, and therapy. Seven months after the diagnosis of extranodal PTCL-NOS, the patient feels well.

3. Discussion

Composite or discordant T- and B-cell lymphomas are uncommon, and T-cell lymphomas associated with CLL/SLL have been only rarely reported. A review of the literature shows 11 cases of CLL/SLL with PTCL-NOS (Table 1). In 6 cases, lymphomas were discordant (CLL/SLL and PTCL-NOS occurrence in separate anatomic sites), and in 5 cases, composite ones (CLL/SLL and PTCL-NOS occurrence in the same anatomical localization). In 4 cases, composite lymphoma was verified by biopsy of the lymph node, and in one case, by bone marrow biopsy. In all cases, CLL/SLL preceded PTCL-NOS, or both lymphomas were diagnosed simultaneously. In our case, SLL preceded the development of PTCL-NOS by 2 years. The rapid growth of an isolated mass in the submandibular region and increase of LDH suggested the development of Richter's syndrome. Histology revealed that the lesion was localized in the submandibular salivary gland. Diffuse infiltration of submandibular salivary gland

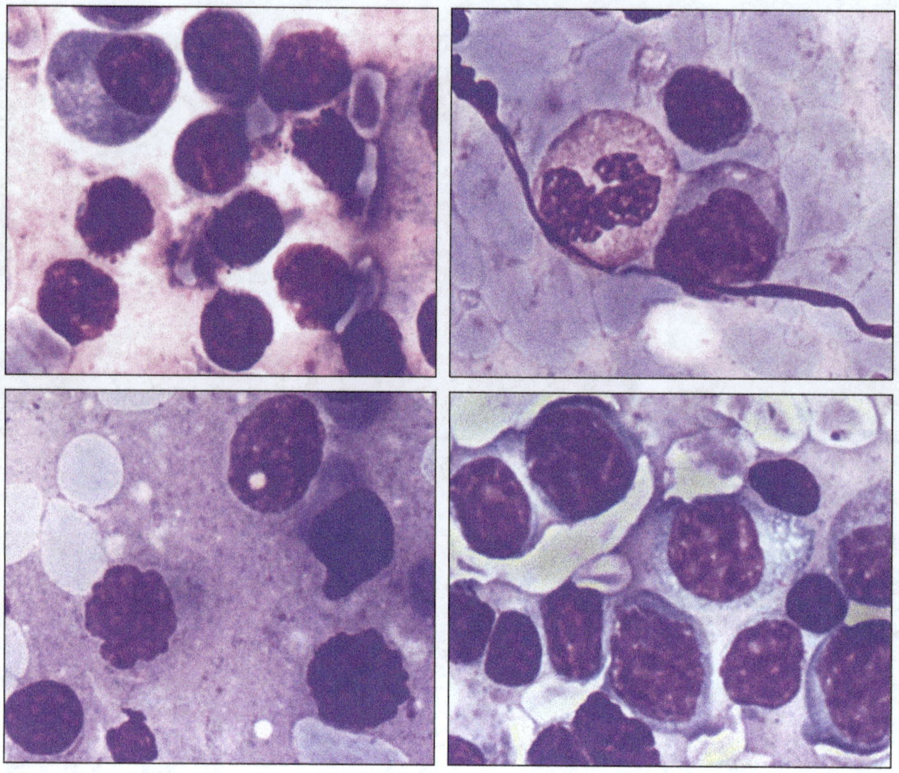

FIGURE 4: The cytology of the imprint of the submandibular salivary gland. Two lymphocyte populations can be detected. Some lymphocytes correspond to the characteristics of CLL/SLL lymphocytes. The others have an irregular shape of the nucleus, and some contain cytoplasmic granules. Romanowsky–Giemsa staining, ×1000.

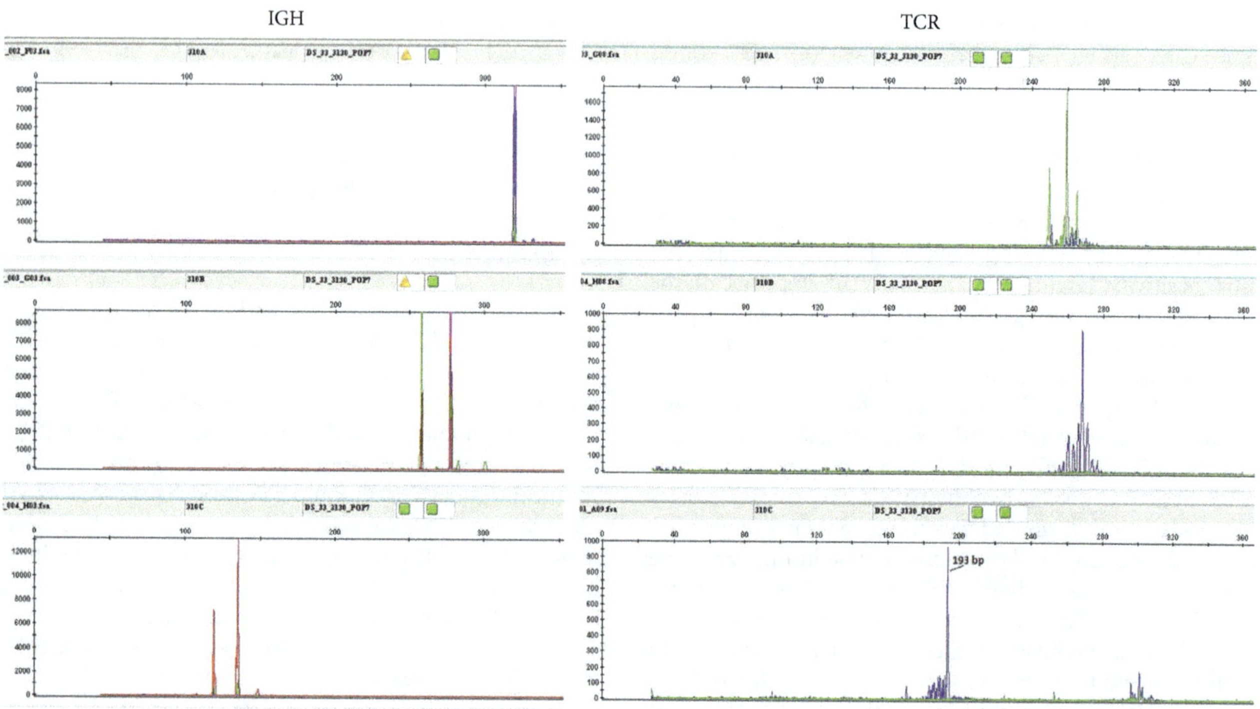

FIGURE 5: Molecular diagnostics of composite lymphoma. Clonality of the B cells and T cells was assessed for IGH and TCRβ gene rearrangements by PCR. Clonal peaks of IGH rearrangement were detected with framework I–III primers. An incomplete rearrangement was revealed of β chain of T-cell receptor: a clonal peak at 193 bp (panel C).

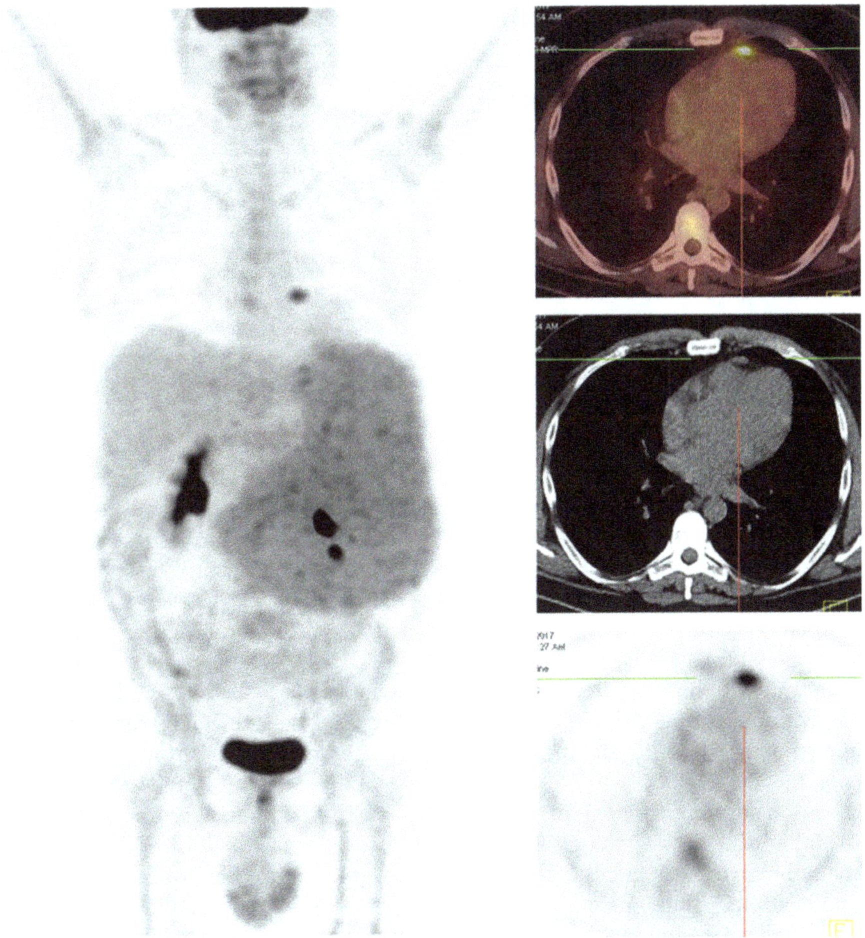

FIGURE 6: Positron emission tomography-computed tomography. Enlarged pericardial lymph node in the anterior mediastinum with SUVmax = 6.1.

TABLE 1: Review of the literature for PTCL-NOS in CLL/SLL patients.

Authors, reference	Age* /sex	Interval, CLL/SLL to PTCL-NOS (mo)	Therapy for CLL/SLL, yes (+)/no (−)	Expression of PTCL-NOS cytotoxic molecules		Discordant lymphoma	Composite lymphoma (localization)
				TIA1	Granzyme B		
Martinez et al. [8]	70/M	156	NA	ND	ND	+	—
Martinez et al. [8]	73/M	ND	NA	+	+	—	+ (LN)
Martinez et al. [8]	59/M	10	+ (PCT)	−	+	+	—
Martinez et al. [8]	73/M	60	+ (IL-4)	+	+	+	—
Martinez et al. [8]	57/M	168	NA	+	+	+	—
Martinez et al. [8]	58/F	ND	NA	+	+	—	+ (LN)
Campidelli et al. [9]	80/M	−	−	+	+	—	+ (LN)
Campidelli et al. [9]	61/M	−	−	ND	+	—	+ (BM)
Buddula and Assad [10]	66/M	72	+ (PCT)	+	+	+	—
Alomari et al. [11]	68/F	84	+ (PCT/RT)	−	+	—	+ (LN)
Boyer et al. [12]	70/M	132	+ (PCT)	ND	+	+	—

*At PTCL-NOS diagnosis; LN: lymph node; BM: bone marrow; PCT: polychemotherapy; RT: radiotherapy; IL-4: interleukin 4; NA: not available; ND: not done; PTCL-NOS: peripheral T-cell lymphoma not otherwise specified; CLL/SLL: chronic lymphocytic leukemia/small lymphocytic lymphoma; TIA1: T-cell intracellular antigen-1.

TABLE 2: Review of the literature for peripheral T-cell lymphomas with aberrant CD79a expression.

Authors, reference	Age/sex	Lymphoma localization		Expression of cytotoxic molecules	
		Lymph node	Extranodal	TIA1	Granzyme B
Blakolmer et al. [19]	77/M	−	Nose	+	+
Blakolmer et al. [19]	63/M	−	Jejunum	+	+
Blakolmer et al. [19]	42/M	−	Jejunum	+	+
Blakolmer et al. [19]	45/M	−	Stomach	+	+
Yao et al. [20]	76/M	−	Left adrenal gland	+	ND
Bo et al. [21]	77/M	+	−	+	+
Matnani et al. [22]	75/M	+	−	ND	ND

ND: not done; TIA1: T-cell intracellular antigen-1.

tissue by small lymphocytes initially suggested SLL origin. Unlike other reports that have described a composite SLL and PTCL-NOS lymphoma [8, 9, 11], in our case, PTCL consisted of small lymphocytes, which precluded histological verification. The discrepancy in the clinical picture (rapid growth of the tumor) and the unspecific histological picture prompted us to conduct further studies. Immunohistochemistry showed a cytotoxic (CD8+, TIA1+, and granzyme B+) T-cell infiltrate with high proliferative activity (70% Ki-67 positivity), with infiltrating B-lymphocytes foci of CLL/SLL immunophenotype showing significantly less proliferative activity (20% Ki-67 positivity). Molecular analysis detected monoclonal rearrangement of the IGH and TCRβ genes in the infiltrating cells. Cytological study of imprints of the submandibular salivary gland revealed two different lymphoid populations. Thus, a combination of immunohistochemistry, molecular, and cytological studies allowed the diagnosis of composite SLL/PTCL-NOS lymphoma of the submandibular salivary gland.

The two lymphomas in the submandibular salivary gland were not clearly delineated, which made it difficult to assess their immunophenotype. Nevertheless, a careful evaluation of the immunohistochemical picture of the composite lymphoma uncovered the aberrant expression of CD79a by T cells of PTCL-NOS. Literature shows 7 cases of peripheral T-cell lymphomas with aberrant CD79a expression [19–22] (Table 2), and in all 6 cases where the expression of cytotoxic molecules was evaluated, tumor T cells had a cytotoxic phenotype. In addition, 5 out of 7 cases were extranodal lymphomas.

Salivary gland lymphomas account for approximately 5% of all extranodal lymphomas [23], 1% to 2% of all salivary gland neoplasms [24], and about 10% of all salivary gland malignancies [25]. Lymphomas of the salivary glands are biologically heterogeneous and inevitably include genuine extranodal lymphomas and nodal-type lymphomas, with the latter arising in intrasalivary lymph nodes [26]. It can be difficult to distinguish between the two types because the lymphoma cells often spill over into the adjacent tissues. The definition of a true primary salivary gland lymphoma is an issue. Schmid et al. reported that if a lesion has no capsule-like structure reminiscent of an expanded lymph node capsule and no lymph nodes, it can be defined as a true primary salivary gland lymphoma [27]. The majority of salivary gland lymphomas are of B-cell lineage. In contrast, primary salivary gland T-cell and NK-cell lymphomas are extremely rare. To the best of our knowledge, only 16 such cases have been reported [28–34]. Nine cases were parotid salivary gland lymphomas (one case with intrasalivary gland lymph nodal origin), 5 were submandibular salivary gland lymphomas, and 2 were sublingual salivary gland lymphomas. Histological subtypes were variable and included PTCL-NOS, ALCL, NK-cell lymphoma, and adult T-cell lymphoma/leukemia. In our case, there was no evidence to suggest that the PTCL-NOS of the submandibular salivary gland developed from an intimately associated submandibular lymph node or PTCL-NOS dissemination.

The pathogenesis of PTCL-NOS lymphoma arising in association with CLL/SLL is not well understood, and several hypotheses may be conceived. It is intriguing that all cases of PTCL-NOS reported in CLL/SLL patients expressed cytotoxic granule proteins (Table 1, except one case where data were unavailable), in contrast to T-cell lymphomas in the general population [35, 36]. In our case, the PTCL-NOS also expressed cytotoxic proteins: TIA1 and granzyme B. Cytotoxic T-cell lymphomas are often associated with chronic antigenic stimulation or chronic immunosuppression [37]. The decreased immunosurveillance accompanying CLL/SLL is well documented, and studies of cellular immunity in CLL/SLL patients have found reduced T-cell function with a paradoxical clonal expansion of CD8+ T cells [8] and increased circulating CD8+ T-cell counts [38]. Theoretically, this could increase the incidence of T-cell large granular leukemia in CLL/SLL patients, but only 2 cases of such an association are described in the literature [4, 5].

The second possibility is the exposure to chemotherapy for CLL/SLL that induces a secondary neoplasm. Information on CLL/SLL therapy before the development of PTCL-NOS was provided for only 7 of 11 patients (Table 1). Four patients received multiagent chemotherapy including fludarabine, one patient received experimental therapy with interleukin 4, and in 2 patients, therapy was not administered (since both lymphomas were diagnosed simultaneously). In our patient, before development of PTCL-NOS, the CLL/SLL therapy was not indicated [39], and we adhered to the wait-and-watch approach.

It is unusual that the patient is feeling well without therapy within seven months after diagnosis of extranodal PTCL. We believe that the total resection of submandibular salivary gland resulted in the complete removal of the primary extranodal T-cell lymphoma. The assumption is supported by the PET-CT. However, we cannot definitively interpret the enlarged pericardial lymph node in the anterior mediastinum with the SUVmax = 6.1. Such an SUV can be observed in the lymph node lesion by both SLL [40] and PTCL as well [41].

We believe this is the first reported case of composite lymphoma (SLL/PTCL-NOS) of the submandibular salivary gland. A feature of this case was the absence of histological signs, indicating the presence of a second lymphoma in the salivary gland initially affected by SLL. The PTCL-NOS consisted of small lymphocytes with a cytotoxic phenotype and aberrant CD79a expression.

Consent

Written informed consent was obtained from the patient for publication of this case report and any accompanying images.

Conflicts of Interest

The authors declare that they have no conflicts of interest.

References

[1] A. M. Tsimberidou and M. J. Keating, "Richter syndrome: biology, incidence, and therapeutic strategies," *Cancer*, vol. 103, no. 2, pp. 216–228, 2005.

[2] T. Liu, M. He, D. L. Carlson, C. Hedvat, and J. Teruya-Feldstein, "ALK-positive anaplastic large cell lymphoma in a patient with chronic lymphocytic leukemia," *International Journal of Surgical Pathology*, vol. 18, no. 5, pp. 424–428, 2008.

[3] G. A. Nai, B. Cabello-Inchausti, and S. Suster, "Anaplastic large cell lymphoma of the spleen," *Pathology–Research and Practice*, vol. 194, no. 7, pp. 517–522, 1998.

[4] J. F. Lesesve, P. Feugier, T. Lamy et al., "Association of B-chronic lymphocytic leukaemia and T-large granular lymphocyte leukaemia," *Clinical and Laboratory Haematology*, vol. 22, no. 2, pp. 121–122, 2000.

[5] A. M. Plata, J. N. Frame, J. Stuelpnagel, T. Juranovic, O. C. Estalilla, and T. M. Jelic, "Development of T-cell large granular lymphocytic leukemia in the course of B-cell chronic lymphocytic leukemia with a causal relationship inferred from a flow cytometric analysis of the bone marrow aspirate," *Pathology Discovery*, vol. 3, no. 1, p. 4, 2015.

[6] J. C. Sluzevich, M. R. Hall, and V. Roy, "Subcutaneous panniculitis-like T-cell lymphoma after rituximab," *Journal of the American Academy of Dermatology*, vol. 67, no. 5, pp. e223–e225, 2012.

[7] J. Guitart, D. D. Weisenburger, A. Subtil et al., "Cutaneous gamma-delta T-cell lymphomas: a spectrum of presentations with overlap with other cytotoxic lymphomas," *American Journal of Surgical Pathology*, vol. 36, no. 11, pp. 1656–1665, 2012.

[8] A. Martinez, S. Pittaluga, N. Villamor et al., "Clonal T-cell populations and increased risk for cytotoxic T-cell lymphomas in B-CLL patients: clinicopathologic observations and molecular analysis," *American Journal of Surgical Pathology*, vol. 28, no. 7, pp. 849–858, 2004.

[9] C. Campidelli, E. Sabattini, M. Piccioli et al., "Simultaneous occurrence of peripheral T-cell lymphoma unspecified and B-cell small lymphocytic lymphoma. Report of 2 cases," *Human Pathology*, vol. 38, no. 5, pp. 787–792, 2007.

[10] A. Buddula and D. Assad, "Peripheral T-Cell lymphoma manifested as gingival enlargement in a patient with chronic lymphocytic leukemia," *Journal of Indian Society of Periodontology*, vol. 15, no. 1, pp. 67–69, 2011.

[11] A. Alomari, P. Hui, and M. Xu, "Composite peripheral T-cell lymphoma not otherwise specified, and B-cell small lymphocytic lymphoma presenting with hemophagocytic lymphohistiocytosis," *International Journal of Surgical Pathology*, vol. 21, no. 3, pp. 303–308, 2013.

[12] D. F. Boyer, N. I. Lindeman, N. L. Harris, and J. A. Ferry, "Peripheral T-cell lymphomas with cytotoxic phenotype in patients with chronic lymphocytic leukemia/small lymphocytic lymphoma," *American Journal of Surgical Pathology*, vol. 38, no. 2, pp. 279–288, 2014.

[13] J. G. Strickler, T. W. Amsden, and P. J. Kurtin, "Small B-cell lymphoid neoplasms with coexisting T-cell lymphomas," *American Journal of Clinical Pathology*, vol. 98, no. 4, pp. 424–429, 1992.

[14] A. Lee, M. E. Skelly, D. W. Kingma, and L. Jeffrey Medeiros, "B-cell chronic lymphocytic leukemia followed by high grade T-cell lymphoma. An unusual variant of Richter's syndrome," *American Journal of Clinical Pathology*, vol. 103, no. 3, pp. 348–352, 1995.

[15] L. V. Abruzzo, L. M. Griffith, M. Nandedkar et al., "Histologically discordant lymphomas with B-cell and T-cell components," *American Journal of Clinical Pathology*, vol. 108, no. 3, pp. 316–323, 1997.

[16] A. Novogrudsky, E. L. Amorosi, and S. R. Gottesman, "High-grade T-cell lymphoma complicating B-cell chronic lymphocytic leukemia: an unusual manifestation of "Richter's syndrome"," *American Journal of Hematology*, vol. 66, no. 3, pp. 203–206, 2001.

[17] J. I. Martin-Subero, R. Siebert, L. Harder et al., "Cytogenetic and molecular characterization of a patient with simultaneous B-cell chronic lymphocytic leukemia and peripheral T-cell lymphoma," *American Journal of Hematology*, vol. 68, no. 4, pp. 276–279, 2001.

[18] S. Swerdlow, E. Campo, N. Harris et al., *WHO Classification Tumours of Haematopoietic and Lymphoid Tissues*, IARC, Lyon, France, 4th edition, 2008.

[19] K. Blakolmer, M. Vesely, J. A. Kummer, W. Jurecka, C. Mannhalter, and A. Chott, "Immunoreactivity of B-cell markers (CD79a, L26) in rare cases of extranodal cytotoxic peripheral T-(NK/T-) cell lymphomas," *Modern Pathology*, vol. 13, no. 7, pp. 766–772, 2000.

[20] X. Yao, J. Teruya-Feldstein, M. Raffeld, L. Sorbara, and E. S. Jaffe, "Peripheral T-cell lymphoma with aberrant expression of CD79a and CD20: a diagnostic pitfall," *Modern Pathology*, vol. 14, no. 2, pp. 105–110, 2001.

[21] W. Bo, K. Mei, W. Zhaoming, Y. Hongtian, B. Yanfeng, and N. Xiaoying, "CD79a positive T cell lymphoma with bone marrow involvement," *Pathology*, vol. 43, no. 7, pp. 737–740, 2011.

[22] R. G. Matnani, R. L. Stewart, J. Pulliam, C. D. Jennings, and M. Kesler, "Peripheral T-cell lymphoma with aberrant expression of CD19, CD20, and CD79a: case report and literature review," *Case Reports in Hematology*, vol. 2013, Article ID 183134, pp. 1–5, 2013.

[23] C. Freeman, J. W. Berg, and S. J. Cutler, "Occurrence and prognosis of extranodal lymphomas," *Cancer*, vol. 29, no. 1, pp. 252–260, 1972.

[24] M. J. Gleeson, M. H. Bennett, and R. A. Cawson, "Lymphomas of salivary glands," *Cancer*, vol. 58, no. 3, pp. 699–704, 1986.

[25] J. J. Sciubba, P. L. Auclari, and G. L. Ellis, *Malignant Lymphomas in Surgical Pathology of the Salivary Glands*, G. L. Ellis, P. L. Auclair, and D. R. Gnepp, Eds., Saunders, Philadelphia, PA, USA, 1991.
[26] P. G. Isaacson and A. J. Norton, *Extranodal Lymphomas*, Churchill Livingstone, Edinburgh, England, 1994.
[27] U. Schmid, D. Helbron, and K. Lennert, "Primary malignant lymphomas localized in salivary glands," *Histopathology*, vol. 6, no. 6, pp. 673–687, 1982.
[28] H. Takahashi, N. Tsuda, F. Tezuka, S. Fujita, and H. Okabe, "Non-Hodgkin's lymphoma of the major salivary gland: a morphologic and immunohistochemical study of 15 cases," *Journal of Oral Pathology and Medicine*, vol. 19, no. 7, pp. 306–312, 1990.
[29] M. James, A. J. Norton, and A. B. Akosa, "Primary T-cell lymphoma of submandibular salivary gland," *Histopathology*, vol. 22, no. 1, pp. 83–85, 1993.
[30] J. K. Chan, W. Y. Tsang, P. K. Hui et al., "T- and T/natural killer-cell lymphomas of the salivary gland: a clinicopathologic, immunohistochemical and molecular study of six cases," *Human Pathology*, vol. 28, no. 2, pp. 238–245, 1997.
[31] S. Wen, Y. Mizugaki, F. Shinozaki, and K. Takada, "Epstein-Barr virus (EBV) infection in salivary gland tumors: lytic EBV infection in nonmalignant epithelial cells surrounded by EBV-positive T-lymphoma cells," *Virology*, vol. 227, no. 2, pp. 484–487, 1997.
[32] W. S. R. Hew, F. A. Carey, N. M. Kernohan, A. D. Heppleston, R. Jackson, and R. F. Jarrett, "Primary T cell lymphoma of salivary gland: a report of a case and review of the literature," *Journal of Clinical Pathology*, vol. 55, no. 1, pp. 61–63, 2002.
[33] T. Miyagi, A. Nagasaki, T. Taira et al., "Extranodal adult T-cell leukemia/lymphoma of the head and neck: a clinicopathological study of nine cases and a review of the literature," *Leukemia & Lymphoma*, vol. 50, no. 2, pp. 187–195, 2009.
[34] N. Yanagawa, M. Osakabe, H. Furuse, K. Maeda, and G. Tamura, "Peripheral T-cell lymphoma arising from an intraglandular lymph node in the parotid gland: a case report and literature review," *Pathology International*, vol. 62, no. 1, pp. 60–64, 2012.
[35] P. Went, C. Agostinelli, A. Gallamini et al., "Marker expression in peripheral T-cell lymphoma: a proposed clinical-pathologic prognostic score," *Journal of Clinical Oncology*, vol. 24, no. 16, pp. 2472–2479, 2006.
[36] E. S. Jaffe, L. Krenacs, and M. Raffeld, "Classification of cytotoxic T-cell and natural killer cell lymphomas," *Seminars in Hematology*, vol. 40, no. 3, pp. 175–184, 2003.
[37] P. Kanavaros, M. L. Boulland, B. Petit, and B. Arnulf, "Expression of cytotoxic proteins in peripheral T-cell and natural killer-cell (NK) lymphomas: association with extranodal site, NK or T gamma-delta phenotype, anaplastic morphology and CD30 expression," *Leukemia & Lymphoma*, vol. 38, no. 3-4, pp. 317–326, 2000.
[38] C. L. Goolsby, M. Kuchnio, W. G. Finn, and L. Peterson, "Expansions of clonal and oligoclonal T cells in B-cell chronic lymphocytic leukemia are primarily restricted to the CD3(+)CD8(+) T-cell population," *Cytometry*, vol. 42, no. 3, pp. 188–195, 2000.
[39] D. Oscier, C. Dearden, E. Erem et al., "Guidelines on the diagnosis, investigation and management of chronic lymphocytic leukaemia," *British Journal of Haematology*, vol. 159, pp. 541–564, 2012.
[40] T. Papajık, M. Myslivecek, R. Urbanova et al., "2-[18F]fluoro-2-deoxy-D-glucose positron emission tomography/computed tomography examination in patients with chronic lymphocytic leukemia may reveal Richter transformation," *Leukemia & Lymphoma*, vol. 55, no. 2, pp. 314–319, 2014.
[41] J. Feeney, S. Horwitz, M. Gönen, and H. Schöder, "Characterization of T-cell lymphomas by FDG PET/CT," *American Journal of Roentgenology*, vol. 195, no. 2, pp. 333–340, 2010.

2

CD56-Negative Aggressive NK Cell Leukemia Relapsing as Multiple Cranial Nerve Palsies

M. Guerreiro,[1] F. Príncipe,[1] M. J. Teles,[2] S. Fonseca,[3] A. H. Santos,[3] E. Fonseca,[4] P. Gomes,[1] C. Marques,[2] and M. Lima[3]

[1]*Department of Clinical Hematology, Centro Hospitalar São João, Alameda Professor Hernâni Monteiro, 4200-319 Porto, Portugal*
[2]*Department of Clinical Pathology, Centro Hospitalar São João, Alameda Professor Hernâni Monteiro, 4200-319 Porto, Portugal*
[3]*Department of Hematology, Laboratory of Cytometry, Hospital de Santo António, Centro Hospitalar do Porto, Rua D. Manuel II, s/n, 4099-001 Porto, Portugal*
[4]*Department of Pathology, Centro Hospitalar São João, Alameda Professor Hernâni Monteiro, 4200-319 Porto, Portugal*

Correspondence should be addressed to M. Lima; mmc.lima@clix.pt

Academic Editor: Kazunori Nakase

Background. Aggressive natural killer cell leukemia (ANKL) is extremely rare and habitually manifests as a systemic disease with multiorgan failure that rapidly evolves to death. The neoplastic natural killer (NK) cells usually harbor the Epstein-Barr virus (EBV) with a latent viral infection pattern type II; they often have a cytoplasmic CD3ε^+ and surface CD3$^-$, CD2$^+$, and CD56$^+$ immunophenotype, and they show complex genetic abnormalities affecting multiple tumor suppressor genes and oncogenes. We present a rare case of CD56-negative ANKL and review the clinical and laboratorial criteria for the diagnosis, as well as the available therapies. *Case Presentation.* A European 36-year-old male presented with acute onset fever, pallor, weakness, and jaundice. He had hepatosplenomegaly, severe pancytopenia, hepatic cytolysis, and very high serum lactic dehydrogenase levels. The bone marrow studies resulted in the diagnosis of an EBV-positive, CD56-negative ANKL. The patient failed to respond to gemcitabine and cisplatin-based polychemotherapy, dying three months later with leukemic meningitis and multiple cranial nerves palsies. *Conclusions.* The diagnosis of ANKL is difficult and requires both clinical suspicion and an extensive laboratorial approach. Absence of CD56 expression on the neoplastic NK cells may impose difficulties in the diagnosis, which requires morphological, immunophenotypic, histopathological, immunohistochemical, cytogenetic, and molecular studies.

1. Background

Natural killer (NK) cell neoplasms are classified by the World Health Organization (WHO) into aggressive NK cell leukemia (ANKL) [1], extranodal NK/T cell lymphoma, nasal type (ENKTL) [2], and chronic lymphoproliferative disorders of NK cells [3], the latter being considered provisionally. ENKTL and ANKL are rare diseases, with higher prevalence in Asia and Central and South America. ENKTL usually present as a destructive tumor affecting the nose and upper aerodigestive tract or any organ or tissue in the body [4, 5]. ANKL is a very rare disease which comprises less than 0.1% of all lymphoid neoplasms [6] and usually manifests as a systemic disease with multiorgan involvement. The histopathological hallmark of these aggressive NK cell tumors is a polymorphic neoplastic infiltrate with angiocentricity, angiodestruction, and tissue necrosis. The tumor cells have cytoplasmic azurophilic granules containing cytotoxic molecules and they usually show a CD45$^+$, CD2$^+$, sCD3$^-$, cytCD3ε^+, CD56$^+$, and CD16$^{-/+}$ immunophenotype and Epstein-Barr virus- (EBV-) encoded membrane proteins; in addition, EBV-encoded small RNAs (EBERs) are usually detected on lymphoma cells by in situ hybridization, and complex chromosomal abnormalities are frequent. The rarity of the NK cell tumors limits our ability to standardize the procedures for the diagnosis and treatment and efforts should be made to encourage multi-institutional registries.

From the review of relevant literature, the patient reported herein is one of the rare cases of ANKL with a CD56-negative immunophenotype, the final event being meningeal infiltration with compromise of multiple cranial nerves; other clinical, laboratory, and biological features were those typically observed in this aggressive NK cell malignancy.

2. Case Presentation

2.1. Disease Presentation. A 36-year-old Caucasian Portuguese male was admitted to the hospital in October 2010, with fever (38°C), pallor, weakness, and jaundice. His medical history revealed chronic alcohol abuse. The physical examination showed hepatosplenomegaly and there were no palpable superficial lymph nodes. Blood counts demonstrated pancytopenia: white blood cells 1.80×10^9/L, neutrophils 0.69×10^9/L, lymphocytes 0.64×10^9/L (no evidence for morphologically abnormal cells), platelets 46×10^9/L, and hemoglobin 6.6 g/dl. Biochemistry analysis revealed markedly increased serum lactate dehydrogenase levels (LDH) 2815 IU/L (135–225 IU/L) and abnormal liver tests: total bilirubin (TB) 1.5 mg/dl (<1.2 mg/dL), aspartate transaminase (AST) 124 IU/L (10–37 IU/L), alanine transaminase (ALT) 62 IU/L (10–31 IU/L) and gama-glutamil transferase (GGT) 107 IU/L (10–49 IU/L); coagulation tests were normal. The abdominal computerized tomography (CT) scan confirmed the hepatosplenomegaly (liver and spleen longitudinal axis of 209 cm and 158 cm, resp.) and did not show other abnormalities (Figure 1(a)).

2.2. Laboratorial Investigation. The bone marrow (BM) aspirate had more than 80% of morphologically immature cells, with a pale or slightly basophilic cytoplasm sometimes with fine azurophilic granules and a nucleus with an immature chromatin, with one or two distinct nucleoli, and the first hypothesis for the diagnosis was that of an acute leukemia (Figure 2).

Flow cytometry (FCM) analysis of the BM aspirate cells using the EuroFlow lymphoid screening tube (LST) and antibody panel for NK cell chronic lymphoproliferative diseases (NK-CLPD) [7], complemented with other cell surface markers, showed that the neoplastic cells were positive for CD45 (high), CD2, CD26, CD38, CD94 (high), and HLA-DR (high, heterogeneous) antigens, and negative for surface CD3, TCR, CD4, CD5, CD7, CD8, CD11b, CD11c, CD16, CD56, CD57, and CD161, as well as for cytoplasmic CD3; in addition, they express intracellular granzyme B and perforin (Figure 3). B cell (CD19, CD20, and CD79a), myeloid (CD13, CD14, CD15, CD64, CD65, and myeloperoxidase), immature (CD34, TdT), and dendritic (CD123) cell associated markers were all negative (data not shown). In the PB there were 10% of phenotypically abnormal $CD45^{+high}$, $CD2^{+}$, $CD16^{+low}$, $CD94^{+high}$, and HLA-DR^{+} NK cells, 19% of which expressed dimly and heterogeneously the CD56 molecule, at levels that were much lower than those observed in normal PB NK cells (data not shown). Flow cytometry propidium iodide based NK cell DNA studies revealed a diploid cell DNA content (DNA index 1.02) and a high proliferative rate (G0/G1 phases: 67.4%; S phase: 31.8%; G2/M phases: 0.8%). Polymerase Chain Reaction (PCR) *TCRG* gene rearrangements studies were consistent with a germ-line configuration.

The BM biopsy revealed a hypercellular marrow infiltrated by $CD45^{+}$, cytoplasmic $CD3\varepsilon^{+}$, $EBER^{+}$ and CD56, CD34, CD20, CD68, myeloperoxidase, and lysozyme-negative atypical lymphoid cells, interpreted individually given rise to the possibility of an immature EBV^{+} T cell leukemia (Figure 4).

The BM karyotype with chromosome banding analysis showed complex aberrancies: 46,add(X)(q27),-Y,i(7q),+8,add(17)(p13),add(19)(q13) (Figure 5).

Infection markers were negative for human immunodeficiency virus types 1 and 2, viral hepatitis B and C, and human T cell lymphotropic virus types 1 and 2. The whole blood EBV load, detected by quantitative PCR for viral DNA, was of 57×10^5 copies/ml.

As no neurologic symptoms were present, central nervous system involvement was not evaluated.

2.3. Diagnosis. In view of these findings and according to the WHO classification of neoplasms of the hematopoietic and lymphoid tissues [1], the final diagnosis was an EBV^{+} ANKL, Ann Arbor stage IVB, high risk NKIPI (NK/T cell lymphoma international prognostic index), ECOG status 4.

2.4. Treatment and Disease Evolution. The patient was treated with a combination of gemcitabine (1 g/m^2 days 1, 8, and 15), cisplatin (100 mg/m^2 day 15), and methylprednisolone (1 g days 1–5) (GEM-P) repeated every 28 days [8].

The first BM reevaluation, performed on day 23 after the first chemotherapy course, revealed 0.5% of phenotypically abnormal ($CD2^{+}$, $CD56^{-}$, $CD94^{+}$, and HLA-DR^{+}) NK cells and a normal karyotype (46, XY). In addition, there was a marked decrease in the EBV load in the PB to 4×10^5 (day 14) persisting at 6.6×10^5 (day 21) copies/ml. Also, the BM aspirate showed 4.1×10^5 EBV copies/ml. These changes correlated with an improvement in clinical status and blood analysis: WBC 5.14×10^9/L, neutrophils 2.78×10^9/L, lymphocytes 0.92×10^9/L, platelets 45×10^9/L, hemoglobin 8.9 g/dl (not dependent on blood or platelet transfusions), TB 1.10 mg/dl, AST 37 IU/L, ALT 39 IU/L, GGT 71 IU/L, and LDH 425 IU/L. A second evaluation of the BM aspirate after the second GEM-P showed only 0.09% of neoplastic NK cells. At that time, the BM biopsy provided evidence for a partial hematopoietic recovery, although intrasinusoidal niches of neoplastic NK cells were still observed; in addition, the BM karyotype was again abnormal, with different chromosomal aberrancies: 77,add(X)(q27),-Y,i(7)(q10),inc[5]/46,XY[15]. Similarly, an increase of the EBV load was observed (42×10^5 copies/ml). Considering the refractoriness to GEM-P, it was decided to change the chemotherapy.

Nearly one month later, when the alternative schema was being discussed, the patient was admitted to urgency reporting loss of vision. At that time, the ophthalmologic and

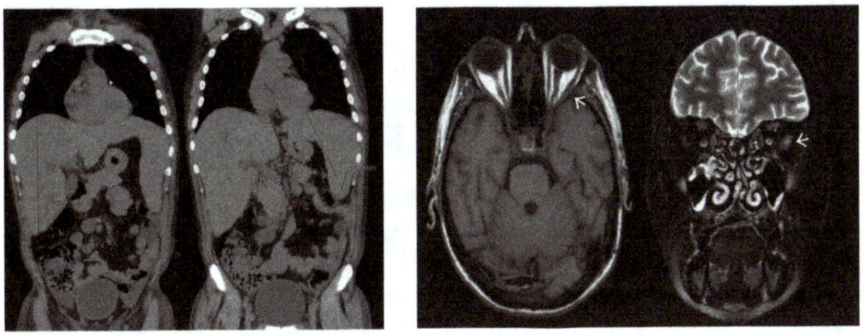

(a) (b)

FIGURE 1: Thoracic-abdominal-pelvic computerized tomography scan showing the hepatosplenomegaly (liver and spleen longitudinal axis of 209 cm and 158 cm, resp.), without other significant abnormalities (a). Cerebral MR images showing swelling of the left lateral rectus muscle on a T2-weighted image, with no other additional findings (b).

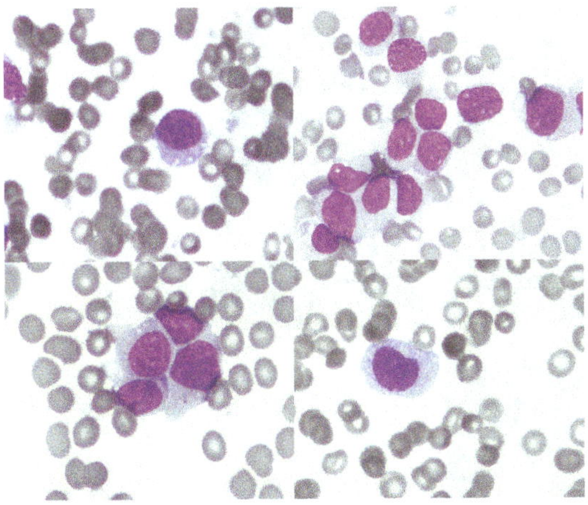

FIGURE 2: Bone marrow cytomorphology findings. Composite image of circulating leukemic cells obtained from Wright-Giemsa-stained peripheral blood smears.

neurological examination revealed an almost total bilateral decline in visual acuity, markedly decreased pupil reflexes, right retinal detachment, and impaired right eye abduction compatible of palsy of the 6th right cranial nerve. Blood analyses were as follows: WBC 4.78×10^9/L, neutrophils 2.14×10^9/L, lymphocytes 1.69×10^9/L, and platelets 155×10^9/L, depending on regular blood transfusions, TB 0.88 mg/dl, AST 34 U/L, ALT 29 U/L, and LDH 429 IU/L. Abnormal NK cells had increased in blood (1.9% by FCM) and there was a marked increment on the EBV load (89×10^5 copies/ml) and on the LDH (1587 IU/L). Head CT revealed a thickening of the right optic nerve, compatible with neoplastic infiltration, without evidence for other abnormalities in brain tissue and structures. Five days later he also developed dysphonia, dysphagia, impaired abduction of the left eye, and left eyelid ptosis and the head MRI showed a thickening of the left lateral rectus muscle (Figure 1(b)). At that time, there was clinical evidence of palsy of multiple cranial nerves (bilateral palsy of the 2nd and 8th left and right cranial pares, left palsy of the 3rd and 5th left cranial pares, and right palsy of the 6th and 7th right cranial pares). The CSF had 262 cells/μl with 88% of atypical mononuclear cells, being consistent with leukemia meningitis. Immunophenotypic characterization was not performed, as on the day of the lumbar puncture flow cytometry was not available at our institution; EBV DNA analysis was not possible due to insufficient sample volume. At this point, no further chemotherapy was administered, and the strategy from here on was best supportive care. Death occurred a few days later, 107 days after the diagnosis.

3. Discussion and Conclusions

ANKL is an extremely rare and aggressive lymphoid neoplasm characterized by a proliferation of EBV-transformed mature NK cells, with a higher incidence in Asia and Central and South America [9]. A review of 73 cases of ANKL published in the English literature, from 1966 to 2003, reported a median age of 37 years at diagnosis and a slight male predominance, alongside acute onset of symptoms and a median survival of 61 days [10]. The largest series were published in 2004 [9] and 2013 [11], and they included only 22 and 43 patients, from Japan and China, respectively. To date, only around one hundred cases have been reported all over the world and the main disease manifestations are in concordance with the patient presented herein. Comparable clinical and pathological features were observed in 3 cases of EBV-negative ANKL that were recently reported [12].

Similarly to that typically found in other ANKL cases, our patient was very ill, with fever, cytopenias, liver function disturbances, and high levels of serum LDH; and, as in other ANKL cases, the disease affected mainly the BM and the PB, as well as the liver and the spleen. During the disease course, disseminated intravascular coagulation and hemophagocytic syndrome (HS) develop frequently, and multiorgan failure finally culminates with death. Unfortunately, the possibility of our patient having a HS was not considered at the diagnosis and, therefore, the criteria for diagnosis of HS were not fully evaluated [13]. Analyzing retrospectively, we verify that although some criteria for HS were present (splenomegaly, periods of fever $\geq 38.5°$, and pancytopenia), some were not

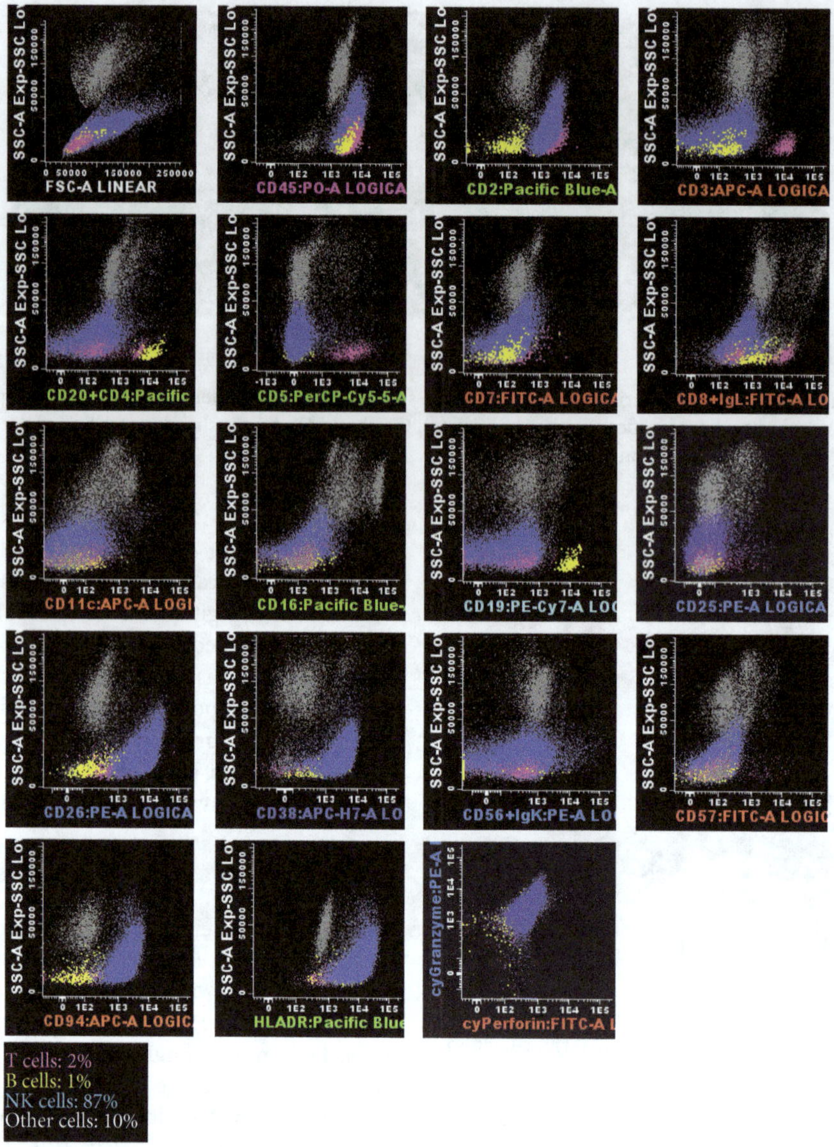

FIGURE 3: Flow cytometry studies in the bone marrow aspirate, using the EuroFlow lymphoid screening tube (LST) and antibody panel for NK cell chronic lymphoproliferative diseases (NK-CLPD), consisting of 8-color combinations of monoclonal antibodies (7), and a FACSCanto II flow cytometer (Becton Dickinson). Data analysis was performed using the Infinicyt software (Cytognos, Spain). Dot-plots illustrate the phenotypic features of the neoplastic NK cells. Blue dots correspond to the neoplastic NK cells whereas pink dots and yellow dots are the normal residual T cells and B cells present in the bone marrow sample. Other cells are represented as gray dots. The abnormal NK cells were positive for surface CD45 (high), CD2, CD26, CD38, CD94 (high), and HLA-DR and cytoplasmic granzyme B and perforin; and they were negative for surface CD3, CD4, CD5, CD7, CD8, CD11c, CD16, CD19, CD20, CD25, CD56, Ig kappa, and lambda chains.

met (fibrinogen < 150 mg/dl and evidence of hemophagocytosis in the BM and liver) and others were not evaluated (ferritin, fasting triglycerides, NK cell activity, and soluble CD25). The available data applied to the HScore proposed by Fardet et al. corresponds to a probability of 30.1% of having HS [14]. In our patient, the final event was leukemic meningitis. Meningeal infiltration may be diffuse or focal, and it may manifest as signals/symptoms of increased intracranial pressure, visual disturbances, or cranial nerves paralysis. It may occur as part of the initial presentation of ANKL was previously documented in two published cases of ANKL with polycranial nerve palsies and peripheral neuropathy and meningitis [15, 16]; more commonly, however, meningeal spread occurs in the form of relapse, as in our patient.

The *immunophenotype* of ANKL cells is indistinguishable from that observed in ENKTL for the majority of the currently used markers, and previously published data would suggest that both diseases originate from $CD56^{+high}$ and $CD16^{-/+low}$ NK cells in most cases [17]. Lack of expression of CD56 observed in this case is uncharacteristic and may indicate a more immature NK cell immunophenotype, as more than 80% of the ANKL and ENKTL cases described to date were found to be $CD56^{+}$; in addition, as in this case,

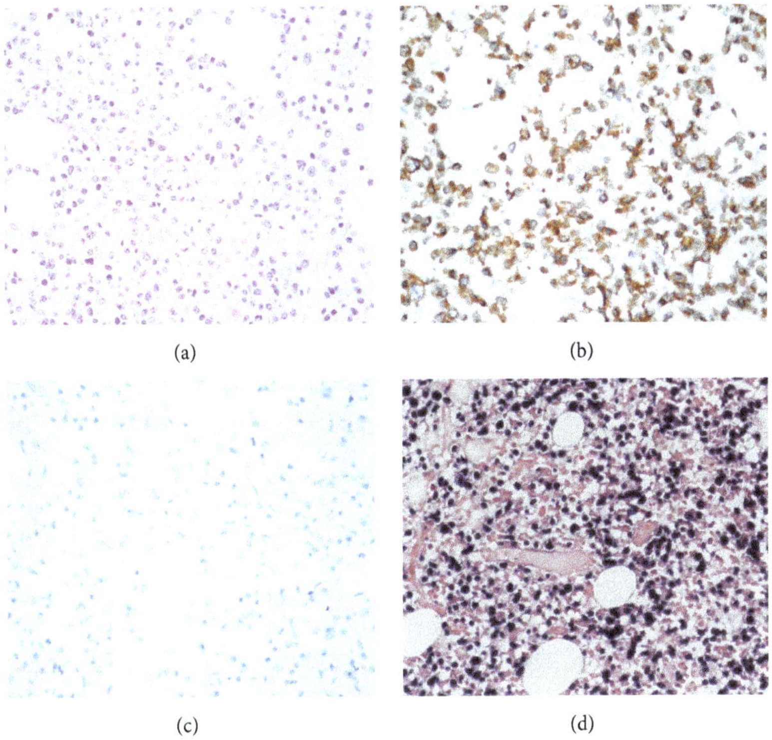

FIGURE 4: Bone marrow histological findings. Bone marrow biopsy section Wright-Giemsa stained (40x) (a). The lymphoid infiltrate is positive for CD3 epsilon (b) and negative for CD56 (c). In situ hybridization showing positivity of the neoplastic cells for EBER (d).

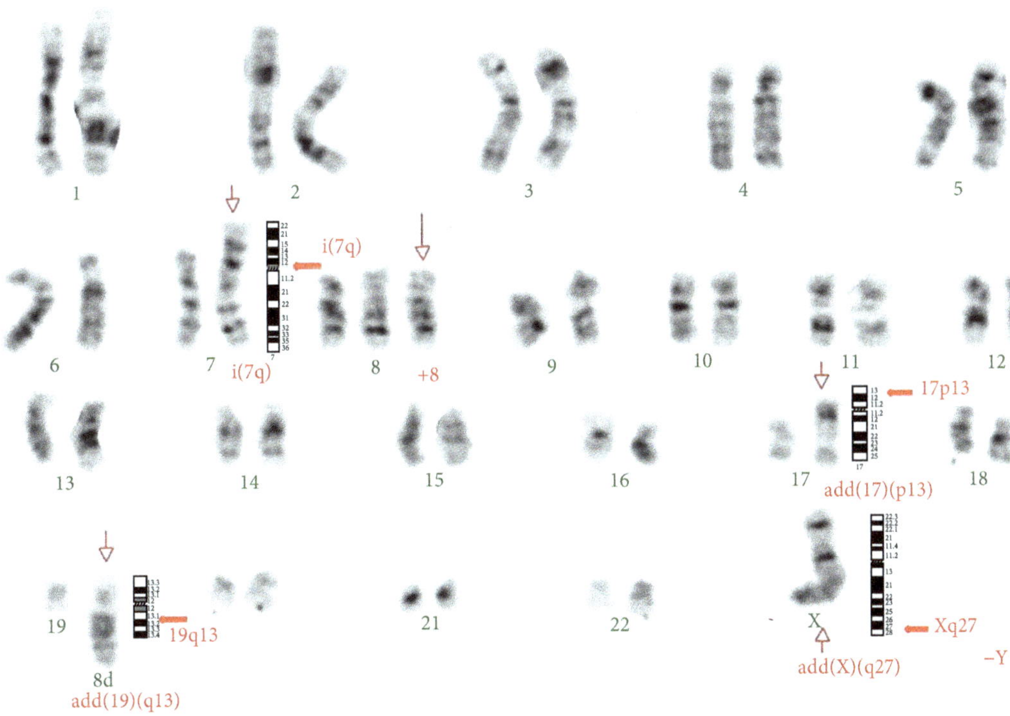

FIGURE 5: Bone marrow karyotype with chromosome banding analysis with complex aberrancies: 46,add(X)(q27),-Y, i(7)(q10),+8,add(17)(p13),add(19)(q13). Arrows indicate the chromosomal abnormalities.

most of the cases tested stained positively for surface CD2, as well as for cytoplasmic (but not surface) CD3ε and cytotoxic granule molecules, and about one-quarter of the ENKTL and half of ANKL cases are CD16$^+$ [17].

A few cases of CD56-negative ENKTL have been reported in the literature [18–25] and case series have included some patients with CD56-negative ENKTL [26–28]. Li et al. found CD56 to be expressed in 90 of 118 (76.3%) patients with ENKTL and that the majority (83.3%) of patients with nasal ENKTL presented with CD56$^+$ lymphoma, whereas patients with extranasal ENKTL of the upper aerodigestive tract were more likely to have CD56-negative tumors (53.6%) [26]. In a large cohort of 288 patients with early-stage ENKTL affecting the upper aerodigestive tract, from which 60 patients (20.8%) were categorized as CD56 negative, Wang et al. observed that CD56-negative ENKTL cases had significantly inferior survival outcomes [28]. In accordance, patients with CD56-negative ENKTL had significantly lower complete remission rates as compared to patients with CD56-positive ENKTL (60.8% versus 80.6%, resp.) and significantly lower 5-year and 10-year progression-free survival (PFS) and overall survival (OS) rates; furthermore, CD56 expression status proved to be an independent prognostic factor for PFS and had a trend to be independently correlated with OS [28].

To the best of our knowledge, so far, no individual cases of CD56 negative ANKL have been previously described in the literature, although a rare case of aggressive T cell large granular lymphocyte leukemia was recently reported [29], and a case series have revealed strong CD56 positivity in all but 5 cases of 43 (88.4%) of ANKL tested by flow cytometry (11). The only case of ANKL published in Portugal was not tested for CD56 expression [30]. Absence of CD56 expression imposes diagnostic difficulties, as the phenotypic criteria routinely used to identify NK cells usually rely on the positivity for CD56. In addition, NK cell neoplasms are sometimes erroneously classified as T cell neoplasms in BM and tissue biopsies, as NK cells frequently have epsilon chains of CD3 in the cytoplasm and, therefore, they may stain positively for CD3 in immunohistochemistry of paraffin sections [31].

The neoplastic NK cells are almost invariably *latently infected with the EBV*, thereby expressing the EBER-1 and EBER-2, the EBV nuclear antigen 1, and, usually, the latent membrane proteins 1 and 2, detected by in situ hybridization or immunohistochemistry on tissue biopsies, respectively. As in the case reported herein, high levels of EBV DNA copies are usually found in the blood [11], and the viral load can be followed up over time using quantitative PCR assays, as previously described for posttransplant lymphoproliferative disorders [32]. Overall, the EBV infection was documented in more than 85% of ANKL cases.

Currently, *genetic abnormalities* specific for ENKTL and ANKL have not yet been identified, although complex chromosomal aberrancies occur in a large fraction of cases [33]. Loss of heterozygosity at chromosomes 6q, 13q, 11q, and 17p is frequent [34], with a recurrent deletion on 6q in the target area 6q21–25 [35]. Consequently, multiple genes are affected, often due to gene deletion, mutation, or methylation, which include tumor suppressor genes and oncogenes [36]. An array-based comparative genomic hybridization study indicates that the genetic aberrancies recurrently observed in ANKL, which include loss of 7p15.1–p22.3 and 17p13.1 and gain of 1q, are different from those found in ENKTL [37]. Among the complex karyotype abnormalities found in our patient, the gain of genetic material on chromosomes 17p13 and 19q13 and the isochromosome 7q might affect genes known to be involved in a wide variety of human cancers. For instance, genes located at 17p13.1 include those codifying for the aurora kinase B (AURKB), a centrosome-associated kinase that plays an important role as regulator of chromosome segregation and cytokinesis, and, for the tumor protein p53, a protein that causes cells with damaged DNA to arrest at the G1 phase of cell cycle (TP53). Deletions on *TP53*, a tumor suppressor gene, are frequently found in neoplastic NK cells and have been associated with more advanced disease, suggesting a secondary oncogenic event rather than a triggering mechanism [38]. In addition, genes located at the 19q13 are the *BAX* and *BCL3* apoptosis related genes [39], genes involved in cell cycle progression that codify for cyclins, such as *CCNE1*, and genes codifying for transcription factors, such as *FOSB* [40], among others [41]. Finally, the isochromosome 7q, the primary cytogenetic abnormality in hepatosplenic gamma/delta T cell lymphoma, where the *TCRB* gene located at 7q35 is affected, was also previously described in 2 cases of ENKTL [42].

Although some treatment algorithms have been proposed for ENKTL and ANKL [43], there is no curative and uniformly accepted approach [44, 45]. Standard anthracycline-based schemas such as CHOP (cyclophosphamide, doxorubicin, vincristine, and prednisone) are known to be ineffective, due to the expression of proteins associated with multidrug resistance [46, 47]. L-Asparaginase, etoposide, and methotrexate based schemas, such as the SMILE regimen (steroids, methotrexate, ifosfamide, L-asparaginase, and etoposide), have shown promising results [48, 49], and a phase II study for evaluating the effectiveness of the association of L-asparaginase, methotrexate, and dexamethasone for relapsing and/or refractory ENKTL has recently been done [50].

This patient was refractory to GEM-P, a gemcitabine and cisplatin-based schema that was previously tested in patients with peripheral T cell lymphoma, with encouraging results and acceptable toxicity [8]. An observational retrospective study on the use of gemcitabine in pretreated/refractory ENKTL has been recently completed, but the results are not yet available so far [51]; in addition two randomized controlled multicenter clinical trials are now evaluating the efficacy of the DDGP (gemcitabine, pegaspargase, cisplatin, and dexamethasone) regimen for patients with ENKTL [52, 53]. The role of stem cell transplantation in the treatment of the NK cell neoplasms has been studied retrospectively by the NK cell Tumor Study Group; results have indicated a possible beneficial effect, but the criteria for transplantation were not uniformly accepted [54]. Investigations on future therapies are under progress and possible targets include survivin [55, 56] and the AURKA (Aurora Kinase A) and NOTCH-1 (Notch Homologue 1) oncogenic pathways [57]; modulation of gene expression with hypomethylating agents [58], immunoconjugates of anti-CD56 monoclonal antibodies [59], and inhibitors of tubule polymerization [42] are other possibilities.

In conclusion, the rarity of the ANKL and its clinical aggressiveness limit our ability to standardize the procedures for the diagnosis and clinical management and efforts should be made to encourage multi-institutional registries and clinical trials. CD56-negative cases impose diagnostic difficulties, being correctly diagnosed only if the immunophenotype of the neoplastic cells is exhaustively studied.

Consent

Written informed consent was obtained from the patient's next of kin for publication of this case report and any accompanying images.

Conflicts of Interest

The authors declare that there are no conflicts of interest regarding the publication of this paper.

Authors' Contributions

M. Lima contributed to flow cytometry data analysis and interpretation, literature review, and manuscript writing, review, and final approval; M. Guerreiro contributed to patient observation and treatment, acquisition of clinical and laboratorial data, and manuscript writing; S. Fonseca contributed to flow cytometry DNA studies and NK cell immunophenotyping; A. H. Santos contributed to flow cytometry NK cell immunophenotyping; M. J. Teles and C. Marques contributed to flow cytometry immunophenotyping; E. Fonseca contributed to histology; P. Gomes contributed to karyotype; F. Príncipe contributed to patient observation and treatment and manuscript review. All authors read and approved the final manuscript.

Acknowledgments

Funds were obtained from the participating institutions. The author thanks are due to the other medical doctors and laboratory technicians from the Departments of Hematology and Pathology of Centro Hospitalar de São João and Centro Hospitalar do Porto, for the support and collaboration concerning the diagnosis and patient care.

References

[1] J. Chan, E. Jan, E. Ralfkiaer et al., "Aggressive NK-cell leukaemia," in *World Health Organization Classification of Tumours of Haematopoietic and Lymphoid Tissues*, S. Swerdlow, E. Campo, N. Harris et al., Eds., pp. 276-267, International Agency for Research on Cancer (IARC) Press, Lyon, France, 4th edition, 2008.

[2] J. Chan, L. Quintanilla-Martinez, J. Ferry et al., "Extranodal NK/T-cell lymphoma, nasal type," in *World Health Organization Classification of Tumours of Haematopoietic and Lymphoid Tissues*, S. Swerdlow, E. Campo, N. Harris et al., Eds., pp. 285–288, International Agency for Research on Cancer (IARC) Press, Lyon, France, 4th edition, 2008.

[3] N. Villamor, L. Chan, and K. Foucar, "Chronic lymphoproliferative disorders of NK cells," in *World Health Organization Classification of Tumours of Haematopoietic and Lymphoid Tissues*, S. Swerdlow, E. Campo, N. Harris et al., Eds., pp. 274-275, International Agency for Research on Cancer (IARC) Press, Lyon, France, 4th edition, 2008.

[4] M. Lima, C. Gonçalves, M. Dos Anjos Teixeira et al., "Aggressive natural-killer cell lymphoma presenting with skin lesions, breast nodule, suprarenal masses and life-threatening pericardial and pleural effusions," *Leukemia and Lymphoma*, vol. 42, no. 6, pp. 1385–1391, 2001.

[5] M. Lima, A. Spínola, S. Fonseca et al., "Aggressive mature natural killer cell neoplasms: report on a series of 12 European patients with emphasis on flow cytometry based immunophenotype and DNA content of neoplastic natural killer cells," *Leukemia & Lymphoma*, vol. 56, no. 1, pp. 103–112, 2015.

[6] J. K. C. Chan, E. S. Jane, E. Ralfkiaer, and Y. H. Ko, "Aggressive NK-cell leukaemia," in *World Health Organization Classification of Tumours of Haematopoieticand Lymphoid Tissues*, S. Swerdlow, E. Campo, N. Harris et al., Eds., pp. 276-277, International Agency for Research on Cancer (IARC) Press, Lyon, France, 4th edition, 2008.

[7] J. J. M. Van Dongen, L. Lhermitte, S. Böttcher et al., "EuroFlow antibody panels for standardized n-dimensional flow cytometric immunophenotyping of normal, reactive and malignant leukocytes," *Leukemia*, vol. 26, no. 9, pp. 1908–1975, 2012.

[8] H.-T. Arkenau, G. Chong, D. Cunningham et al., "Gemcitabine, cisplatin and methylprednisolone for the treatment of patients with peripheral T-cell lymphoma: the Royal Marsden Hospital experience," *Haematologica*, vol. 92, no. 2, pp. 271-272, 2007.

[9] R. Suzuki, J. Suzumiya, S. Nakamura et al., "Aggressive natural killer-cell leukemia revisited: Large granular lymphocyte leukemia of cytotoxic NK cells," *Leukemia*, vol. 18, no. 4, pp. 763–770, 2004.

[10] A. K. Ruskova, R. Thula, and G. T. C. Chan, "Aggressive natural killer-cell leukemia: Report of five cases and review of the literature," *Leukemia and Lymphoma*, vol. 45, no. 12, pp. 2427–2438, 2004.

[11] N.-G. Jiang, Y.-M. Jin, Q. Niu, T.-T. Zeng, J. Su, and H.-L. Zhu, "Flow cytometric immunophenotyping is of great value to diagnosis of natural killer cell neoplasms involving bone marrow and peripheral blood," *Annals of Hematology*, vol. 92, no. 1, pp. 89–96, 2013.

[12] J. Gao, A. Behdad, P. Ji, K. L. Wolniak, O. Frankfurt, and Y. Chen, "EBV-negative aggressive NK-cell leukemia/lymphoma: a clinical and pathological study from a single institution," *Modern Pathology*, vol. 30, no. 8, pp. 1100–1115, 2017.

[13] J.-I. Henter, A. Horne, M. Aric, and M. Aricó, "HLH-2004: diagnostic and therapeutic guidelines for hemophagocytic lymphohistiocytosis," *Pediatric Blood Cancer*, vol. 48, no. 2, pp. 124–131, 2007.

[14] L. Fardet, L. Galicier, O. Lambotte et al., "Development and validation of the HScore, a score for the diagnosis of reactive hemophagocytic syndrome," *Arthritis & Rheumatology*, vol. 66, no. 9, pp. 2613–2620, 2014.

[15] S. Taniguchi, M. Machi, and Y. Ohno, "Epstein-Barr virus-associated CD3- large granular lymphocyte leukemia presenting with polycranial nerve palsies [5]," *Blood*, vol. 87, no. 11, pp. 4914-4915, 1996.

[16] D. Lackowski, J. L. Koberda, T. G. DeLoughery, and Y. So, "Natural killer cell leukemia as a cause of peripheral neuropathy and meningitis: Case report," *Neurology*, vol. 51, no. 2, pp. 640-641, 1998.

[17] M. Lima, "Extranodal NK/T cell lymphoma and aggressive NK cell leukaemia: Evidence for their origin on CD56+bright CD16-/+dim NK cells," *Pathology*, vol. 47, no. 6, pp. 503–514, 2015.

[18] B. H. Chang, L. Stork, and G. Fan, "A unique case of adolescent CD56-negative extranodal NK/T-cell lymphoma, nasal type," *Pediatric and Developmental Pathology*, vol. 11, no. 1, pp. 50–54, 2008.

[19] B. Chang, L. Stork, and G. Fan, "A unique case of Adolescent CD56-negative nasal extranodal NK/T-cell Lymphoma," *Pediatric and Developmental Pathology*, vol. 11, no. 4, article 325, 2006.

[20] P. Katsaounis, A. Alexopoulou, S. P. Dourakis et al., "An extranodal NK/T cell lymphoma, nasal type, with specific immunophenotypic and genotypic features," *International Journal of Hematology*, vol. 88, no. 2, pp. 202–205, 2008.

[21] M. X. Lan, Z. X. Zhen, and W. H. Ming, "CD56-negative extranodal nasal type of natural killerT-cell lymphoma with extranasal skin involvement," *Leukemia and Lymphoma*, vol. 50, no. 10, pp. 1715–1717, 2009.

[22] R. R. Miles, Z. Afify, and H. Yaish, "CD56-negative extranodal nasal type NK/T-cell lymphoma," *Pediatric Blood Cancer*, vol. 55, no. 1, pp. 186–189, 2010.

[23] R. R. Pine, J. D. Clark, and J. A. Sokol, "CD56 negative extranodal NK/T-cell lymphoma of the orbit mimicking orbital cellulitis," *Orbit*, vol. 32, no. 1, pp. 45–48, 2013.

[24] Y.-S. Baek, S.-H. Shin, H.-G. Yi et al., "Cardiac involvement in CD56 negative primary pancreatic extranodal NK/T-cell lymphoma, nasal type, presenting with ventricular tachycardia during the early stages of chemotherapy," *Internal Medicine*, vol. 53, no. 20, pp. 2333–2336, 2014.

[25] H. J. Kim, S. H. Kim, and S. H. Oh, "CD56-negative extranodal NK/T-cell lymphoma, nasal type, with extranasal cutaneous involvement," *Annals of Dermatology*, vol. 27, no. 5, pp. 618–620, 2015.

[26] Y.-X. Li, H. Wang, X.-L. Feng et al., "Immunophenotypic characteristics and clinical relevance of CD56+ and CD56- extranodal nasal-type natural killer/T-cell lymphoma," *Leukemia and Lymphoma*, vol. 52, no. 3, pp. 417–424, 2011.

[27] T. Pongpruttipan, T. Kummalue, A. Bedavanija et al., "Aberrant antigenic expression in extranodal NK/T-cell lymphoma: A multi-parameter study from Thailand," *Diagnostic Pathology*, vol. 6, no. 1, article 79, 2011.

[28] L. Wang, Z. Wang, Z.-J. Xia, Y. Lu, H.-Q. Huang, and Y.-J. Zhang, "CD56-negative extranodal NK/T cell lymphoma should be regarded as a distinct subtype with poor prognosis," *Tumor Biology*, vol. 36, no. 10, pp. 7717–7723, 2015.

[29] M. T. Sylvia, S. E. Jacob, and D. Basu, "CD56 Negative Aggressive T Cell Large Granular Lymphocytic Leukemia," *Indian Journal of Hematology Blood Transfusion*, vol. 32, pp. 121–124, 2016.

[30] J. Sousa, L. Cabezuelo, and S. Almeida, "Aggressive NK/T cell leukemia/lymphoma associated with EBV," *Acta Médica Portuguesa*, vol. 24, supplement 3, pp. 649–652, 2011.

[31] K. Gaal, N. C. J. Sun, A. M. Hernandez, and D. A. Arber, "Sinonasal NK/T-cell lymphomas in the United States," *American Journal of Surgical Pathology*, vol. 24, no. 11, pp. 1511–1517, 2000.

[32] M. L. Gulley and W. Tang, "Using epstein-barr viral load assays to diagnose, monitor, and prevent posttransplant lymphoproliferative disorder," *Clinical Microbiology Reviews*, vol. 23, no. 2, pp. 350–366, 2010.

[33] X. Liang and D. K. Graham, "Natural killer cell neoplasms," *Cancer*, vol. 112, no. 7, pp. 1425–1436, 2008.

[34] L. L. Siu, V. Chan, J. K. Chan, K. Wong, R. Liang, and Y. Kwong, "Consistent Patterns of Allelic Loss in Natural Killer Cell Lymphoma," *The American Journal of Pathology*, vol. 157, no. 6, pp. 1803–1809, 2000.

[35] H. S. Sun, I.-J. Su, Y.-C. Lin, J.-S. Chen, and S.-Y. Fang, "A 2.6 Mb interval on chromosome 6q25.2-q25.3 is commonly deleted in human nasal natural killer/T-cell lymphoma," *British Journal of Haematology*, vol. 122, no. 4, pp. 590–599, 2003.

[36] Y. Huang, A. de Reyniès, L. de Leval et al., "Gene expression profiling identifies emerging oncogenic pathways operating in extranodal NK/T-cell lymphoma, nasal type," *Blood*, vol. 115, no. 6, pp. 1226–1237, 2010.

[37] Y. Nakashima, H. Tagawa, R. Suzuki et al., "Genome-wide array-based comparative genomic hybridization of natural killer cell lymphoma/leukemia: different genomic alteration patterns of aggressive NK-cell leukemia and extranodal NK/T-cell lymphoma, nasal type," *Genes Chromosomes and Cancer*, vol. 44, no. 3, pp. 247–255, 2005.

[38] L. Quintanilla-Martinez, M. Kremer, G. Keller et al., "p53 mutations in nasal natural killer/t-cell lymphoma from mexico: Association with large cell morphology and advanced disease," *American Journal of Pathology*, vol. 159, no. 6, Article ID 63061, pp. 2095–2105, 2001.

[39] F. Llambi and D. R. Green, "Apoptosis and oncogenesis: give and take in the BCL-2 family," *Current Opinion in Genetics Development*, vol. 21, no. 1, pp. 12–20, 2011.

[40] R. Eferl and E. F. Wagner, "AP-1: a double-edged sword in tumorigenesis," *Nature Reviews Cancer*, vol. 3, no. 11, pp. 859–868, 2003.

[41] "Cancer Genetics Web," http://www.cancer-genetics.org.

[42] A. L. Feldman, M. Law, K. L. Grogg et al., "Incidence of TCR and TCL1 gene translocations and isochromosome 7q in peripheral T-cell lymphomas using fluorescence in situ hybridization," *American Journal of Clinical Pathology*, vol. 130, no. 2, pp. 178–185, 2008.

[43] E. Tse and Y.-L. Kwong, "Treatment algorithms for mature T-cell and natural killer-cell neoplasms," *Future Oncology*, vol. 7, no. 9, pp. 1101–1112, 2011.

[44] K. Oshimi, "Progress in understanding and managing natural killer-cell malignancies," *British Journal of Haematology*, vol. 139, no. 4, pp. 532–544, 2007.

[45] R. Suzuki, "Treatment of advanced extranodal NK/T cell lymphoma, nasal-type and aggressive NK-cell leukemia," *International Journal of Hematology*, vol. 92, no. 5, pp. 697–701, 2010.

[46] A. Saglam, M. Hayran, and A. H. Uner, "Immunohistochemical expression of multidrug resistance proteins in mature T/NK-cell lymphomas," *APMIS*, vol. 116, no. 9, pp. 791–800, 2008.

[47] W.-T. Huang, C.-C. Huang, S.-W. Weng, and H.-L. Eng, "Expression of the multidrug resistance protein MRP and the lung-resistance protein LRP in nasal NK/T cell lymphoma: Further exploring the role of P53 and WT1 gene," *Pathology*, vol. 41, no. 2, pp. 127–132, 2009.

[48] M. Yamaguchi, Y.-L. Kwong, W. S. Kim et al., "Phase II study of SMILE chemotherapy for newly diagnosed stage IV, relapsed, or refractory extranodal Natural Killer (NK)/T-cell lymphoma, nasal type: The NK-cell tumor study group study," *Journal of Clinical Oncology*, vol. 29, no. 33, pp. 4410–4416, 2011.

[49] Y.-L. Kwong, W. S. Kim, S. T. Lim et al., "SMILE for natural killer/T-cell lymphoma: analysis of safety and efficacy from the Asia Lymphoma Study Group," *Blood*, vol. 120, no. 15, pp. 2973–2980, 2012.

[50] "Association of L-asparaginase-Methotrexate-Dexamethasone for Nasal and Nasal-type Natural Killer (NK)-T-cell Lymphoma," ClinicalTrials.gov identifier:NCT00283985, 2017, https://clinicaltrials.gov/ct2/show/NCT00283985.

[51] "Gemcitabine in NK/T Cell Lymphoma," ClinicalTrials.gov identifier: NCT01660568, 2017, https://clinicaltrials.gov/ct2/show/NCT01660568.

[52] "Treatment of Natural Killer/T Cell Lymphoma-I/II (CTTNKTL-I/II)," ClinicalTrials.gov identifier: NCT01501136, 2017, https://clinicaltrials.gov/ct2/show/NCT01501136.

[53] "Treatment of Natural Killer/T Cell Lymphoma-III/IV (CTTNKTL-III/IV)," ClinicalTrials.gov Identifier: NCT01501149, 2017, https://clinicaltrials.gov/ct2/show/ NCT01501149.

[54] R. Suzuki, J. Suzumiya, S. Nakamura et al., "Hematopoietic stem cell transplantation for natural killer-cell lineage neoplasms," *Bone Marrow Transplantation*, vol. 37, no. 4, pp. 425–431, 2006.

[55] X. Liu, L. Ryland, J. Yang et al., "Targeting of survivin by nanoliposomal ceramide induces complete remission in a rat model of NK-LGL leukemia," *Blood*, vol. 116, no. 20, pp. 4192–4201, 2010.

[56] S.-B. Ng, V. Selvarajan, G. Huang et al., "Activated oncogenic pathways and therapeutic targets in extranodal nasal-type NK/T cell lymphoma revealed by gene expression profiling," *Journal of Pathology*, vol. 223, no. 4, pp. 496–510, 2011.

[57] J. Iqbal, D. D. Weisenburger, A. Chowdhury et al., "Natural killer cell lymphoma shares strikingly similar molecular features with a group of non-hepatosplenic $\gamma\delta$ T-cell lymphoma and is highly sensitive to a novel aurora kinase A inhibitor in vitro," *Leukemia*, vol. 25, no. 2, pp. 348–358, 2010.

[58] B. J. Schmiedel, V. Arélin, F. Gruenebach, M. Krusch, S. M. Schmidt, and H. R. Salih, "Azacytidine impairs NK cell reactivity while decitabine augments NK cell responsiveness toward stimulation," *International Journal of Cancer*, vol. 128, no. 12, pp. 2911–2922, 2011.

[59] K. Ishitsuka, S. Jimi, V. S. Goldmacher, O. Ab, and K. Tamura, "Targeting CD56 by the maytansinoid immunoconjugate IMGN901 (huN901-DM1): A potential therapeutic modality implication against natural killer/T cell malignancy," *British Journal of Haematology*, vol. 141, no. 1, pp. 129–131, 2008.

Immune Thrombocytopenia and JAK2V617F Positive Essential Thrombocythemia

M. A. Sobas,[1] T. Wróbel,[1] K. Zduniak,[2] M. Podolak-Dawidziak,[1] J. Rybka,[1] M. Biedroń,[1] M. Sawicki,[1] J. Dybko,[1] and K. Kuliczkowski[1]

[1] *Department of Haematology, Blood Neoplasms and Bone Marrow Transplantation, Medical University of Wrocław, Wrocław, Poland*
[2] *Department of Pathology, Medical University of Wrocław, Wrocław, Poland*

Correspondence should be addressed to M. A. Sobas; marta.sobas@gmail.com

Academic Editor: Eduardo Arellano-Rodrigo

We present the case where immune thrombocytopenia (ITP) and essential thrombocythemia (ET) sequentially appeared in the space of twenty-one years of follow-up. Impaired platelet production is present in both diseases, but clinical presentation and treatment are different. On the basis of this case history a possible role of autoimmunity as a predisposing factor to myeloproliferation has been discussed.

1. Introduction

Primary immune thrombocytopenia previously called idiopathic thrombocytopenic purpura or immune thrombocytopenic purpura (ITP) is characterized by autoimmune-mediated platelet destruction and suppression of megakaryocyte platelet production [1]. ITP is a diagnosis of exclusion. The definition of primary ITP by the International Working Group is platelet count less than 100 G/L without other reasons to explain thrombocytopenia [2].

Essential thrombocythemia (ET) is a clonal expansion of multipotential stem cells. Clonal thrombocytosis is a part of ET and is found also in 50% of patients with polycythemia vera and 35% of patients with chronic myeloid leukemia. Similarly to ITP, ET is also a diagnosis of exclusion once other thrombocytoses such as reactive thrombocytosis, myelodysplastic syndrome (MDS), and other myeloproliferative neoplasms (MPN) have been eliminated. JAK2 V617F mutation was found in 50% of ET patients, CALR in 25%, and MPL in few %, and only about 15% of ET patients do not harbor any of driver mutations (triple negative cases) [3, 4].

Some data shows that autoimmune disorders, including immune thrombocytopenia, may precede the development of myeloproliferative neoplasms [5–8]. Others did not find any associations between autoimmune disorders and MPN Ph(−) but proved one with myelodysplastic syndrome (MDS) and acute myeloid leukemia (AML) [6].

Here we present a case report of a patient with ITP who was diagnosed with ET, after 21 years of follow-up.

2. Case Report

The female patient was initially presented at the age of 45 in July 1992 with ecchymoses in the skin over limbs and arms and hemorrhagic bullae on oral mucous membrane. She admitted having menorrhagia and single ecchymoses a few weeks earlier. In 1987 she had an incidental mild asymptomatic thrombocytopenia but no other history of personal or family bleeding. There was no history of long term medication or any preceding infection. No constitutional symptoms, for example, weight loss, bone pain, or night sweats, were present. The lymph nodes, liver, and spleen were not enlarged. Gynecological examination was normal. Laboratory results shown isolated thrombocytopenia with platelet count 14 G/L as her hemoglobin level was 14 g/dL and white blood cell count was 8.6 G/L. There were no abnormalities in peripheral blood smear. Coagulation tests, C-protein level, and liver and kidney tests were normal. Tests for viral hepatitis B and hepatitis C, CMV, and HIV were all negative. Test for

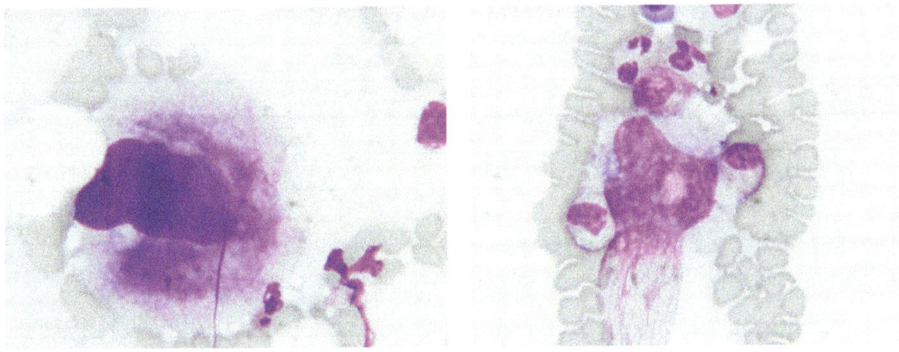

FIGURE 1: Bone marrow aspiration showed increased number of megakaryocytes, particularly those with hypolobulated nuclei. There was not any other abnormality in the bone marrow smear.

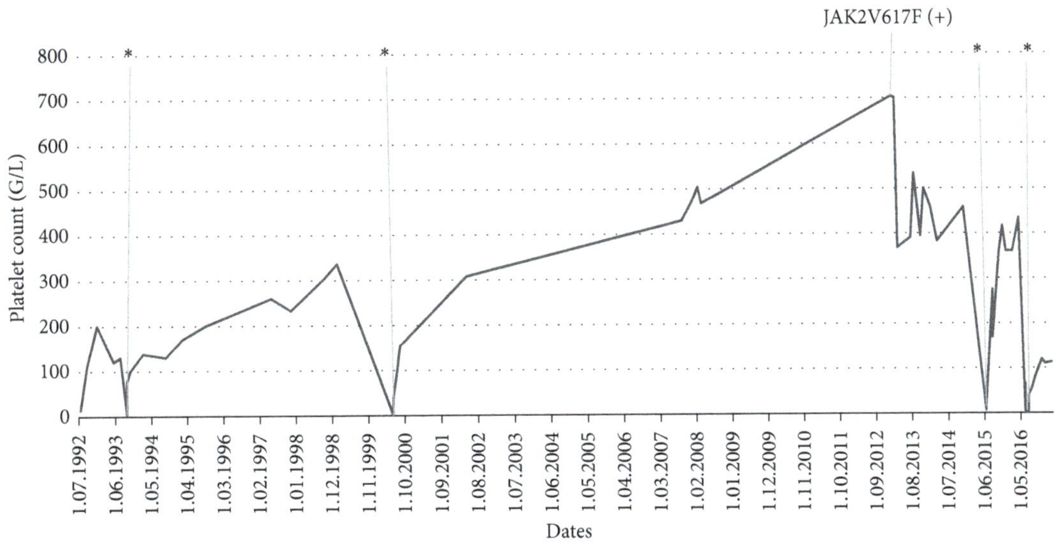

FIGURE 2: Kinetics of a platelet count during the follow-up of ITP-ET patient. *ITP relapse.

Helicobacter pylori was not performed. Antiplatelet antibodies examined by immunoenzymatic method (MAIPA) and ANA (antinuclear antibodies) were negative. Bone marrow aspirated biopsy (Figure 1) confirmed a peripheral thrombocytopenia. She was diagnosed as having immune thrombocytopenia (ITP). Prednisone in doses of 1 mg/kg of body weight was administered for six weeks, and platelet count rose above 100 G/L. No further medication was given and her platelet count was monitored closely. First relapse of ITP was observed in August 1993 and the second one in June 2000, and at both patient responded well to corticosteroids. Platelet counts remained stable till 2007 when they started to increase slowly and reached 704 G/L in January 2013 (Figure 2), while hemoglobin level was 15.4 g/dL and leukocytes were 5.85 G/L. The JAK2 V617F mutation was found (performed in DNA from peripheral blood leukocytes by PCR ARMS method). According to WHO 2008 diagnostic criteria, bone marrow biopsy was done, and it was compatible with ET (Figure 3). The patient had no previous incidents of thrombosis or hemorrhage; however as she was older than 65 years cytoreductive therapy with hydroxyurea (HU) has been introduced. The complete response was achieved, and platelet counts were stable until June 2015 when severe thrombocytopenia suddenly appeared (platelet count was 4.0 G/L). HU was stopped. A central thrombocytopenia was excluded on the basis of a picture of bone marrow aspirate. The presence of JAK2 V617F mutation was confirmed. The third relapse of ITP was diagnosed, and corticosteroids were restarted, but this time there was no response and IVIG in the dose 0.4 mg/kg/daily were given for five days with good effect. To maintain the response, azathioprine (AZT) was added (150 mg/day), and it was tapering slowly until stopped after four months, in November 2015. A month later patient had platelet count 466 G/L and HU was reintroduced in the dose 500 mg every second day. Platelet count remained stable till June 2016 when patient had a gastrointestinal infection and there was a severe thrombocytopenia with platelets 1.0 G/L. After exclusion of central thrombocytopenia in bone marrow the fourth ITP relapse was diagnosed. This time patient did not respond to corticosteroids or to IVIG. However, we decided to put her on

Table 1: MPN Ph(−) and ITP case reports.

Case number	1	2	3
Authors	Huang CE et al. [9]	Farhat et al. [10]	Sobas et al. [this report]
Sex	Female	Female	Female
ITP diagnosis	January 2009 (14 y.o.)	October 2001	July 1992 (45 y.o.)
ITP treatment	(1) DXM × 5 (2) Splenectomy (Aug. 2012)	(1) DXM × 4 (2) Igs (no data about doses)	(1) PD 1 mg/kg × 3 (1st and 2nd relapse) (2) After ET dgn: (i) 3rd ITP relapse: Igs 0,4 mg/kg × 5 days + AZT (ii) 4th ITP relapse: PD + AZT
ET diagnosis	August 2012: highly probable	March 2001	January 2013
JAK2 mutation	Positive: 11% allele burden	Positive	Positive
BM biopsy	Not done (patient refused)	Compatible with ET (2001)	Compatible with ET (2013)
MPN – ITP latency	Not known	ITP diagnosed 8 months after ET diagnosis (in 1994 patient was diagnosed with TTP)	ET diagnosed after 21 years of follow-up
Splenomegaly	No	No	No
ET treatment	No data	(1) Aspirin and ANA for 2 months, no response (2) HU	HU

Bone marrow (BM) biopsy, dexamethasone (DXM) 40 mg/day × 4 days, immunoglobulins (Igs), TTP (thrombotic thrombocytopenic purpura), ANA (anagrelide), HU (hydroxyurea), prednisone (PD), and azathioprine (AZT).

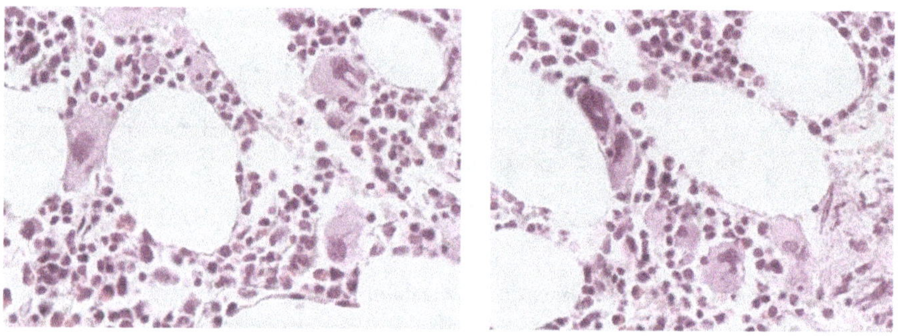

(a) (b)

Figure 3: Trephine biopsy revealed normocellular bone marrow without fibrosis with normal differentiation of granulocytic and erythroid lineage. A marked increase in megakaryocytic density was present. Megakaryocytes presented with moderate pleomorphism, most cells showing nuclear hyposegmentation with normal nuclear to cytoplasmic ratio (a) and a few myeloproliferative hypersegmented and atypical forms. Moreover megakaryocytic lineage displayed focal aggregation (b).

low dose of prednisone (20 mg/day) plus AZT (150 mg/day). After one month on such a therapy platelet count increased up to 26.0 G/L, in August 2016 it was 47 G/L, and prednisone was slowly tapered off. Since September 2016 she was only on AZT, which was stopped in December 2016 when platelet count reached 110 G/L. The last control was performed in February 2017, and patient was in good condition with platelet count 113 G/L without any medication (Figure 2).

3. Discussion

We present a case where immune thrombocytopenic purpura and essential thrombocythemia were diagnosed in the space of eleven years. Interrelationship between autoimmunity and myeloproliferation is quite complex and not wholly understood. Table 1 showed characteristic of our patient in comparison to two other cases in whom ITP was followed by ET [9, 10].

According to the literature, certain treatments for autoimmune conditions, such as azathioprine, could increase the risk of developing MDS or AML [11, 12]. There are also suggestions that chronic inflammation may drive clonal myeloproliferation [7, 8]. Autoimmune/inflammatory diseases may precede or develop during the course of MPNs [5, 7, 8]. Kristinsson et al., in a large population-based study performed on a cohort of 11,039 MPN patients versus 43,550 matched controls, found that a prior history of MPN development [odds ratio (OR) 1.2, 95% confidence interval

(CI) 1.0–1.3, and $p = 0.021$], specifically ITP, Crohn's disease, rheumatic polymyalgia, giant cell arteritis, Reiter's syndrome, and aplastic anaemia, was associated with the risk of MPN [5]. In a study by Anderson et al. [6] conducted on an American population with 13.486 myeloid malignancy patients and 160.086 controls, association between any prior autoimmune disease and the risk of myelodysplastic syndrome (MDS) and acute myeloid leukemia (AML) was reported. This relation was not seen in MPN. Based on a potent anti-inflammatory effects of JAK2-inhibitors, Hasselbalch postulated that their early introduction in treatment of MPN patients, especially in case of patients with myelofibrosis, may change the course of the disease [7, 8]. The sequential occurrence of two different types of platelet disorder is rarely reported in the literature [9, 10]. Autoimmune disorders can act as possible predisposing factors for myeloproliferative neoplasms development [5–8].

It can only be speculated that autoimmunity may interact with the JAK/STAT signaling pathway and could possibly participate in the development of neoplastic essential thrombocythemia in female with recurrent immune thrombocytopenia.

Conflicts of Interest

The authors declare that there are no conflicts of interest regarding the publication of this paper.

References

[1] T. Gernsheimer, "Chronic idiopathic thrombocytopenic purpura: mechanisms of pathogenesis," *Oncologist*, vol. 14, no. 1, pp. 12–21, 2009.

[2] F. Rodeghiero, R. Stasi, T. Gernsheimer et al., "Standardization of terminology, definitions and outcome criteria in immune thrombocytopenic purpura of adults and children: report from an international working group," *Blood*, vol. 113, no. 11, pp. 2386–2393, 2009.

[3] D. A. Arber, A. Orazi, R. Hasserjian et al., "The 2016 revision to the World Health Organization classification of myeloid neoplasms and acute leukemia," *Blood*, vol. 127, no. 20, pp. 2391–2405, 2016.

[4] T. Klampfl, H. Gisslinger, A. S. Harutyunyan et al., "Somatic mutations of calreticulin in myeloproliferative neoplasms," *The New England Journal of Medicine*, vol. 369, no. 25, pp. 2379–2390, 2013.

[5] S. Y. Kristinsson, O. Landgren, J. Samuelsson, M. Björkholm, and L. R. Goldin, "Autoimmunity and the risk of myeloproliferative neoplasms," *Haematologica*, vol. 95, no. 7, pp. 1216–1220, 2010.

[6] L. A. Anderson, R. M. Pfeiffer, O. Landgren, S. Gadalla, S. I. Berndt, and E. A. Engels, "Risks of myeloid malignancies in patients with autoimmune conditions," *British Journal of Cancer*, vol. 100, no. 5, pp. 822–828, 2009.

[7] H. C. Hasselbalch, "Perspectives on chronic inflammation in essential thrombocythemia, polycythemia vera, and myelofibrosis: is chronic inflammation a trigger and driver of clonal evolution and development of accelerated atherosclerosis and second cancer?" *Blood*, vol. 119, no. 14, pp. 3219–3225, 2012.

[8] A. L. Sørensen and H. C. Hasselbalch, "Antecedent cardiovascular disease and autoimmunity in Philadelphia-negative chronic myeloproliferative neoplasms," *Leukemia Research*, vol. 41, pp. 27–35, 2016.

[9] C.-E. Huang, Y.-Y. Chen, J.-L. Liu, H.-Y. Ho, C.-P. Li, and C.-C. Chen, "JAK2V617F mutation in immune thrombocytopenia," *Thrombosis Research*, vol. 144, pp. 149–151, 2016.

[10] M. H. Farhat, P. Kuriakose, M. Jawad, and A. Hanbali, "Sequential occurrence of thrombotic thrombocytopenic purpura, essential thrombocythemia, and idiopathic thrombocytopenic purpura in a 42-year-old African-American woman: a case report and review of the literature," *Journal of Medical Case Reports*, vol. 6, article 93, 2012.

[11] E. Alexson and K. D. Brandt, "Acute leukemia after azathioprine treatment of connective tissue disease," *The American Journal of the Medical Sciences*, vol. 273, no. 3, pp. 335–340, 1977.

[12] Y. L. Kwong, W. Y. Au, and R. H. S. Liang, "Acute myeloid leukemia after azathioprine treatment for autoimmune diseases: Association with -7/7q-," *Cancer Genetics and Cytogenetics*, vol. 104, no. 2, pp. 94–97, 1998.

4

Waldenstrom's Macroglobulinemia: A Report of Two Cases, One with Severe Retinopathy and One with Renal Failure

Naoko Kudo,[1] Masakatsu Usui,[2] Yukiharu Nakabo,[3] Ken-ichi Yoshida,[4] Kenji Miki,[2] Takashi Osafune,[5] Keisuke Nishimura,[6] and Shinsaku Imashuku[1,7]

[1]*Division of Hematology, Takasago-seibu Hospital, Takasago 676-0812, Japan*
[2]*Department of Internal Medicine, Uji-Tokushukai Medical Center, Uji 611-0042, Japan*
[3]*The Center for Hematological Diseases, Takeda General Hospital, Kyoto 601-1495, Japan*
[4]*Division of Ophthalmology, Takasago-seibu Hospital, Takasago 676-0812, Japan*
[5]*Department of Urology, Uji-Tokushukai Medical Center, Uji 611-0042, Japan*
[6]*Department of Pathology, Uji-Tokushukai Medical Center, Uji 611-0042, Japan*
[7]*Department of Laboratory Medicine, Uji-Tokushukai Medical Center, Uji 611-0042, Japan*

Correspondence should be addressed to Shinsaku Imashuku; shinim95@mbox.kyoto-inet.or.jp

Academic Editor: Sergio Storti

We report here two cases of Waldenstrom's macroglobulinemia (WM), one with central nervous system (CNS) symptoms and severe retinopathy and one with renal failure. In both cases, the serum IgM levels exceeded 3,000 mg/dL and monoclonal IgM-kappa was observed in the blood. At onset, Case 1, a 63-year-old female, developed CNS symptoms—namely, drowsiness and syncope. Case 2, a 58-year-old male, had nausea and dysgeusia on admission associated with renal failure, which is quite rare in patients with WM. Both patients exhibited hyperviscosity-related retinopathy, but it was particularly severe in Case 1: she suddenly lost her vision after admission. However, her vision recovered completely during treatment. Case 2 required hemodialysis immediately after admission. Needle biopsy of his kidney revealed tubulointerstitial nephritis with marked infiltration with CD20-positive lymphoplasmacytic lymphoma cells. After treatment, Case 1 has been in a remission longer than 8 years, but Case 2 died of pneumonia in 6 months. Since the initial symptoms of WM are ambiguous and vary significantly and hyperviscosity-related ophthalmological problems or severe renal dysfunction can arise, it is essential to promptly measure serum IgM levels and to institute appropriate care immediately when WM is confirmed in a patient.

1. Introduction

Waldenstrom's macroglobulinemia (WM) is a lymphoplasmacytic lymphoma (LPL) that is characterized by high levels of monoclonal immunoglobulin M (IgM) protein in the blood. WM is one of low-grade B-cell lymphomas [1, 2]. The incidence of LPL in Japan is very rare. In 1998, it was reported that 22 (0.7%) of all 3,194 malignant lymphomas diagnosed in Japan were LPLs. Since the vast majority of LPLs are WM, this indicates that WM is exceedingly uncommon in Japan [3]. A diagnosis of WM is made when the monoclonal IgM-kappa protein that associates with ≥10% clonal LPL cells in the bone marrow is detected [1]; however, this 10% cutoff seems not to be mandatory, because there are a number of patients with <10% bone marrow involvement with high-serum IgM and viscosity levels, necessitating therapy [1, 2]. Also, it is often difficult to diagnose WM morphologically because the lymphoplasmacytoid LPL cells in the bone marrow can resemble mature lymphocytes or plasma cells [4, 5]. In terms of immunophenotype, lymphoplasmacytoid LPL cells generally express CD19, CD20, and kappa light chain. In addition, CD38 and/or CD138 can be used to identify plasmacytoid lymphocytes [6]. Recent studies have shown that there are several genomic abnormalities that are characteristic for WM: the most common are the L265P mutation in MYD88 (found in 95–97% of patients with WM) and a somatic mutation in CXCR4 (found in 30–40% of patients with WM) [7]. These mutations (MYD88 and CXCR4) were mentioned to have the impact on treatment decisions on WM [8].

The symptoms of WM range from vague general symptoms such as fatigue, weight loss, and anorexia to more specific symptoms—namely, anemia/thrombocytopenia (due to LPL cell infiltration in the bone marrow), hyperviscosity (due to elevated serum levels of a high molecular weight IgM pentamer), and hyperviscosity-related neurological, vascular, and hemorrhagic symptoms. The neurological symptoms include dizziness, ataxia, paresthesia, and coma. The hemorrhagic symptoms include epistaxis, gingival and gastrointestinal hemorrhage, and menorrhagia: these symptoms arise from vascular disturbances [1, 2]. A particularly characteristic finding in WM is retinopathy (specifically, dilated retinal veins, retinal hemorrhage, and papilledema) [9, 10]. In addition, WM occasionally associates with nephropathy (it appears to be much more common in multiple myeloma). Nephropathy can arise via various mechanisms, including the infiltration of the kidneys with LPL cells [11]. Several prognostic risk factors have been identified for WM—namely, an *older* age, presence of anemia or thrombocytopenia, high levels of serum β_2 microglobulin, and *high* monoclonal IgM concentrations. It is recommended to adjust the treatment for WM according to the presence of these risk factors [1, 2, 8]. In terms of eventual outcome, a number of highly effective therapeutic agents are now available for WM, and the prognosis is not as dire as it once was, but it still remains incurable [1, 12, 13]. We report here two cases of WM; one with CNS symptoms and severe retinopathy, and one with renal failure.

2. Case Report

2.1. Case 1. A 63-year-old Japanese female was referred with complaints of lightheadedness and drowsiness. In the 2 weeks prior to admission, she had episodes of fainting at the shopping mall and in the bathroom at home. When she attended the clinic near her home, she was found to have high levels of serum IgM. On admission in our hospital, she was alert with no disorientation but exhibited slight consciousness impairment (Japan Coma Scale; I-1). Her BP was 130/86 mmHg, HR was 61 bpm, SpO_2 was 95% (room air), and RR was 20/min. Her laboratory data are summarized in Table 1. A peripheral blood smear clearly exhibited rouleaux formation (Figure 1(a)). Bone marrow was only available as a clot: smear preparations could not be obtained because of rapid coagulation at the time of bone marrow aspiration. As shown in Figure 2, the bone marrow was infiltrated with LPL cells that were diffusely positive for CD20 but only sporadically positive for CD38. The karyotypes of the bone marrow were not available. After admission and diagnosis of WM, the patient remained drowsy on and off. A week after admission, she developed a sudden loss of vision due to severe retinopathy (Figure 3(a)) in association with nasal and genital hemorrhages. In the first 8 weeks after admission, Case 1 was given one course of double-filtration plasmapheresis, four courses of plasma exchange, and three doses of rituximab (375 mg/m^2/dose, drip) associated with two courses of 2-chloro-2′-deoxyadenosine (2-CDA; 0.1 mg/kg/day × 5 days, drip) chemotherapy. This initial treatment was followed by monthly rituximab treatment. Fortunately, while on the initial treatment, the patient's vision recovered completely (4 weeks after the patient reported having loss of vision). Her serum IgM levels dropped gradually but constantly in response to the initial treatment and the following monthly rituximab treatment. After 6 months, her serum IgM levels were <500 mg/dL, and we started oral thalidomide (100 mg/day, daily) combined with rituximab every 4 months as the maintenance treatment. Eight years after the WM diagnosis, the patient has been in

Table 1: Clinical features and laboratory data.

	Case 1	Case 2
Age (yrs)/gender	63/F	58/M
Chief complaints	Lightheadedness Drowsiness Blurred vision	Nausea Dysgeusia Oliguria
Major clinical features	Retinopathy (group 3*)	Renal failure (group 3**)
Laboratory data on admission		
WBC (/μL)	6,900	8,200
Hb (g/dL)	7.9	8.2
Platelet counts (/μL)	124,000	107,000
PB smear	Rouleaux formation	Rouleaux formation
CRP (mg/dL)	0.19	1.15
LDH (U/L)	174	102
Total protein (g/dL)	9.2	9.3
Albumin (g/dL)	2.1	3.2
Serum BUN (mg/dL)	20.9	124.4
Creatinine (mg/dL)	1.25	11.1
Na (mmol/L)	135	137
K (mmol/L)	4.3	7.6
Cl (mmol/L)	98	112
IgG (mg/dL)	427	473
IgA (mg/dL)	137	20
IgM (mg/dL)	6,080	3,603
Beta-2-MG (mg/dL)	4.0	36.5
sIL-2R (U/L)	767	NT
Monoclonal protein	IgM-kappa	IgM-kappa
Proteinuria	2+	2+
MYD88	NT	NT
Treatment		
Initial management and chemotherapy induction	DFPP/PE/ rituximab/2-CDA	Hemodialysis Rituximab/ bendamustine
Maintenance	Rituximab/thalidomide	None
Outcome		
Alive (yrs)	8+	0.5***

*Defined by Menke et al. [14]; **defined by Chauvet et al. [21], Vos et al. [11], and Audard et al. [20]; ***died of severe pneumonia after the sixth cycle of rituximab/bendamustine. NT = not tested, MYD88 = myeloid differentiation 88, DFPP = double-filtration plasmapheresis, PE = plasma exchange, 2-CDA = 2-chloro-2′-deoxyadenosine.

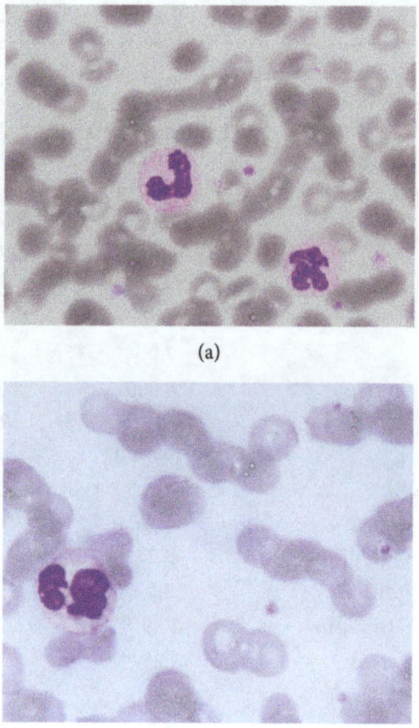

(a)

(b)

FIGURE 1: Peripheral blood smears from (a) Case 1 and (b) Case 2, which exhibit rouleaux formation of the red blood cells.

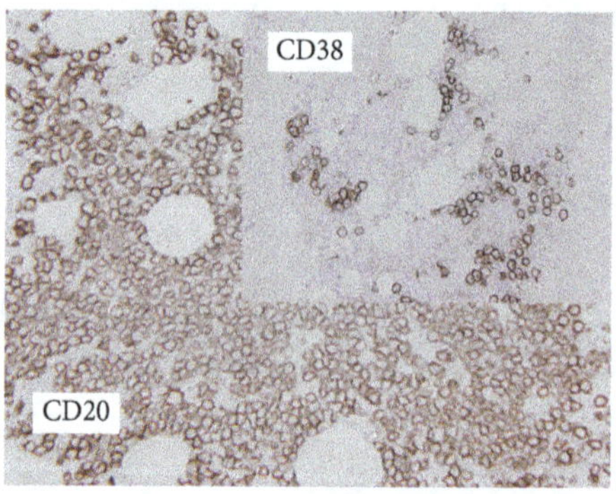

FIGURE 2: Immunostaining of lymphoplasmacytic lymphoma (LPL) cells in the bone marrow clot preparation from Case 1. The LPL cells were diffusely positive for CD20 but only sporadically positive for CD38 (original magnification, ×400).

remission without any symptoms. She has normal serum IgM levels, a normal free light chain kappa/lambda ratio with residually detectable M protein in her blood.

2.2. Case 2. A 58-year-old Japanese male was transferred to the clinic near his home due to renal failure. Eight months prior to admission, his renal function was normal (serum BUN 14 mg/dL and creatinine 0.87 mg/dL) and he was not anemic (Hb 10.0 g/dL). One month prior to admission, the patient complained of nausea, loss of appetite, decreased water intake, dysgeusia, watery diarrhea, and oliguria. On admission, he was alert and afebrile, with a BP of 118/59 mmHg, a HR of 67 bpm, a SpO_2 of 99% (room air), and a RR of 16/min. His laboratory data are summarized in Table 1. A peripheral blood smear clearly exhibited rouleaux formation (Figure 1(b)). His bone marrow was infiltrated with LPL cells (32% of NCC) that were positive for CD19

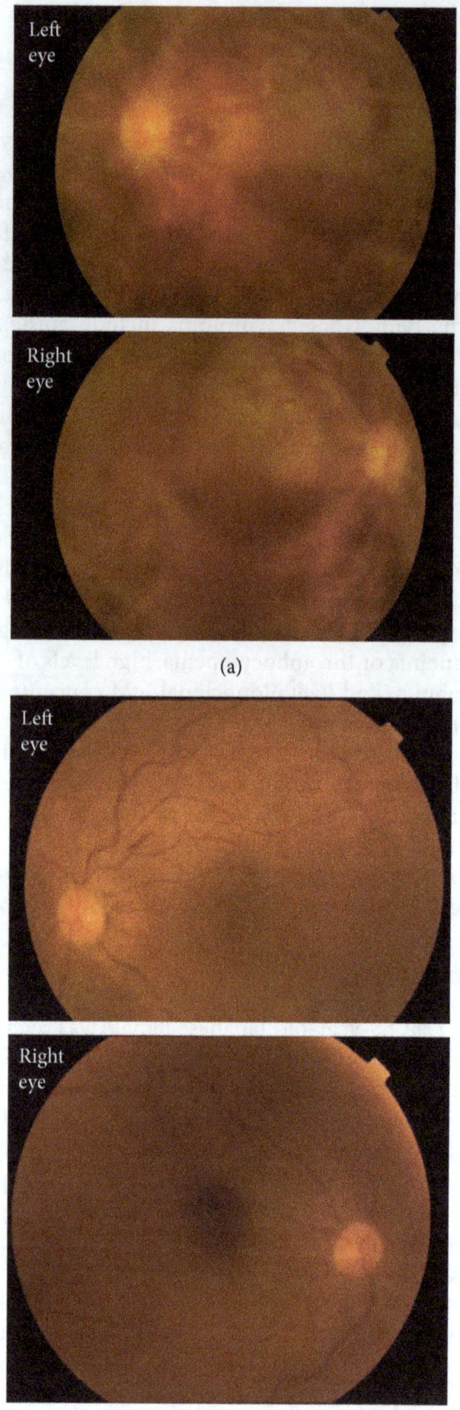

(a)

(b)

FIGURE 3: Fundoscopic findings. (a) Case 1 exhibited bilateral central retinal vein occlusion (CRVO) and optic nerve head edema with diffuse peripheral and central retinal hemorrhages that were accompanied by a large vitreous hemorrhage. (b) Case 2 exhibited bilateral tortuous blood vessels with a rod-like retinal hemorrhage (left eye) without macular edema.

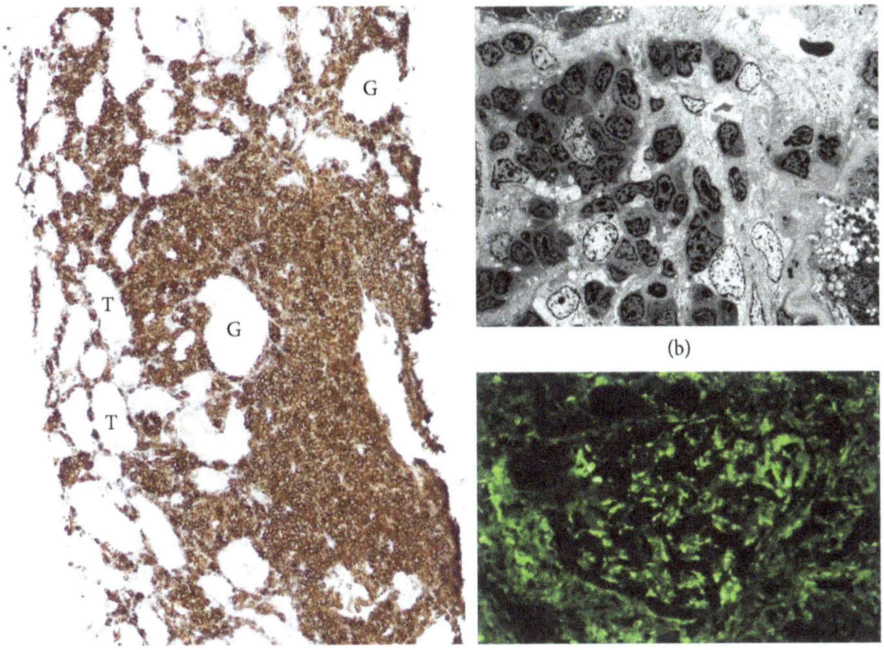

(a) (b) (c)

FIGURE 4: Histopathology findings of the biopsied tissue of the right kidney of Case 2. (a) Light microscopy revealed tubulointerstitial nephritis with marked infiltration by lymphoplasmacytic lymphoma (LPL) cells that were diffusely positive for CD20 (G: glomerulus; T: tubules; original magnification, ×100). (b) Electron microscopy showed that the renal tissue was infiltrated by LPL cells (original magnification, ×1,000). (c) Fluorescence microscopy revealed dot-like IgM depositions in the mesangial region (there were no depositions for IgG, IgA, or C3c). Significant morphological glomerular changes were not noted (photos not shown).

(26.4%), CD20 (28.3%), and kappa light chain (38.3%). The bone marrow clot section contained aggregates of LPL cells that were positive for CD20 and CD138 (data not shown). The bone marrow karyotype was 46, XY (20/20). Other laboratory data, including the collagen disease markers for systemic lupus erythematosus, were all negative. Although the patient did not complain of vision problems, fundoscopy revealed bilateral tortuous blood vessels with a few hemorrhages but no macular edema (Figure 3(b)). The patient's main problem was renal failure that was characterized by high serum levels of BUN (124.4 mg/dL), creatinine (11.1 mg/dL), and beta-2-microglobulin (beta-2-MG; 36.5 mg/dL). Given that the renal failure had led to hyperkalemia (7.6 mmol/L), oliguria, and metabolic acidosis (pH 7.110; BE: −17.9 mmol/dL), hemodialysis (three days a week) was introduced immediately. In addition, to clarify the pathogenesis of the renal failure, a needle biopsy of the right kidney was performed on day 12 of admission. Light and electron microscopic studies of the biopsied kidney tissue revealed massive interstitial LPL cell infiltration, while the fluorescence microscopic study revealed mild dot-like mesangial IgM depositions (Figure 4). Given his relatively young age and presumed poor outcome, the patient was sent to a tertiary referral center for renal failure care and chemotherapy. At the referral center, BR chemotherapy, a combination of rituximab (375 mg/m^2, drip, day 1) and bendamustine (90 mg/m^2, drip, days 2 and 3) q 4 weeks, was started with continuation of hemodialysis. After 3 courses of a total of 6 courses of BR chemotherapy planned, the patient's condition was stable with serum creatinine 4.57 mg/dL and IgM 1,246 mg/dL, showing gradual improvement in renal function; however, considering the reduction rate of serum creatinine, it seemed not to be possible for the patient to make a successful hemodialysis withdrawal. Unfortunately, the patient died of severe pneumonia during maintenance dialysis after the sixth cycle of rituximab/bendamustine chemotherapy.

3. Discussion

The clinical features of WM vary from anemia/thrombocytopenia that is due to LPL infiltration in the bone marrow to CNS symptoms that are due to the hyperviscosity, which is caused by the high serum IgM concentrations. In particular, the thickened blood causes poor brain circulation, which leads to CNS problems such as confusion, dizziness, and syncope: these CNS symptoms were all apparent in our Case 1. Another sign of the hyperviscosity that characterizes WM is vision problem such as blurred vision or blindness: this reflects the fact that hyperviscosity impairs the circulation in the retina and causes hemorrhages around the small retinal vessels [9, 10, 14]. In addition, although renal problems are uncommon in WM (~5%) (unlike in multiple myeloma, where it occurs in 30–40% of patients), nephropathy (namely, nephrotic syndrome, renal failure, and uremic encephalopathy) can arise in patients with WM [11, 15]. Below, we will discuss three issues—namely, WM-related retinopathy, WM-related nephropathy, and the recent progress in the management of WM.

WM-related eye diseases vary from bilateral simultaneous central retinal vein occlusion (CRVO) [9, 10] and bilateral serous macular detachment [16] to LPL infiltration of the optic nerve [17]. However, vision loss in WM is mostly caused by bilateral simultaneous CRVO that is caused by hyperviscosity: it is estimated to affect 15–17% of all patients with WM [9, 18]. Notably, when Menke et al. studied the funduscopic findings in 46 patients with WM, they were able to classify them into three groups depending on the degree of the retinopathy. Thus, group 1 had no signs of retinopathy (52%), group 2 exhibited dilated retinal veins with peripheral retinal hemorrhages (39%), and group 3 had optic disc edema, peripheral and central retinal hemorrhages, and venous sausaging (9%). Menke et al. found that the mean serum IgM level associated with the first retinal changes in WM was 5,442 mg/dL (range: 2,950–8,440 mg/dL) [14]. Indeed, our Case 1, who developed blindness due to the group 3–type renal damage defined by Menke et al., had IgM levels of 6,080 mg/dL at the time the blindness arose. Moreover, our Case 2 showed mild retinopathy when his serum IgM level was 3,603 mg/dL. These observations suggest that when patients exhibit bilateral simultaneous CRVO and hyperviscosity, their serum IgM levels must be determined. In addition, when a patient with WM is diagnosed, they should undergo routine funduscopic evaluation. It is possible to reverse retinopathy and reduce the abnormal venous dilatation in WM by plasmapheresis [19]. However, it has been noted that even when multiple plasmapheresis treatments are given, serous macular detachments can persist [16]. Nevertheless, in our Case 1, her severe retinopathy was successfully cured by her treatment, which consisted of four courses of plasma exchange, rituximab, and 2-CDA chemotherapy.

Various monoclonal IgM-secreting lymphoproliferative diseases, including WM, are associated with renal lesions [11, 20, 21]. According to Vos et al., the cumulative incidence of renal involvement in WM is 5.1% in 15 years [11]. Recently, Chauvet et al. [21] examined 35 patients with renal damage that related to B-cell lymphoproliferative disease involving monoclonal IgM secretion. Of the 35 patients, 26 had WM. Chauvet et al. were able to divide the 35 patients into three groups on the basis of their renal pathology. Thus, group 1 had glomerular AL amyloidosis (31.4%), group 2 had non-amyloid glomerulopathies (42.8%), and group 3 had tubulointerstitial nephropathies (25.7%: this included three cases of LPL infiltration). The study of Vos et al. on the WM-related nephropathy also showed three major similar groups on the basis of their renal pathology; 25% had group 1–type renal damage (amyloidosis), 23% had group 2–type renal damage (monoclonal IgM deposition disease/cryoglobulinemia), and 18% had group 3–type renal damage (tubulointerstitial LPL infiltration), and the remaining consisted of other types of renal damage [11]. In addition, in an analysis of eight cases of WM nephropathy by Audard et al. [20], three patients had tubulointerstitial LPL infiltration (i.e., group 3–type renal damage; 37.5%). In terms of symptoms, Chauvet et al. [21] reported that nephrotic syndrome was mostly observed in groups 1 and 2, whereas acute kidney injury and/or proximal tubular dysfunction were noted in group 3. In our Case 1, nephropathy did not arise despite the fact that she had proteinuria on admission. In our Case 2, it was difficult to determine whether he had acute renal failure or not. However, the kidney damage did progress quite rapidly: he had normal kidney function only 8 months prior to his admission for renal failure. The main cause of his renal failure was tubulointerstitial LPL infiltration (i.e., he had group 3–type renal damage; Figure 4). However, the impact of the mild mesangial IgM deposition that was observed is unknown. In terms of response to therapy by patients with biopsy-confirmed monoclonal IgM nephropathy, Chauvet et al. [21] reported that five of ten evaluable group 1 patients, nine of fifteen evaluable group 2 patients, and five of eight evaluable group 3 patients exhibited a renal response to first-line treatment. In addition, Vos et al. [11] showed that the median overall survival of WM patients with nephropathy was 11.5 years, which was shorter than the overall survival of the WM patients without nephropathy (16 years, $P = 0.03$). However, the patients with nephropathy whose renal function remained stable or improved after treatment had better overall survival than those whose nephropathy worsened despite treatment ($P = 0.05$). Unfortunately, in our Case 2, the renal damage was progressed prior to the initiation of chemotherapy; thus, it seemed not to be possible for the patient to make a successful hemodialysis withdrawal.

Regarding the management of WM, it was proposed that initiation of therapy can be based on symptoms such as recurrent fever, night sweats, fatigue, anemia, or weight loss rather than on the serum IgM levels. In addition, symptoms due to hyperviscosity syndrome, renal insufficiency, or symptomatic cryoglobulinemia may also be indications for therapy initiation [22]. Besides effective plasmapheresis in the management of hyperviscosity [19], chemotherapy with a combination of rituximab and 2-chloro-2′-deoxyadenosine (2-CDA), or of rituximab and bendamustine, has been proven effective for WM [23–25]. This was confirmed by the success of rituximab/2-CDA combination therapy in our Case 1 as well as a partial response of rituximab/bendamustine therapy in our Case 2. We also successfully managed Case 1 during the maintenance therapy with a combination of rituximab and thalidomide. More recent treatment recommendations in the international consensus paper for WM include other novel and promising agents such as ofatumumab, lenalidomide, bortezomib, and the BTK inhibitor ibrutinib. [8]. However, because of his early death, our Case 2 lost the chance of receiving such novel therapeutic measures.

In summary, we presented two cases of WM; one with CNS symptoms and severe retinopathy, and one with renal failure that was due to tubulointerstitial infiltration of LPL cells (as confirmed by renal biopsy). To obtain excellent outcomes in patients with WM, it is essential that ophthalmological and/or renal problems are early diagnosed and appropriately managed.

Conflicts of Interest

The authors declare no conflicts of interest.

Acknowledgments

The authors thank Drs. Yoshio Akagi and Ken-ichi Kai for their ophthalmological management and Dr. Shin-ichi Kotani for his helpful discussion and advice in Case 2.

References

[1] M. A. Gertz, "Waldenström macroglobulinemia: 2017 update on diagnosis, risk stratification, and management," *American Journal of Hematology*, vol. 92, no. 2, pp. 209–217, 2017.

[2] J. J. Castillo, R. Garcia-Sanz, E. Hatjiharissi et al., "Recommendations for the diagnosis and initial evaluation of patients with Waldenström macroglobulinaemia: a task force from the 8th International Workshop on Waldenström macroglobulinaemia," *British Journal of Haematology*, vol. 175, no. 1, pp. 77–86, 2016.

[3] Lymphoma Study Group of Japanese Pathologists, "The World Health Organization classification of malignant lymphomas in Japan: incidence of recently recognized entities," *Pathology International*, vol. 50, no. 9, pp. 696–702, 2000.

[4] W. G. Morice, D. Chen, P. J. Kurtin, C. A. Hanson, and E. D. McPhail, "Novel immunophenotypic features of marrow lymphoplasmacytic lymphoma and correlation with Waldenström's macroglobulinemia," *Modern Pathology*, vol. 22, no. 6, pp. 807–816, 2009.

[5] F. Berger, A. Traverse-Glehen, P. Felman et al., "Clinicopathologic features of Waldenstrom's macroglobulinemia and marginal zone lymphoma: are they distinct or the same entity?," *Clinical Lymphoma*, vol. 5, no. 4, pp. 220–224, 2005.

[6] M. C. Kyrtsonis, G. Levidou, P. Korkolopoulou et al., "CD138 expression helps distinguishing Waldenström's macroglobulinemia (WM) from splenic marginal zone lymphoma (SMZL)," *Clinical Lymphoma Myeloma Leukemia*, vol. 11, no. 1, pp. 99–102, 2011.

[7] Z. R. Hunter, G. Yang, L. Xu, X. Liu, J. J. Castillo, and S. P. Treon, "Genomics, signaling, and treatment of Waldenström macroglobulinemia," *Journal of Clinical Oncology*, vol. 35, no. 9, pp. 994–1001, 2017.

[8] V. Leblond, E. Kastritis, R. Advani et al., "Treatment recommendations from the Eighth International Workshop on Waldenström's macroglobulinemia," *Blood*, vol. 128, no. 10, pp. 1321–1328, 2016.

[9] P. Alexander, D. Flanagan, K. Rege, A. Foss, and M. Hingorani, "Bilateral simultaneous central retinal vein occlusion secondary to hyperviscosity in Waldenstrom's macroglobulinaemia," *Eye*, vol. 22, no. 8, pp. 1089–1092, 2008.

[10] B. Chanana, N. Gupta, and R. V. Azad, "Case report: bilateral simultaneous central retinal vein occlusion in Waldenström's macroglobulinemia," *Optometry*, vol. 80, no. 7, pp. 350–353, 2009.

[11] J. M. Vos, J. Gustine, H. G. Rennke et al., "Renal disease related to Waldenström macroglobulinaemia: incidence, pathology and clinical outcomes," *British Journal of Haematology*, vol. 175, no. 4, pp. 623–630, 2016.

[12] J. J. Castillo, A. J. Olszewski, S. Kanan, K. Meid, Z. R. Hunter, and S. P. Treon, "Overall survival and competing risks of death in patients with Waldenström macroglobulinaemia: an analysis of the Surveillance, Epidemiology and End Results database," *British Journal of Haematology*, vol. 169, no. 1, pp. 81–89, 2015.

[13] J. P. Abeykoon, U. Yanamandra, and P. Kapoor, "New developments in the management of Waldenström macroglobulinemia," *Cancer Management Research*, vol. 9, pp. 73–83, 2017.

[14] M. N. Menke, G. T. Feke, J. W. McMeel, A. Branagan, Z. Hunter, and S. P. Treon, "Hyperviscosity-related retinopathy in Waldenstrom macroglobulinemia," *Archives of Ophthalmology*, vol. 124, no. 11, pp. 1601–1606, 2006.

[15] M. A. Dimopoulos, E. Terpos, A. Chanan-Khan et al., "Renal impairment in patients with multiple myeloma: a consensus statement on behalf of the International Myeloma Working Group," *Journal of Clinical Oncology*, vol. 28, no. 33, pp. 4976–4984, 2010.

[16] A. F. Pilon, P. S. Rhee, and L. V. Messner, "Bilateral, persistent serous macular detachments with Waldenström's macroglobulinemia," *Optometry and Vision Science*, vol. 82, no. 7, pp. 573–578, 2005.

[17] H. Nishida, R. Hashida, M. Hatano, M. Hori, and K. Obara, "Optic nerve involvement of Waldenström's macroglobulinemia: with autopsy findings," *Neurological Sciences*, vol. 35, no. 8, pp. 1299–1302, 2014.

[18] G. Merlini, L. Baldini, C. Broglia et al., "Prognostic factors in symptomatic Waldenström's macroglobulinemia," *Seminars in Oncology*, vol. 30, no. 2, pp. 211–215, 2003.

[19] M. N. Menke, G. T. Feke, J. W. McMeel, and S. P. Treon, "Effect of plasmapheresis on hyperviscosity-related retinopathy and retinal hemodynamics in patients with Waldenstrom's macroglobulinemia," *Investigative Ophthalmology & Visual Science*, vol. 49, no. 3, pp. 1157–1160, 2008.

[20] V. Audard, B. Georges, P. Vanhille et al., "Renal lesions associated with IgM-secreting monoclonal proliferations: revisiting the disease spectrum," *Clinical Journal of American Society of Nephrology*, vol. 3, no. 5, pp. 1339–1349, 2008.

[21] S. Chauvet, F. Bridoux, L. Ecotière et al., "Kidney diseases associated with monoclonal immunoglobulin M-secreting B-cell lymphoproliferative disorders: a case series of 35 patients," *American Journal of Kidney Diseases*, vol. 66, no. 5, pp. 756–767, 2015.

[22] R. A. Kyle, S. P. Treon, R. Alexanian et al., "Prognostic markers and criteria to initiate therapy in Waldenstrom's macroglobulinemia: consensus panel recommendations from the Second International Workshop on Waldenstrom's Macroglobulinemia," *Seminars in Oncology*, vol. 30, no. 2, pp. 116–120, 2003.

[23] M. A. Dimopoulos, E. Kastritis, M. Roussou et al., "Rituximab-based treatments in Waldenström's macroglobulinemia," *Clinical Lymphoma and Myeloma*, vol. 9, no. 1, pp. 59–61, 2009.

[24] D. Laszlo, G. Andreola, L. Rigacci et al., "Rituximab and subcutaneous 2-chloro-2′-deoxyadenosine combination treatment for patients with Waldenstrom macroglobulinemia: clinical and biologic results of a phase II multicenter study," *Journal of Clinical Oncology*, vol. 28, no. 13, pp. 2233–2238, 2010.

[25] M. Varettoni, E. Marchioni, M. Bonfichi et al., "Successful treatment with rituximab and bendamustine in a patient with newly diagnosed Waldenström's macroglobulinemia complicated by Bing-Neel syndrome," *American Journal of Hematology*, vol. 90, no. 8, pp. E152–E153, 2015.

5

Sarcoidosis and Monoclonal Gammopathy of Undetermined Significance (MGUS): A True Association or Just a Coincidence?

Mohamed Hassanein, Lilit Karapetyan, Afshan Khan, and Supratik Rayamajhi

Michigan State University, Clinical Center, 788 Service Road, East Lansing, MI 48824, USA

Correspondence should be addressed to Mohamed Hassanein; mohamed.hassanein@hc.msu.edu

Academic Editor: Alessandro Gozzetti

Sarcoidosis is a systemic inflammatory disease characterized by the presence of noncaseating granulomas in different organs. Sarcoidosis associated with monoclonal gammopathy of undetermined significance (MGUS) is a rare finding with only 10 cases reported to date. We describe a 79-year-old male patient who presented with dry mouth for 4 months. Lip biopsy done prior to admission showed nonnecrotizing epithelioid cell granulomas. On admission, laboratory analysis was significant for elevated calcium, decreased parathyroid hormone, increased erythrocyte sedimentation rate, undetectable parathyroid hormone-related peptide (PTHrp), mildly decreased 25-hydroxyvitamin D, elevated 1,25-dihydroxyvitamin D, elevated angiotensin converting enzyme, and positive Bence Jones protein in the urine. Serum protein electrophoresis showed an elevated gamma globulin level at 38% and an IgG monoclonal gammopathy with an M-spike of 1.47. Bone marrow biopsy was consistent with MGUS. The patient showed significant improvement with steroids and was discharged with close follow-up from nephrology and oncology. Salivary gland involvement in patients with sarcoidosis is a rare finding. Our case is a valuable addition to the small number of cases described in the literature supporting an association between plasma cell disorders and sarcoidosis. Larger prospective studies are needed to determine if a true association between the two diseases exists.

1. Introduction

Sarcoidosis is a systemic inflammatory disease characterized by the presence of noncaseating granulomas in different organs. The most common affected sites include the lungs, skin, and lymph nodes. Patients may be asymptomatic or may have a wide variety of clinical manifestations depending on the organs involved. Persistent cough, generalized weakness, fever, night sweats, peripheral lymphadenopathy, erythema nodosum, fatigue, and incidental chest radiograph abnormalities are the most common disease manifestations. The nonspecific clinical picture of sarcoidosis often leads to a late diagnosis of the disease [1].

An association between sarcoidosis and malignant neoplasms has been described in the literature [2]. Sarcoidosis-lymphoma syndrome is characterized by the development of lymphoproliferative disorders following the diagnosis of sarcoidosis, with Hodgkin's lymphoma being the most common type [3, 4]. Sarcoidosis association with monoclonal gammopathy of undetermined significance (MGUS) is a rare finding with only 10 cases reported until date [5–13].

We describe a patient who presented with dry mouth and was later found to have concurrent sarcoidosis and MGUS.

2. Case Presentation

A 79-year-old male with a past medical history of hypothyroidism and benign prostatic hyperplasia presented with dry mouth for four months. Family history was significant for the presence of Crohn's disease and systemic lupus erythematosus (SLE) in his sister. He was initially referred to an oral surgeon who performed a lip biopsy two weeks prior to admission revealing nonnecrotizing epithelioid cell granulomas. The patient was prescribed a mouthwash solution containing diphenhydramine, nystatin, lidocaine, hydrocortisone, and tetracycline. He was referred to a rheumatologist.

His xerostomia significantly worsened prior to his appointment with rheumatology so he decided to go to the emergency department (ED). He presented to the ED with generalized weakness and decreased oral intake secondary to mouth pain resulting in a 30-pound weight loss over four months. Physical exam was remarkable for dry oropharyngeal mucosa. Laboratory analysis revealed an elevated serum calcium of 12.71 mg/dL (reference range: 8.4–10.7 mg/dL), an increased ionized calcium of 1.9 mmoL/L (reference range: 1.10–1.30 mmoL/L), an increased creatinine level of 3.81 mg/dL (reference range: 0.7–1.3 mg/dL), a decreased parathyroid hormone level of 6.5 pg/mL (reference range: 15–65 pg/mL), and an increased erythrocyte sedimentation rate (ESR) of 55 mm/hr (reference range: 0–15 mm/hr). Despite adequate fluid hydration, his calcium level remained elevated. Further workup for hypercalcemia revealed undetectable parathyroid hormone-related peptide (PTHrp), mildly decreased 25-hydroxyvitamin D at 18.1 ng/ml (reference range: 20–100 ng/ml), and an elevated 1,25-dihydroxyvitamin D at 72 pg/ml (reference range: 18–64 pg/ml).

Further workup for hypercalcemia showed an elevated angiotensin-converting enzyme at 91 U/L (reference range: 18–53 U/L). Bence Jones protein revealed free lambda light chains in the urine. Serum protein electrophoresis showed an elevated gamma globulin level of 38% and an IgG monoclonal gammopathy with an M-spike of 1.47. Immunoglobulin free light chain revealed elevated kappa free light chains at 5.79 and elevated lambda free light chains at 14.1 with a kappa to lambda ratio of 0.4. A bone marrow biopsy was done and was sent for pathology.

Further workup for dry mouth showed positive antinuclear antibody (ANA) at a titer of 1 : 160, and the other rheumatologic workup was negative.

The constellation of findings prompted further workup for sarcoidosis. Chest radiograph (CXR) showed minimal hilar lymphadenopathy which was more pronounced on the right side, bibasilar infiltrates and mild bilateral pleural effusions. High-resolution computerized tomography (HRCT) of the chest showed prominent hilar densities, ground glass opacities, and bilateral pleural effusions (Figure 1). He was started on prednisone 40 mg/day and noticed immediate symptomatic improvement. His calcium level normalized, and his acute kidney injury resolved. Bone marrow biopsy results revealed lambda-restricted plasma cell neoplasm with 5%–6% of bone marrow cellularity consistent with MGUS. The patient was discharged with a one-month follow-up from nephrology and oncology.

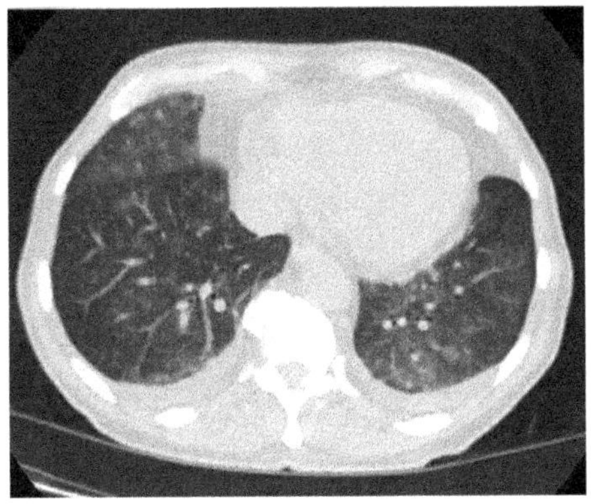

Figure 1: High-resolution CT showing bilateral ground glass opacities and bilateral pleural effusion.

Table 1: Stages of Sarcoidosis according to chest X-ray findings.

Stage	Chest X-ray findings
0	Normal chest X-ray
1	Mediastinal lymphadenopathy
2	Mediastinal lymphadenopathy with parenchymal lesions
3	Parenchymal lesions only
4	Pulmonary fibrosis

3. Discussion

Sarcoidosis is a chronic inflammatory disease of unknown etiology. It is thought to occur secondary to exaggerated immunologic response to environmental factors in genetic susceptible patients. The diagnosis is made by clinical and radiological criteria, histopathological finding of noncaseating granulomas, and absence of alternative diagnoses. The pathophysiology involves activation of different arms of the immune system including lymphocytes, macrophages, and antigen-presenting cells [14]. Upon exposure to different antigens, antigen-presenting cells produce tissue necrosis factors alpha (TNF-α) and several interleukins that stimulate cluster of differentiation 4 (CD4) T cells to differentiate into T1 helper- (TH1-) and T2 helper- (TH2-) like cells, which secrete various interleukins and interferon gamma, leading to the formation of granulomas [15].

The presentation of sarcoidosis in our patient was atypical in several ways. Sarcoidosis most commonly affects patients between 20–40 years of age. Persistent cough, generalized weakness, fever, night sweats, peripheral lymphadenopathy, erythema nodosum, fatigue, and incidental chest radiograph abnormalities are the most common disease manifestations. Our patient was 79 years old and presented with dry mouth, both of which are atypical for sarcoidosis. Orofacial sarcoidosis is a rare finding. Common orofacial symptoms of sarcoidosis include pain, nasal obstruction, loosening of the teeth, swelling of the mandible, and localized swelling and ulcers of the oral cavity. A few case series reported oral involvement as an initial presentation of the disease [16–18]. In addition, a case-control study by Baughman et al. reported a 3.9% involvement of the salivary glands in 736 patients with biopsy-proven sarcoidosis [19].

Sarcoidosis is divided into 5 stages based on CXR findings (Table 1) [20]. In our case, the minimal hilar lymphadenopathy with bilateral infiltrates and pleural effusions on CXR is nonspecific for sarcoidosis. HRCT is used to confirm CXR findings and can detect parenchymal abnormalities not evident on CXR. The most common radiologic findings of sarcoidosis on HRCT include lymphadenopathy, perilymphatic micronodules, interstitial thickening, and pulmonary fibrosis [20, 21]. Bilateral ground glass opacities are a rare finding of sarcoidosis. In our case,

Table 2: Cases with sarcoidosis and MGUS reported in the literature.

Author	Year, country	Age/sex	Ethnicity/race	First Dx (Sarcoidosis/MGUS)?	Latency	Monoclonal protein type	Progression to MM?	Prognosis/outcome
Antela Lopez [5]	1992, Spain	68 F	UNK	Sarcoidosis	3 YRS	IgM	UNK	Treated with prednisone, diagnosed with NHL 3 YRS later, treated with chemotherapy ⟶ complete remission
Sharma et al. [6]	1992, USA	53 F	AA	Sarcoidosis	17 YRS	IgG	N	Stable 16 YRS later
Sharma et al. [6]	1992, USA	69 F	Caucasian	Diagnosed same time	UNK	IgG	N	UNK
Berner et al [7]	1999, Germany	67 M	UNK	Diagnosed same time. Diagnosed with renal sarcoidosis	UNK	IgG	N	Normalization of kidney function with prednisolone therapy
Sen et al [8]	2002, USA	49 F	AA	Diagnosed same time	UNK	IgG	Y (4 YRS)	Stable 30 MS later
Saad et al. [9]	2009, Israel	67 F	ME/Egyptian	Sarcoidosis	3 YRS	IgG	UNK	UNK
Ghafour and Almakki [10]	2014, USA	69 M	UNK	MGUS. Later diagnosed with renal sarcoidosis	1 YRS	IgG	N	UNK
Guboutan et al. [11]	2016, USA	57 F	Caucasian	MGUS	4 YRS	UNK	N	Treated with steroid taper for 4 MS. Resolution of symptoms 2 YRS later
Abdulai and Englert [12]	2016, USA	58 M	Caucasian	MGUS. Later diagnosed with neurosarcoidosis	2 MS	IgG	N	UNK
Armaral et al. [13]	2017, Brazil	54 F	UNK	Diagnosed same time	UNK	IgG	N	UNK

Abbreviations: M: male; F: female; AA: African American; ME: Middle Eastern; UNK: unknown; not mentioned. Y: yes; N: no; YRS: years; MS: months; NHL: non-Hodgkin's lymphoma. MGUS: Monoclonal gammopathy of undetermined significance.

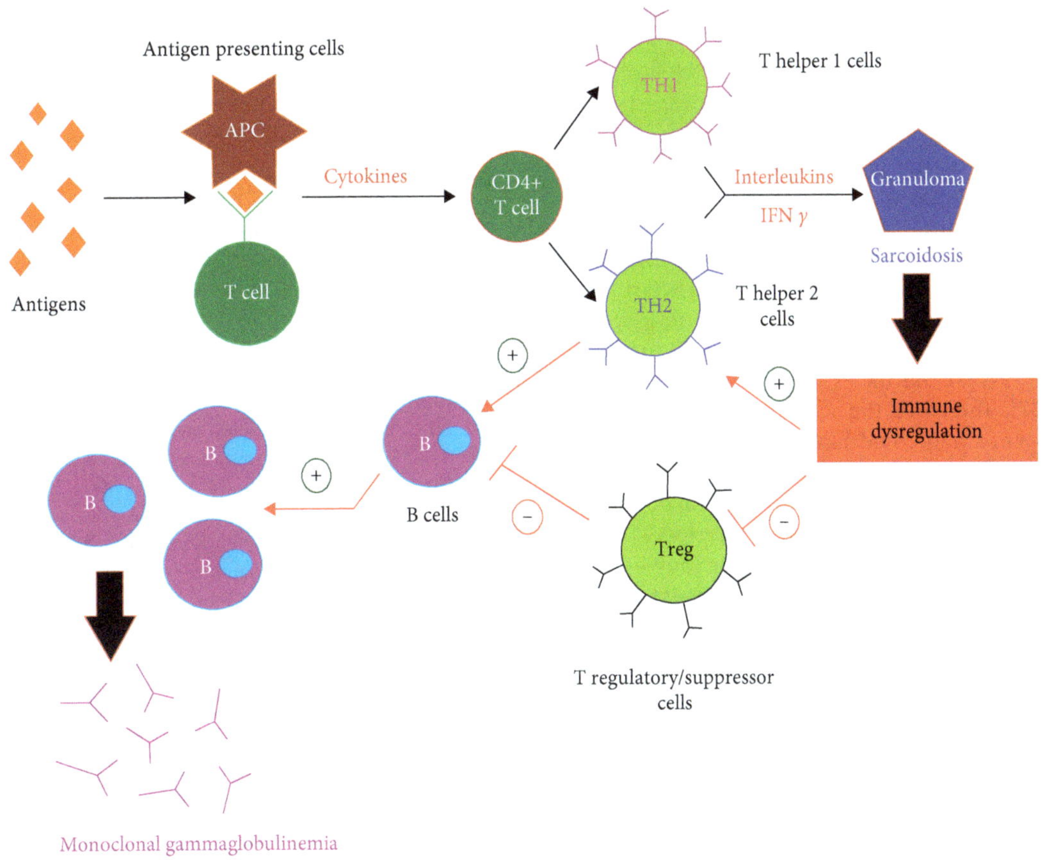

FIGURE 2: Proposed pathogenesis of MGUS in patients with sarcoidosis. Abbreviations: APC (Antigen-presenting cells), T cell (T lymphocytes), CD4+ T cell (cluster differentiation 4 positive T cell), TH1 (T Helper 1 cells), TH2 (T Helper 2 cells), IFN γ (Interferon gamma), Treg (Regulatory T cells), B Cells (B lymphocytes).

the presence of bilateral ground glass opacities with prominent hilar densities is atypical for sarcoidosis. Pleural effusion in sarcoidosis is also rare and most commonly occurs in stages 1 and 2 [22]. Without thoracentesis and thoracoscopy with pleural biopsy, a definite diagnosis of pleural sarcoidosis cannot be made. In our case, the pleural fluid was minimal and insufficient for thoracentesis, posing a risk of pneumothorax. The diagnosis was strongly supported by the patient's presentation of dry mouth, elevated calcium, 1,25-dihydroxyvitamin D, ACE, the pathological finding of noncaseating granulomas on lip biopsy, and the drastic improvement on steroids. One positive biopsy result is usually sufficient for diagnosis. An elevated ACE level is present in approximately 60% of patients at the time of diagnosis, but it lacks both sensitivity and specificity. Inflammatory biomarkers similar to interleukin-2 receptor, neopterin, chitotriosidase, lysozyme, KL-6, and amyloid A might be a better option to assess disease activity. Positive ANA is detected in 29% of patients with sarcoidosis. Hypercalciuria is detected in 40% of patients, and hypercalcemia is seen in 11% of patients. Hypercalcemia can lead to intrarenal calcium deposition and renal failure [1, 15, 23].

Patients with sarcoidosis have an increased risk for developing cancer of the lung, stomach, small intestine, liver, and lymphoid tissues. The relative risk of developing lymphoid malignancies was found to be 13.2% in patients with sarcoidosis [24, 25].

The simultaneous occurrence of sarcoidosis and plasma cell disorders is a rare finding. To the best of our knowledge, only 10 cases have been reported thus far (Table 2). The cases described in the literature show a median latency period of four years between the diagnosis of sarcoidosis and MGUS. In 30% of cases, sarcoidosis was the initial diagnosis, and in another 30%, MGUS was the initial diagnosis. Five cases, including ours, report simultaneous presentation of MGUS and sarcoidosis at the same time. The median age of onset in these patients was 61, and 70% were female. 80% had elevated IgG monoclonal protein, as was seen in our patient.

There are no epidemiologic data to our knowledge to support the increased risk of plasma cell disorders in patients with sarcoidosis. It is suggested that dysregulation of the immune system may induce development of autonomous plasma cell clones and result in the uncontrolled production of the monoclonal immunoglobulins. Activation of CD4 positive T helper cells, suppression of CD8 positive T regulatory/suppressor cells, and increased cytokine production may contribute to the continuous stimulation of B cells, causing monoclonal or polyclonal hypergammaglobulinemia (Figure 2) [8]. This hypothesis was supported by Hunninghake and Crystal, who found increased numbers of IgG- and IgM-secreting cells in the blood in untreated patients with pulmonary sarcoidosis, compared to normal individuals [26]. Moreover, they extracted T lymphocytes from the lungs of patients with high and low proportions of T lymphocytes and cocultured each of the T lymphocyte samples with blood mononuclear cells of normal individuals. T lymphocytes from the group with high proportion of T lymphocytes induced differentiation of the cocultured mononuclear cells into immunoglobulin-secreting cells. On the other hand, the diagnosis of MGUS in patients with sarcoidosis could be a coincidence. Dispenzieri et al. studied the prevalence of MGUS in a retrospective population-based cohort of 18,357 patients. The prevalence of MGUS in 79-year-old males was found to be approximately 7% [27]. Therefore, the occurrence of MGUS in our 79-year-old gentleman could have occurred by chance.

The annual risk of progression of MGUS to multiple myeloma (MM) is approximately 1% in general population. Up to 16% of patients with MGUS may develop MM after >30 years. Risk factors for progression per Mayo Criteria include an M-protein level >1.5 g/dL, Non-IgG isotype (IgA or IgM), and an abnormal Kappa-Lambda free light chain ratio (<0.26 or >1.65). Monitoring for progression to MM depends on the number of risk factors present. Patients with no risk factors are recommended to repeat serum protein electrophoresis (SPEP) in 6 months and every 2-3 years thereafter. Patients with 1 or more risk factors are recommended to check serum LDH, B2 microglobulin, C-reactive protein, and bone marrow biopsy at time of diagnosis, in addition to a CT abdomen for patients with IgM subtype to rule out Waldenström's macroglobulinemia. If all tests are unremarkable, these patients should monitor complete blood count (CBC), SPEP and creatinine in 6 months and then, yearly for life [28]. Patients with MGUS and sarcoidosis might be associated with an increased risk of development of MM. Indeed, in patients with sarcoidosis, MGUS is thought to progress to MM more rapidly than in the general population [8]. We suggest monitoring these patients with CBC, SPEP, and creatinine 6 months after diagnosis and annually for life similar to those with the risk factors mentioned previously to early detect and possibly prevent complications of progression to MM.

4. Conclusion

In conclusion, we describe a patient who presented with dry mouth and was diagnosed simultaneously with MGUS and sarcoidosis. Salivary gland involvement in patients with sarcoidosis is a rare finding. Our patient was treated with steroids which resulted in symptomatic improvement. Our case is one of few others in the literature describing concurrent plasma cell disorders and sarcoidosis. Larger prospective studies are needed to determine if an association between the two diseases exists and define the nature of association and whether causality exists.

Consent

The patient's written consent was obtained.

Conflicts of Interest

The authors declare that there are no conflicts of interest regarding the publication of this article.

References

[1] C. C. Leung, I. T. S. Yu, and W. Chen, "Sarcoidosis," *The Lancet*, vol. 379, no. 9830, pp. 2008–2018, 2012.

[2] M. Bonifazi, F. Bravi, S. Gasparini et al., "Sarcoidosis and cancer risk; systematic review and meta-analysis of observational studies," *Chest*, vol. 147, no. 3, pp. 778–791, 2015.

[3] H. Brincker, "The sarcoidosis-lymphoma syndrome," *British Journal of Cancer*, vol. 54, no. 3, pp. 467–473, 1986.

[4] N. Suvajdzic, B. Milenkovic, M. Perunicic, J. Stojsic, and S. Jankovic, "Two cases of sarcoidosis-lymphoma syndrome," *Medical Oncology*, vol. 24, pp. 469–471, 2007.

[5] A. Antela López, "Association of sarcoidosis, diffuse centroblastic-centrocytic lymphoma and IgM monoclonal gammopathy in the same female patient," *Medicina Clínica*, vol. 98, no. 9, pp. 342–344, 1992.

[6] A. M. Sharma, J. Fried, and O. P. Sharma, "Monoclonal gammopathy of undetermined significance in sarcoidosis. Two case reports," *Sarcoidosis*, vol. 9, no. 1, pp. 70–72, 1992.

[7] B. Berner, E. Schulz, U. Wieneke, M. A. Reuss-Borst, B. Sattler, and G. A. Müller, "Rasch progrediente Niereninsuffizienz als Primärmanifestation einer systemischen Sarkoidose," *Medizinische Klinik*, vol. 94, no. 12, pp. 690–694, 1999.

[8] F. Sen, K. P. Mann, and L. J. Medeiros, "Multiple myeloma in association with sarcoidosis—a case report and review of the literature. Archives of pathology and laboratory medicine," *Archives of Pathology & Laboratory Medicine*, vol. 126, no. 3, pp. 365–368, 2002.

[9] T. Saad, N. Agmon-Levin, and Y. Shoenfeld, "Chronic stimulation of the immune system in sarcoidosis and monoclonal gammopathy of undetermined significance," *Harefuah*, vol. 148, no. 12, pp. 809-810, 2009.

[10] A. Ghafoor and A. Almakki, "Renal confined sarcoidosis: natural history and diagnostic challenge," *Avicenna Journal of Medicine*, vol. 4, no. 2, pp. 44–47, 2014.

[11] J. Gubatan, X. Wang, A. Louissaint, A. Mahindra, and J. Vanderpool, "Hypercalcemia associated with isolated bone marrow sarcoidosis in a patient with underlying monoclonal gammopathy of undetermined significance: case report and review of literature," *Biomarker Research*, vol. 4, no. 1, p. 18, 2016.

[12] R. Abdulai and J. A. Englert, "Sarcoid-associated with mgus: an atypical presentation," *American Journal of Respiratory and Critical Care Medicine*, vol. 193, 2016.

[13] A. F. Amaral, M. R. Oliveira, F. E. Arimura et al., "Association of sarcoidosis, monoclonal gammopathy of undetermined significance and cardiac amyloidosis: a case report," *American Journal of Respiratory and Critical Care Medicine*, vol. 195, p. A3385, 2017.

[14] S. Saidha, E. S. Sotirchos, and C. Eckstein, "Etiology of sarcoidosis: does infection play a role?," *Yale Journal of Biology and Medicine*, vol. 85, no. 1, pp. 133–141, 2012.

[15] M. C. Iannuzzi, B. A. Rybicku, and A. S. Teirstein, "Sarcoidosis," *New England Journal of Medicine*, vol. 357, no. 21, pp. 2153–2165, 2007.

[16] L. Suresh and L. Radfar, "Oral sarcoidosis: a review of literature," *Oral Diseases*, vol. 11, no. 3, pp. 138–145, 2005.

[17] A. E. Kolokotronis, M. A. Belazi, G. Haidemenos, T. K. Zaraboukas, and D. Z. Antoniades, "Sarcoidosis: oral and perioral manifestations," *Hippokratia*, vol. 13, no. 2, pp. 119–121, 2009.

[18] A. Bouaziz, J. Le Scanff, C. Chapelon-Abric et al., "Oral involvement in sarcoidosis: Report of 12 cases," *QJM*, vol. 105, no. 8, pp. 755–767, 2012.

[19] R. P. Baughman, A. S. Teirstein, M. A. Judson et al., "Clinical characteristics of patients in case control study of sarcoidosis," *American Journal of Respiratory and Critical Care Medicine*, vol. 164, no. 10, pp. 1885–1889, 2001.

[20] F. G. Greco, P. Spagnolo, M. Muri et al., "The value of chest radiograph and computed tomography in pulmonary sarcoidosis," *Sarcoidosis, Vasculitis, and Diffuse Lung Diseases*, vol. 31, no. 2, pp. 108–116, 2014.

[21] M. Fontecha Ortega, S. J. Rodríguez Alvarez, and J. L. García Satué, "Pleural effusion: a rare manifestation of sarcoidosis," *Archivos de Bronconeumología*, vol. 53, no. 3, pp. 170-171, 2017.

[22] E. Criado, M. Sánchez, J. Ramírez et al., "Pulmonary sarcoidosis: typical and atypical manifestations at high-resolution CT with pathologic correlation," *Radiographics*, vol. 30, no. 6, pp. 1567–1586, 2010.

[23] R. Heinle and C. Chang, "Diagnostic criteria for sarcoidosis," *Autoimmunity Reviews*, vol. 13, no. 4-5, pp. 383–387, 2014.

[24] P. R. Cohen and R. Kurzrock, "Sarcoidosis and malignancy," *Clinics in Dermatology*, vol. 25, no. 3, pp. 326–333, 2007.

[25] L. Gooneratne, W. Nagi, Z. Lim et al., "Sarcoidosis and haematological malignancies: Is there an association?," *British Journal of Haematology*, vol. 141, no. 2, pp. 260–262, 2008.

[26] G. W. Hunninghake and R. G. Crystal, "Pulmonary sarcoidosis: a disorder mediated by excess helper T-lymphocyte activity at sites of disease activity," *New England Journal of Medicine*, vol. 305, no. 8, pp. 429–434, 1981.

[27] A. Dispenzieri, J. A. Katzmann, R. A. Kyle et al., "Prevalence and risk of progression of light-chain monoclonal gammopathy of undetermined significance: a retrospective population-based cohort study," *The Lancet*, vol. 375, no. 9727, pp. 1721–1728, 2010.

[28] S. V. Rajkumar, "Serum free light chain ratio is an independent risk factor for progression in monoclonal gammopathy of undetermined significance," *Blood*, vol. 106, no. 3, pp. 812–817, 2005.

6

Sickle Cell Beta-Plus Thalassemia with Subcapsular Hematoma of the Spleen

Suyash Dahal,[1] Sumit Dahal,[2] Dipesh K. C. Ghimire,[2] Ebad Ur Rahman,[2] and Eliza Sharma[3]

[1]*KIST Medical College and Teaching Hospital, Lalitpur, Nepal*
[2]*Interfaith Medical Center, Brooklyn, NY, USA*
[3]*Maimonides Medical Center, Brooklyn, NY, USA*

Correspondence should be addressed to Sumit Dahal; sumit.dahal@gmail.com

Academic Editor: Marie-Christine Kyrtsonis

While splenic complications like hypersplenism, sequestration crisis, and infarction are commonly reported in sickle cell variants like sickle cell beta-plus thalassemia, splenic rupture with hematoma is rare. We present a case of a 32-year-old young male who presented with dull left upper quadrant pain who was found to have multiple subcapsular splenic lacerations and hematoma on abdominal imaging. Hemoglobin electrophoresis confirmed sickle cell beta-plus thalassemia in the patient. There was no history of trauma, and rest of the workup for possible cause of spontaneous rupture of spleen was negative. With the patient refusing splenectomy, he was managed conservatively. Clinicians need to be aware of this rare complication of sickle cell variants.

1. Introduction

Sickle cell disease (SCD) refers to a group of autosomal recessive disorders characterized by hemoglobin S variant of the beta-globin gene. It affects millions of people worldwide and is particularly most prevalent in people whose ancestors came from sub-Saharan Africa, Central America, South America, Saudi Arabia, India, and Mediterranean countries. Centers for Disease Control and Prevention estimates approximately 100,000 Americans to be affected by SCD, with occurrences of about 1 in every 365 births in African Americans and about 1 in every 16,300 births in Hispanic Americans [1].

Beta-thalassemia is an inherited hemoglobinopathy caused by beta-globin gene mutations that impair the production of one or both beta-globin chains. Depending on the degree of reduction in beta-globin synthesis, it is divided into beta-thalassemia major, beta-thalassemia intermedia, and beta-thalassemia minor. It is most prevalent in Mediterranean and Southeast Asian countries [2]. Newborn screening in California estimated its incidence to be 1.8 per 100,000 infants [3].

Sickle cell beta-thalassemia is a sickle cell variant syndrome and is characterized by the compound heterozygosity for sickle and beta-thalassemia genes. It is divided into sickle cell beta^{+} thalassemia and sickle cell beta^{0} thalassemia based on a decrease or complete absence of beta-globin synthesis respectively. The gene frequency of hemoglobin S and beta-thalassemia in African Americans are estimated to be 0.04 and 0.004, respectively [4]. Newborn screening for hemoglobinopathies in California between 1998 and 2006 found the incidence of sickle cell beta^{+} thalassemia and sickle cell beta^{0} thalassemia to be 1.4 per 100,000 infants and 0.8 per 100,000 infants respectively [3]. The symptoms in patients with sickle cell beta^{+} thalassemia are less frequent and less severe than those in patients with homozygous sickle cell disease or sickle cell beta^{0} thalassemia [5, 6]. Splenic complications like hypersplenism, sequestration crisis, and infarction have been reported frequently in patients with SCD and its variants, including in sickle cell beta-plus thalassemia [7, 8]. Splenic hematoma, however, has rarely been described before. Here, we present a case of a young man with sickle cell beta-plus thalassemia who presents with spontaneous splenic rupture with multiple subcapsular hematomas.

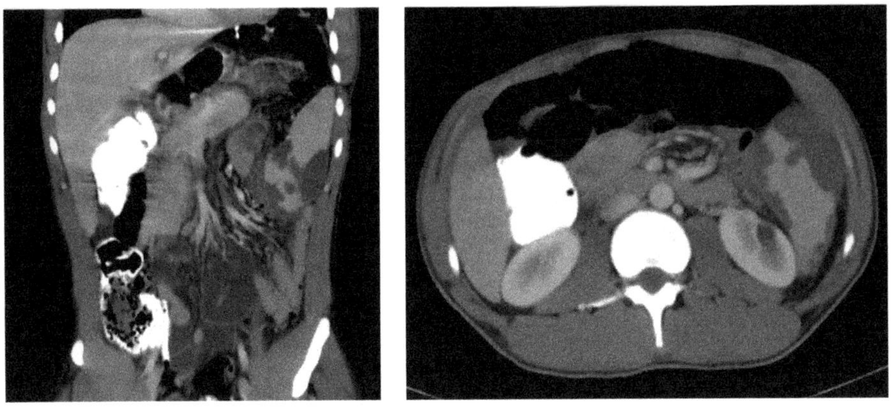

(a) (b)

Figure 1: Coronal (a) and transverse (b) sections of the abdominal computed tomography scan showing multiple subcapsular hematoma in the spleen.

2. Case Report

Our patient was a 32-year-old male who came to the hospital complaining of dull left upper quadrant pain of 2 days duration. He denied any recent trauma. He had no fever, chills, sore throat, malaise, arthralgia, skin rash, or bleeding from the gums or any other site. The rest of the review of symptoms was negative. His past medical history was significant for an unclear sickling disorder. The patient himself reported having sickle cell trait and getting exchange transfusions as a child. His family history was significant for SCD in mother.

His vitals were stable at presentation. Physical examination was significant for splenomegaly and mild tenderness at the left upper quadrant of the abdomen with no icterus, hepatomegaly, or lymphadenopathy. Laboratory tests showed a leukocyte count of 10,400/μL (normal 4,500–11,000/μL), hemoglobin of 13.4 gm/dL (normal 13.5–17.5 gm/dL), hematocrit of 41% (normal 41%–53%) with mean corpuscular volume of 66.8 fL (normal 80–100 fL), platelet count of 78,000/μL (normal 130,000–400,000/μL), activated partial thromboplastin time of 35.7 seconds (normal 24.9–35.9 seconds), serum blood urea nitrogen of 13 mg/dL (normal 8–20 mg/dL), serum creatinine of 1 mg/dL (normal 0.4–1.3 mg/dL), total bilirubin of 2.2 mg/dL (normal 0.3–1.2 mg/dL), aspartate aminotransferase of 28 IU/L (normal 15–41 IU/L), alanine aminotransferase of 33 IU/L (normal 17–63 IU/L), and serum alkaline phosphatase of 56 IU/L (normal 32–91 IU/L). Further workup for microcytic anemia showed a reticulocyte count of 1.96% (normal 0.5%–2%), serum haptoglobin of 62 mg/dL (normal 34–200 mg/dL), serum lactate dehydrogenase of 245 IU/L (normal 98–192 IU/L), serum iron of 33 ug/dL (normal 38–169 ug/dL), iron saturation of 16% (normal 15%–55%), serum ferritin of 269 ng/mL (normal 30–400 ng/mL), and a positive sickle cell screen. Subsequent hemoglobin electrophoresis revealed 17.5% of hemoglobin A (normal 94%–98%), 7.2% of hemoglobin A2 (normal 0.7%–3.1%), 73.8% of hemoglobin S (normal 0%), and 1.5% of hemoglobin F (normal 0–2%), which was suggestive of sickle cell beta-plus thalassemia. Computed tomography (CT) scans of the abdomen showed splenomegaly with multiple splenic subcapsular lacerations and hematomas (Figure 1). No other possible cause for spontaneous splenic rupture was found in the patient. His symptomatology, physical examination, and initial lab tests were not consistent with the common causes of splenic rupture like hematological malignancies, hemophilia, or malaria. Tests for Epstein–Barr virus, cytomegalovirus, human immunodeficiency virus, and hepatitis A, B, and C viruses returned negative. So, with the diagnosis of spontaneous splenic rupture with multiple subcapsular hematomas in a patient with sickle cell beta-plus thalassemia, the patient was initially managed conservatively with bed rest, analgesia, multivitamin, folic acid, and pneumococcal and meningococcal vaccinations with plans for splenectomy going forward.

However, on the fourth day of admission, the patient started to have cough, productive of yellowish sputum and palpitation. He had low-grade fever, tachycardia, and tachypnea. Repeat CT scan of the chest showed new bilateral lower lobe infiltrates. Arterial blood gas analyses in room air showed a pH of 7.46 (normal 7.35–7.45), pCO_2 of 37 mmHg (normal 35–45 mmHg), pO_2 of 100 mmHg (normal 75–100 mmHg), and HCO_3 of 26.2 mmol/L (normal 18–24 mmol/L). So, with the possible diagnosis of acute chest syndrome and/or hospital-acquired pneumonia, the patient underwent exchange transfusion with 2.8 liters of leukocyte-reduced red blood cell and broad-spectrum antibiotics. Subsequently his symptoms resolved, and his vital signs stabilized. The patient, however, refused splenectomy during his hospital stay. And with his hematological parameters stable, he was discharged home with a leukocyte count of 7,400/μL, hemoglobin of 10.7 gm/dL, hematocrit of 32.5%, and platelets count of 263,000/μL at discharge.

3. Discussion

Splenic rupture and hematoma are mostly seen with blunt abdominal trauma. However nontraumatic cases in patients with splenomegaly or underlying hematological disorders have been described [9–11]. The most common causes of spontaneous rupture of spleen include infections like

Epstein–Barr virus, malaria, human immunodeficiency virus, and hepatitis virus and hematological malignancies like leukemia and lymphoma [10, 12–17]. Cases of spontaneous rupture in patients with underlying hematological disorders like hemophilia have also been reported [18, 19].

Spleen is also commonly involved in different hemoglobinopathies and usually manifest with splenomegaly, hypersplenism, acute splenic sequestration, and splenic infarction [7, 8]. Sickle cell beta-thalassemia is a sickle cell variant and is characterized by the compound heterozygosity for sickle and beta-thalassemia genes. Depending on the reduction or complete absence of beta-globin synthesis, they are divided into sickle cell beta$^+$ thalassemia and sickle cell beta^0 thalassemia. Patients with sickle cell beta-plus thalassemia have reduced synthesis of beta-globin chains rather than a complete absence and tend to have a more benign clinical course than those with sickle cell beta^0 thalassemia or homozygous sickle cell disease [5, 20–22]. Splenic involvement occurs earlier and more frequently in patients with HbSS and sickle cell beta^0 thalassemia as compared to sickle cell beta$^+$ thalassemia [8]. There have been a few reported cases of spontaneous rupture of spleen in patients with sickle cell disease and trait [23, 24]. However, cases of sickle cell beta-plus thalassemia presenting with spontaneous splenic rupture and splenic hematoma has rarely been described before our case [25]. Mukhopadhyay et al. described a similar case of splenic hematoma, which was possibly triggered by cocaine-induced vasospasm with acute splenic infarction and subsequent hemorrhage into the infarct. Our patient, however, had no clear triggers for the hematoma. It may have resulted from spontaneous bleed into chronic splenic infarcts that our patient was predisposed to due to his underlying hemoglobinopathy. Sickled red blood cells with irregular shape and propensity to adhere to blood vessels tend to clog blood vessels and lead to congestive splenomegaly and splenic infarcts [26, 27]. This hypercoagulable state and the splenic effect may be synergized by the coexisting thalassemia [28].

In conclusion, splenic rupture and hematoma mimicking acute abdomen may rarely be the only presenting feature in patients with sickle cell disease and its variants like sickle cell beta$^+$ thalassemia as seen in our case. Clinicians, therefore, need to be aware of this rare complication and consider hemoglobin electrophoresis a part of the workup for unexplained cases of nontraumatic splenic hematoma.

Conflicts of Interest

The authors declare that there are no conflicts of interest regarding the publication of this paper.

References

[1] *Sickle Cell Disease (SCD), (2016, August 31)*, November 2017, https://www.cdc.gov/ncbddd/sicklecell/data.html.

[2] J. Flint, R. M. Harding, A. J. Boyce, and J. B. Clegg, "1 The population genetics of the haemoglobinopathies," *Baillière's Clinical Haematology*, vol. 11, no. 1, pp. 1–51, 1998.

[3] J. Michlitsch, M. Azimi, C. Hoppe et al., "Newborn screening for hemoglobinopathies in California," *Pediatric Blood and Cancer*, vol. 52, no. 4, pp. 486–490, 2009.

[4] A. G. Motulsky, "Frequency of sickling disorders in U.S. blacks," *New England Journal of Medicine*, vol. 288, no. 1, pp. 31–33, 1973.

[5] G. R. Serjeant and B. E. Serjeant, "Comparison of sickle cell beta o-thalassemia and sickle cell beta +-thalassemia in black populations," *Birth Defects Original Article Series*, vol. 18, no. 7, pp. 223–229, 1982.

[6] F. M. Gill, L. A. Sleeper, S. J. Weiner et al., "Clinical events in the first decade in a cohort of infants with sickle cell disease. Cooperative Study of Sickle Cell Disease," *Blood*, vol. 86, no. 2, pp. 776–783, 1995.

[7] A. Ashley-Koch, Q. Yang, and R. S. Olney, "Sickle hemoglobin (HbS) allele and sickle cell disease: a HuGE review," *American Journal of Epidemiology*, vol. 151, no. 9, pp. 839–845, 2000.

[8] H. A. Pearson, D. Gallagher, R. Chilcote et al., "Developmental pattern of splenic dysfunction in sickle cell disorders," *Pediatrics*, vol. 76, no. 3, pp. 392–397, 1985.

[9] M. E. Lieberman and M. A. Levitt, "Spontaneous rupture of the spleen: a case report and literature review," *American Journal of Emergency Medicine*, vol. 7, no. 1, pp. 28–31, 1989.

[10] S. J. Rhee, Y. Sheena, and C. Imber, "Spontaneous rupture of the spleen: a rare but important differential of an acute abdomen," *American Journal of Emergency Medicine*, vol. 26, no. 6, pp. 733.e5–733.e6, 2008.

[11] T. Drapanas, A. J. Yates, R. Brickman, and M. Wholey, "The syndrome of occult rupture of the spleen," *Archives of Surgery*, vol. 99, no. 3, pp. 298–306, 1969.

[12] M. Papesch and R. Watkins, "Epstein-Barr virus infectious mononucleosis," *Clinical Otolaryngology and Allied Sciences*, vol. 26, no. 1, pp. 3–8, 2001.

[13] H. E. Hynes, M. N. Silverstein, and K. J. Fawcett, "Spontaneous rupture of the spleen in acute leukemia. Report of 2 cases," *Cancer*, vol. 17, no. 10, pp. 1356–1360, 1964.

[14] T. W. Bauer, G. E. Haskins, and J. O. Armitage, "Splenic rupture in patients with hematologic malignancies," *Cancer*, vol. 48, no. 12, pp. 2729–2733, 1981.

[15] J. Zieren, M. Paul, M. Scharfenberg, and J. M. Müller, "The spontaneous splenic rupture as first manifestation of mantle cell lymphoma, a dangerous rarity," *American Journal of Emergency Medicine*, vol. 22, no. 7, pp. 629–631, 2004.

[16] H. I. Saba, W. Garcia, and R. C. Hartmann, "Spontaneous rupture of the spleen: an unusual presenting feature in Hodgkin's lymphoma," *Southern Medical Journal*, vol. 76, no. 2, pp. 247–249, 1983.

[17] S. B. Van Landingham, D. E. Rawls, and J. W. Roberts, "Pathological rupture of the spleen associated with hepatitis A," *Archives of Surgery*, vol. 119, no. 2, pp. 224-225, 1984.

[18] J. Brook and P. E. Newnam, "Spontaneous rupture of the spleen in hemophilia," *Archives of Internal Medicine*, vol. 115, no. 5, pp. 595–597, 1965.

[19] G. Mariani, V. Ziparo, G. de Rossi et al., "Spontaneous splenic haematoma in haemophilia. Report of a case and review of the literature (author's transl)," *Haematologica*, vol. 59, no. 2, pp. 205–211, 1974.

[20] O. S. Platt, B. D. Thorington, D. J. Brambilla et al., "Pain in sickle cell disease. Rates and risk factors," *New England Journal of Medicine*, vol. 325, no. 1, pp. 11–16, 1991.

[21] O. S. Platt, W. Rosenstock, and M. A. Espeland, "Influence of sickle hemoglobinopathies on growth and development," *New England Journal of Medicine*, vol. 311, no. 1, pp. 7–12, 1984.

[22] E. W. Smith and C. L. Conley, "Clinical features of the genetic variants of sickle cell disease," *Bulletin of the Johns Hopkins Hospital*, vol. 94, no. 6, pp. 289–318, 1954.

[23] D. Sharma, "Sub capsular splenectomy for delayed spontaneous splenic rupture in a case of sickle cell anemia," *World Journal of Emergency Surgery*, vol. 4, p. 17, 2009.

[24] M. T. Shoemaker, A. C. Pitney, D. J. Harford, and J. A. Barker, "Acute splenic rupture in an adult with homozygous sickle cell anemia treated with chronic transfusions," *Journal of Pediatric Hematology/Oncology*, vol. 26, no. 12, pp. 849–851, 2004.

[25] S. Mukhopadhyay, S. Mukhopadhyay, and R. Malhotra, "Splenic hematoma in Hb S-beta+thalassemia," *American Journal of Hematology*, vol. 74, no. 3, pp. 224-225, 2003.

[26] N. J. Wandersee, R. C. Punzalan, M. P. Rettig et al., "Erythrocyte adhesion is modified by alterations in cellular tonicity and volume," *British Journal of Haematology*, vol. 131, no. 3, pp. 366–377, 2005.

[27] A. H. Al-Salem, Z. Naserullah, S. Qaisaruddin, H. Al-Abkari, A. Al-Faraj, and Y. M. Yassin, "Splenic complications of the sickling syndromes and the role of splenectomy," *Journal of Pediatric Hematology/Oncology*, vol. 21, no. 5, pp. 401–406, 1999.

[28] A. T. Taher, Z. K. Otrock, I. Uthman, and M. D. Cappellini, "Thalassemia and hypercoagulability," *Blood Reviews*, vol. 22, no. 5, pp. 283–292, 2008.

7

Erdheim-Chester Disease with No Skeletal Bone Involvement and Massive Weight Loss

Hind Salama,[1] Suleiman Kojan,[2,3] Shaima Abdulrahman,[4] Fahad Azzumeea,[3,4] and Ayman Alhejazi[1,3]

[1]*Division of Hematology and HSCT, Department of Oncology, King Abdulaziz Medical City, Riyadh, Saudi Arabia*
[2]*Department of Neurology, King Abdulaziz Medical City, Riyadh, Saudi Arabia*
[3]*College of Medicine, King Saud bin Abdulaziz University for Health Science, Riyadh, Saudi Arabia*
[4]*Department of Medical Imaging, King Abdulaziz Medical City, Riyadh, Saudi Arabia*

Correspondence should be addressed to Hind Salama; hindahmed161@hotmail.com

Academic Editor: Neelam Giri

Erdheim-Chester disease (ECD) is a rare type of non-Langerhans cell histiocytosis, with only 550 cases reported worldwide. ECD is characterized by diffuse histiocytic infiltration of multiorgans. The age of presentation of this disease is typically between 40 and 70 years. Bone disease is the most common symptom, as unique radiological findings of long bone sclerosis occur in 96% of cases. Furthermore, BRAF V600E mutation is detected in 60% of ECD cases. In this manuscript, we are describing a unique case of ECD; the patient is younger than most reported cases and has no bone pain or any skeletal involvement. This patient has unintentionally lost about 50% of his body mass and is suffering from progressive cerebellar manifestations with radiological evidence of cerebellar atrophy, in contrast to the usual ECD manifestation of cerebellar infiltration. In addition, the patient has cardiac, retroperitoneal, and perinephric involvement, but he retains his sexual drive and fertility. A tissue biopsy from the retroperitoneal mass displayed typical morphological and immunohistochemical features of ECD, and BRAF V600E mutation was detected. He was treated with pegylated interferon alpha, but his disease progressed and the treatment was changed to vemurafenib to which he had an excellent response at 6 weeks.

1. Introduction

ECD was first described in 1930 by William Chester and Jacob Erdheim. Since ECD is quite uncommon and is clinically diverse, diagnosis is frequently delayed and is possibly only confirmed at the autopsy. Diagnosis is usually based on radiological features and diffuse foamy histiocytic infiltrations of involved organs. The histiocytes are positive for CD68 and CD1a, but S100 is rarely positive. The presence of the BRAF V600E mutation further supports the diagnosis.

We are describing a unique case who presented with multisystem involvement mainly cerebellar, retroperitoneal, cardiac, and skin involvement, with no skeletal involvement and massive weight loss.

2. Case Presentation

We are reporting a case of a 34-year-old male who presented with a history of progressive unsteadiness, weakness, and slurred speech for the last three years. He reported bilateral arm weakness and difficulty in walking, getting out of chair, and standing up. He had rare episodes of choking. Although he claimed no loss of appetite, he lost 90 kilograms (kg) in the previous 3 years, and his baseline weight was 200 kg with a height of 180 cm. He also complained of polyuria and polydipsia but denied any visual impairment, headache, erectile dysfunction, palpitations, or orthostatic dizziness. He is working as a farmer. He is married and has one child and seven normal siblings.

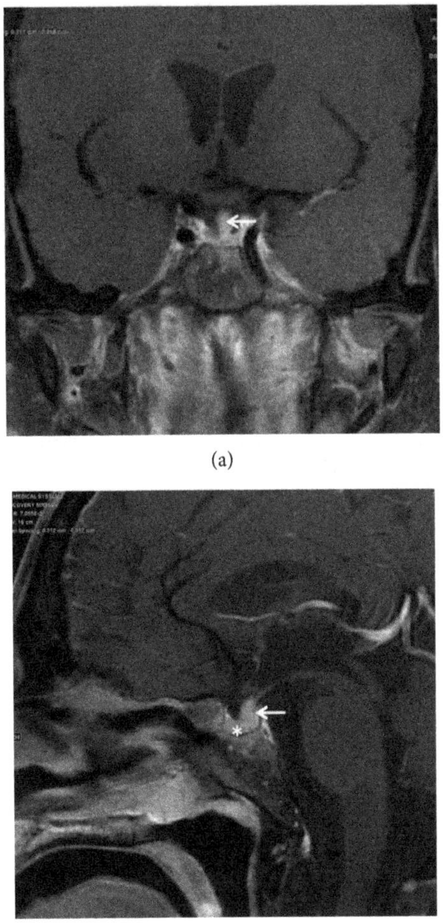

(a)

(b)

FIGURE 1: (a) Coronal and (b) sagittal pituitary MRI images post-gadolinium contrast show thickened enhancing pituitary stalk (arrow). It measures 4.7 mm at the level of the optic chiasm. The pituitary gland is within normal limits (asterisk).

A detailed examination revealed xanthelasmas around his right eye and anterior chest and abdominal wall. He has normal visual acuity and no Kayser-Fleischer ring or exophthalmos. Neurological examination showed normal cognitive function and normal cranial nerves. However, he presented with dysarthria, impaired coordination, and mild symmetrical weakness of the proximal arms and legs, and he needed assistance to get out of a chair. Laboratory investigations including a complete blood count as well as liver, renal, and thyroid function were within normal limits.

Given the history of polyuria and polydipsia, diabetes insipidus (DI) was suspected. Diabetes insipidus is a shared feature of ECD and Langerhans cell histiocytosis, occurring in 25% of ECD patients. Further investigations to confirm cranial DI revealed serum osmolality of 324 mOsm/kg, serum sodium 140 mmol/L, urine osmolality 167 mOsm/kg, and Copeptin-proAVP(s) 2.4 Pmol/L, which are suggestive of central DI. The level of prolactin, LH, and FSH was normal. Pituitary magnetic resonance imaging (MRI) showed mild thickening of the pituitary stalk (Figure 1), diagnosis of cranial DI

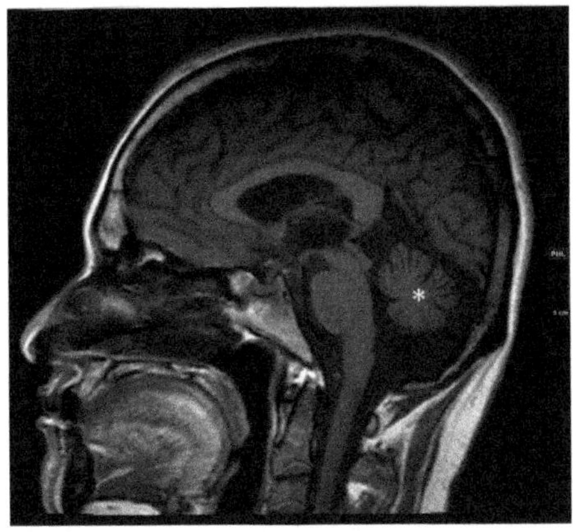

FIGURE 2: T1-weighted sagittal MRI of the brain shows uniform cerebellar loss.

was confirmed, and he was started on desmopressin sublingually which dramatically improved his polyuria and polydipsia.

A brain MRI revealed mild cerebellar volume loss and T2 hyperintensity predominantly in the right more than in the left cerebellar hemisphere and tegmental pons. There was symmetrical volume loss of the normally formed cerebellum associated with few bilateral confluent white matter T2/FLAIR hyperintensities involving the superior cerebellar and, to a lesser extent, the middle cerebellar peduncles, without diffusion restriction or enhancement (Figure 2). No infiltrative lesions were seen.

Computed tomography scan (CT) revealed bilateral perinephric soft tissue infiltration (hairy kidney sign), soft tissue thickening at the right atrioventricular sulcus, and infiltrative mass on the anterior abdominal wall (Figure 3(a)) as well as soft tissue thickening overlying the right atrium posteriorly (Figure 4). A cardiac MRI further confirmed a mass overlying the right atrium posteriorly which extended to the atrioventricular groove.

The orbit MRI was normal. A bone scan did not show abnormalities as well as X-rays of both femurs. The positron emission tomography (PET) (Figure 3(b)) showed intense hypermetabolic uptake in the muscles and skin of the anterior chest and abdominal wall and left axillary and inguinal lymph nodes as well as perinephric and cerebellar uptake.

A biopsy from the anterior abdominal wall muscle showed infiltration with xanthomatous histiocytes and Touton multinucleated giant cells, positive for CD68 and negative for S100 and CD1a indicating xanthogranuloma (Figure 5). The tissue was sent to the bioreference laboratory (Gen Path) in the United States of America for sequencing of *BRAF* gene, and the BRAF V600E mutation was detected.

In conclusion, a young man with a three-year history of progressive weakness and unsteadiness was found to have cerebellar dysfunction, proximal muscle weakness, weight loss, and xanthelasmas as well as radiological and histological findings consistent with the diagnosis of ECD.

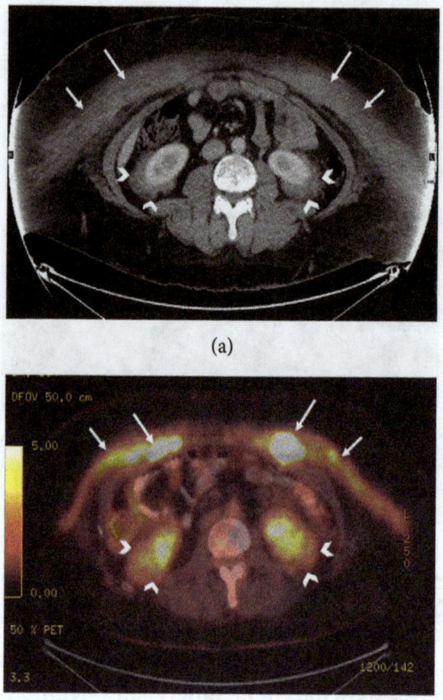

(a)

(b)

Figure 3: (a) Axial contrast-enhanced CT image of the abdomen and pelvis at the level of the kidneys shows bilateral rind-like perirenal soft tissue infiltrations, giving the appearance of "hairy kidney" (arrowheads). Anterior abdominal wall infiltration is also seen (arrows). (b) Corresponding PET/CT image shows intense FDG uptake in the same areas.

3. Discussion

ECD is an extremely rare type of non-Langerhans cell histiocytosis characterized by infiltration of multiple organs including the bones, central nervous system (CNS), heart, lungs, retroperitoneum, and skin. Skeletal involvement is the most frequent manifestation, with 96% of the patients having characteristic radiological findings of bilateral symmetric long bone sclerosis involving the diaphysis and metaphysis with sparing of the epiphysis [1]. Our patient had no skeletal involvement or bone pain.

CNS involvement is found in 30% of the patients [1], the most frequent sites involved are cerebellum and pons; however, cerebellar atrophy without infiltration as described in our case is also reported. Orbital infiltration and exophthalmos as well as pituitary infiltration and DI can also occur [2]. Our patient's MRI showed evidence of significant cerebellar atrophy. Laboratory investigations indicated features of DI.

Cardiac manifestations are also common but are often asymptomatic [10] and only discovered during routine imaging. The presence of cardiac involvement correlates with poor prognosis. The most frequent manifestation is the coated aorta which is visualized on CT as circumferential soft tissue sheathing of the thoracic and abdominal aorta. Other cardiac manifestations include pericardial effusions, pseudotumor of the right atrium in 30% of the cases, myocardial infarction, and pulmonary hypertension [3, 4].

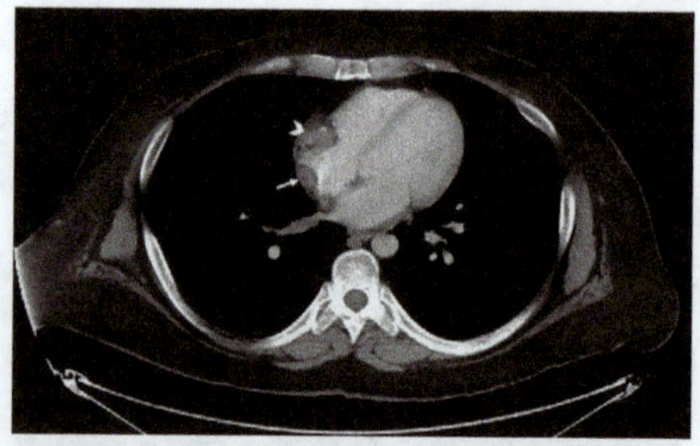

Figure 4: Axial contrast-enhanced CT image of the chest shows nodular soft tissue thickening overlying the right atrium posteriorly (arrow) and extending to the atrioventricular groove (arrowhead).

Infiltration of perinephric tissue ("hairy kidney sign"), hydronephrosis, and retroperitoneal soft tissue lesions may occur. Liver and spleen involvement is rare, but if present, it correlates with a poor outcome [5]. Lung involvement occurs in 50% of patients in the form of pulmonary infiltration, pleural effusion, and a restrictive pattern when doing a pulmonary function test. Bronchoalveolar lavage usually contains macrophages and foamy histiocytes. Our patient had no CT findings, suggestive of lung involvement [6]. Skin xanthelasmas, mainly as eyelid plaques, can also involve the face, neck, axilla, trunk, and groin. Histologically, there is proliferation of foamy lipid-laden histiocytes and surrounding Touton giant cells. The results of immunohistochemical (IHC) staining for CD68, CD163, and FACTOR XIII are positive, with CD1a and Langerin testing being negative. S100 is rarely weakly positive. ECD histiocytes are morphologically and immunohistochemically identical to those in juvenile xanthogranuloma (JXG). ECD is considered as a variant of JXG. The BRAF V600E mutation is present in more than 50% of cases, with other mutations such as *N/KRAS* and *PIK3CA* described in *BRAF*-negative ECD [7].

Our patient had CNS, cardiac, skin, and retroperitoneal involvement without skeletal, orbital, or pulmonary involvement. The tissue biopsy supported ECD, and the BRAF V600E mutation was detected.

He developed his symptoms shortly after his marriage; however, he maintained his libido, erectile function, and fertility. He has a one-year-old healthy son. There is limited literature about fertility and ECD, although erectile dysfunction and gonadotropin insufficiency are possible complications [5, 8]. Most ECD patients remain undiagnosed for many years due to the rarity of the disease and diverse presentation. Our patient was diagnosed less than a year from his presentation to the subspecialty clinic.

Various treatment options have been used in ECD with limited success. Interferon alpha and pegylated interferon alpha are currently the therapeutic modalities supported by many clinical trials, with higher doses needed for those with CNS and cardiac involvement [5, 9]. Anticytokine-directed therapies such as anakinra and infliximab as well as corticosteroids and imatinib have been tried with a lower success

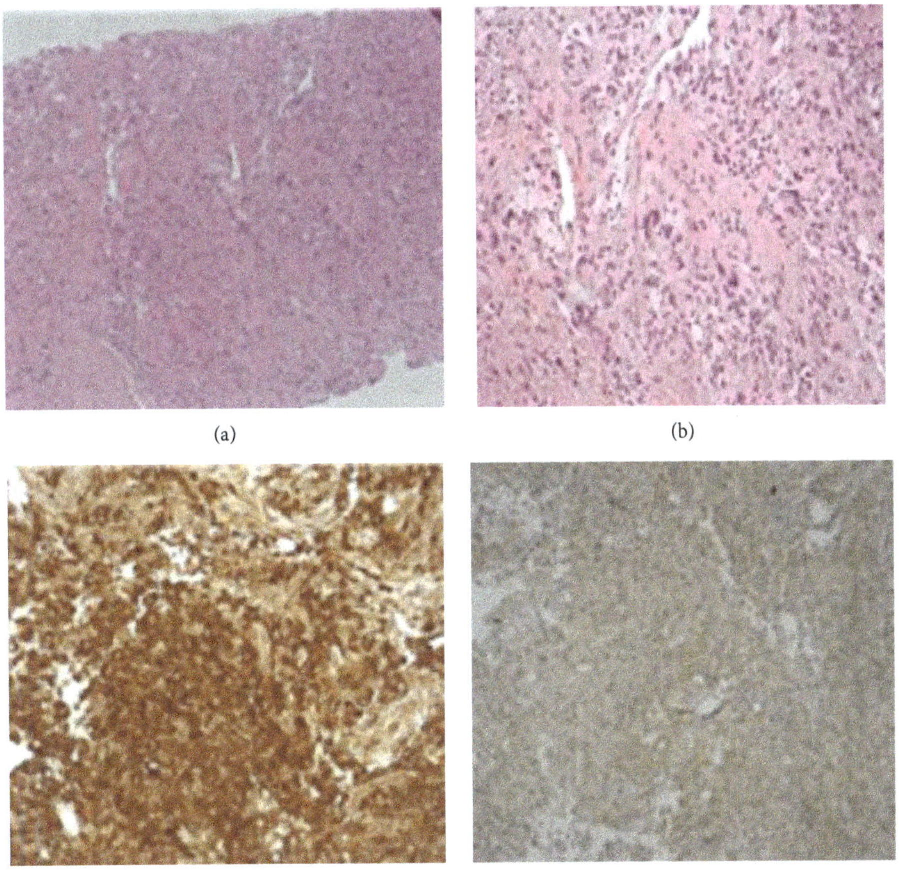

(a) (b) (c) (d)

Figure 5: Histologically, the hematoxylin and eosin (H&E) stain shows infiltration by histiocytes (a), 100X. The infiltrate is composed of bland-looking histiocytes with foam-cell and giant-cell forms (b), 200X. The histiocytes stain positive for CD68 immunostain (c) and negative for S100 immunostain (d).

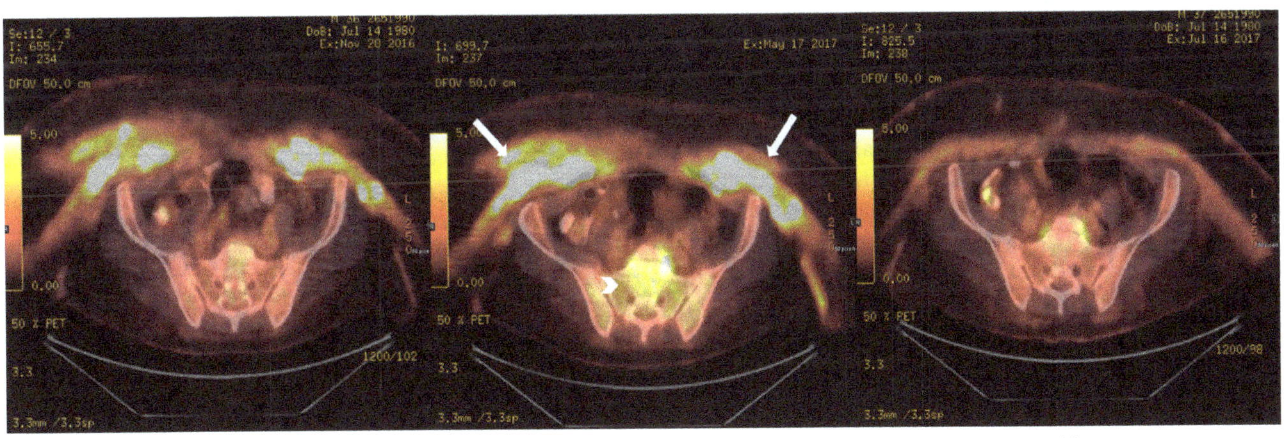

(a) (b) (c)

Figure 6: Series of FDG-PET/CT images of the abdomen and pelvis at the level of the sacrum throughout the management course. (a) Initial PET scan at the time of presentation (November 2016). (b) Progression of anterior abdominal wall involvement (arrows) and new sacral involvement (arrowhead) while on pegylated interferon (May 2017). (c) Significant interval regression of sacral and anterior abdominal wall involvement after starting vemurafenib (July 2017).

rate than interferon [5]. Vemurafenib, an inhibitor of BRAF V600E, has shown an excellent response in *BRAF*-mutated ECD refractory to interferon. It resulted in radiological and clinical improvement and should be considered as a second line of treatment for patients with detected *BRAF* mutation [4, 5].

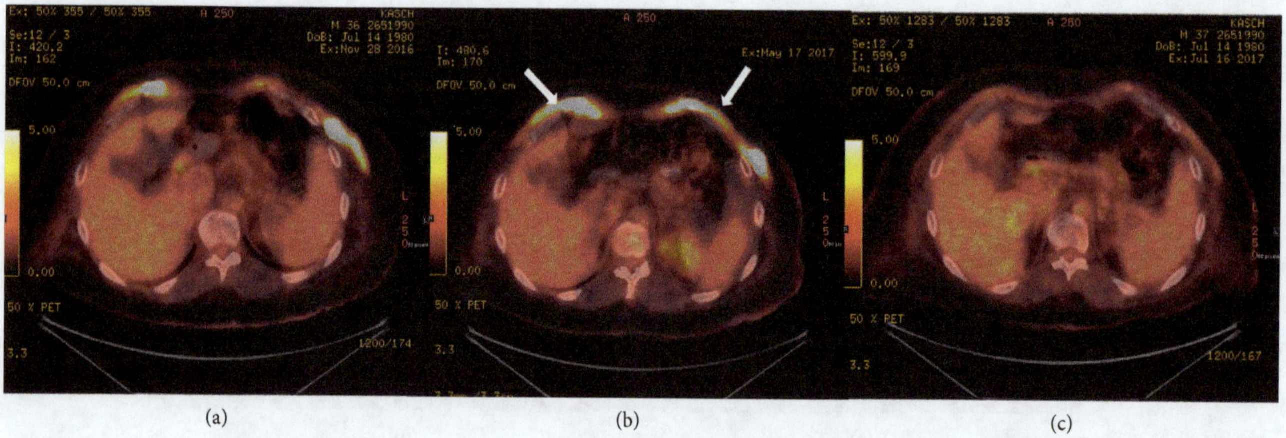

FIGURE 7: Series of FDG-PET/CT images of the chest at the level of T11 throughout the same period. (a) Initial PET scan at the time of presentation (November 2016). (b) Progression of lower anterior chest wall involvement (arrows) (May 2017). (c) Interval regression of lower anterior chest wall involvement after starting vemurafenib (July 2017).

Based on a study performed on 80 patients with ECD in France, those who are *NRAS* or *PIK3CA* mutated present with multiorgan involvement compared to patients with mutated *BRAF* or the wild-type *BRAF/NRAS/PIK3CA*, although a larger number of patients are required to confirm this result [7].

ECD patients with *RAS* mutations might benefit from anti-MEK therapy such as binimetinib or trametinib. Combinations of anti-BRAF and anti-MEK have benefited patients with advanced melanoma who are *RAS* mutant [7, 11]. Future studies targeting this pathway in ECD are needed.

Cladribine has been studied and found effective in refractory patients who lack the *BRAF* mutation [6]. Our patient was started on pegylated interferon alpha at a dose of 180 micrograms weekly. Unfortunately, after three months, his cardiac mass remained the same on cardiac MRI while repeated PET scan showed interval increase in metabolic activity of the anterior abdominal and chest wall muscles (Figure 6), as well as development of new axillary lymphadenopathy. A brain MRI showed significant cerebellar atrophy. He was then started on vemurafenib 480 mg twice per day. After six weeks of therapy, he showed clinical and radiological improvement. A repeated PET scan after six weeks of vemurafenib (Figures 6 and 7) showed significant interval regression in the cutaneous lesions and perinephric lesions as well as the disappearance of the axillary lymphadenopathy and slight regression in the right atrial soft tissue thickening. Our plan is to continue on vemurafenib until disease progression.

4. Conclusion

ECD is an extremely rare disease, with heterogeneous and diverse clinical manifestations. Atypical presentation can be challenging.

This case is unique for many reasons: the patient had severe constitutional symptoms manifested as weight loss of 90 kg, no skeletal involvement, and cerebellar atrophy without clear infiltrations at presentation. He preserved his fertility and libido, and lastly, he is younger than currently reported cases with typical age presentation of 40–70 years.

Without treatment, ECD is fatal. The estimated survival is 3 years. Even with therapy, the outcome is poor especially in patients with CNS manifestations. Clinical trials are needed to explore improved therapeutic options.

Conflicts of Interest

The authors declare that they have no conflicts of interest.

References

[1] R. D. Mazor, M. Manevich-Mazor, and Y. Shoenfeld, "Erdheim-Chester disease: a comprehensive review of the literature," *Orphanet Journal of Rare Diseases*, vol. 8, p. 137, 2013.

[2] R. A. Wright, R. C. Hermann, and J. E. Parisi, "Neurological manifestations of Erdheim-Chester disease," *Journal of Neurology, Neurosurgery, and Psychiatry*, vol. 66, no. 1, pp. 72–75, 1999.

[3] A. Ponsiglione, M. Puglia, L. Barbuto et al., "Cardiac involvement in Erdheim-Chester disease: MRI findings and literature revision," *Acta Radiologica Open*, vol. 4, no. 9, 2015.

[4] J. Haroche, F. Cohen-Aubart, J.-F. Emile et al., "Dramatic efficacy of vemurafenib in both multisystemic and refractory Erdheim-Chester disease and Langerhans cell histiocytosis harboring the BRAF V600E mutation," *Blood*, vol. 121, no. 9, pp. 1495–1500, 2013.

[5] E. L. Diamond, L. Dagna, D. M. Hyman et al., "Consensus guidelines for the diagnosis and clinical management of Erdheim-Chester disease," *Blood*, vol. 124, no. 4, pp. 483–492, 2014.

[6] N. Azadeh, H. D. Tazelaar, M. B. Gotway, F. Mookadam, and R. Fonseca, "Erdheim Chester disease treated successfully with cladribine," *Respiratory Medicine Case Reports*, vol. 18, pp. 37–40, 2016.

[7] J.-F. Emile, E. L. Diamond, Z. Hélias-Rodzewicz et al., "Recurrent RAS and PIK3CA mutations in Erdheim-Chester disease," *Blood*, vol. 124, no. 19, pp. 3016–3019, 2014.

[8] N. Tritos, S. Weinrib, and T. Kaye, "Endocrine manifestations of Erdheim–Chester disease (a distinct form of histiocytosis)," *Journal of Internal Medicine*, vol. 244, no. 6, pp. 529–535, 1998.
[9] F. Braiteh, C. Boxrud, B. Esmaeli, and R. Kurzrock, "Successful treatment of Erdheim-Chester disease, a non–Langerhans-cell histiocytosis, with interferon-α," *Blood*, vol. 106, no. 9, pp. 2992–2994, 2005.
[10] M. A. Nicolazzi, A. Carnicelli, M. Fuorlo, A. M. Favuzzi, and R. Landolfi, "Cardiovascular involvement in Erdheim–Chester disease: a case report and review of the literature," *Medicine*, vol. 94, no. 43, p. e1365, 2015.
[11] Z. Eroglu and A. Ribas, "Combination therapy with BRAF and MEK inhibitors for melanoma: latest evidence and place in therapy," *Therapeutic Advances in Medical Oncology*, vol. 8, no. 1, pp. 48–56, 2016.

8

KIT D816V Positive Acute Mast Cell Leukemia Associated with Normal Karyotype Acute Myeloid Leukemia

Marta Lopes,[1] Maria dos Anjos Teixeira,[1,2,3] Cláudia Casais,[1] Vanessa Mesquita,[1] Patrícia Seabra,[1] Renata Cabral,[1,3] José Palla-García,[4] Catarina Lau,[1,2,3] João Rodrigues,[1,3,5,6] Maria Jara-Acevedo,[7,8,9] Inês Freitas,[3,10] Jose Ramón Vizcaíno,[4] Jorge Coutinho,[1] Luis Escribano,[8,11,12,13] Alberto Orfao,[8,9,11,12,13] and Margarida Lima[1,2,3]

[1]*Serviço de Hematologia Clínica, Hospital de Santo António (HSA), Centro Hospitalar do Porto (CHP), Porto, Portugal*
[2]*Laboratório de Citometria, Serviço de Hematologia Clínica, Hospital de Santo António (HSA), Centro Hospitalar do Porto (CHP), Porto, Portugal*
[3]*Unidade Multidisciplinar de Investigação Biomédicas, Instituto de Ciências Biomédicas Abel Salazar da Universidade do Porto (UMIB/ICBAS/UP), Porto, Portugal*
[4]*Serviço de Anatomia Patológica, Hospital de Santo António (HSA), Centro Hospitalar do Porto (CHP), Porto, Portugal*
[5]*Laboratório de Genética Molecular, Serviço de Hematologia Clínica, Centro Hospitalar do Porto (CHP), Porto, Portugal*
[6]*Unidade de Biologia Molecular, Hospital de Santo António (HSA), Centro Hospitalar do Porto (CHP), Porto, Portugal*
[7]*Sequencing Service (NUCLEUS), University of Salamanca, Salamanca, Spain*
[8]*Institute of Biomedical Research of Salamanca (IBSAL), Salamanca, Spain*
[9]*Biomedical Research Networking Centre Consortium (CIBER-CIBERONC), Madrid, Spain*
[10]*Serviço de Hematologia Laboratorial, Hospital de Santo António (HSA), Centro Hospitalar do Porto (CHP), Porto, Portugal*
[11]*Cytometry Service (NUCLEUS), University of Salamanca, Salamanca, Spain*
[12]*Cancer Research Centre (IBMCC, USAL-CSIC), University of Salamanca, Salamanca, Spain*
[13]*Department of Medicine, University of Salamanca, Salamanca, Spain*

Correspondence should be addressed to Margarida Lima; mmc.lima@clix.pt

Academic Editor: Stephen Langabeer

Introduction. Mast cell (MC) leukemia (MCL) is extremely rare. We present a case of MCL diagnosed concomitantly with acute myeloblastic leukemia (AML). *Case Report.* A 41-year-old woman presented with asthenia, anorexia, fever, epigastralgia, and diarrhea. She had a maculopapular skin rash, hepatosplenomegaly, retroperitoneal adenopathies, pancytopenia, 6% blast cells (BC) and 20% MC in the peripheral blood, elevated lactate dehydrogenase, cholestasis, hypoalbuminemia, hypogammaglobulinemia, and increased serum tryptase (184 μg/L). The bone marrow (BM) smears showed 24% myeloblasts, 17% promyelocytes, and 16% abnormal toluidine blue positive MC, and flow cytometry revealed 12% myeloid BC, 34% aberrant promyelocytes, a maturation blockage at the myeloblast/promyelocyte level, and 16% abnormal CD2−CD25+ MC. The BM karyotype was normal, and the *KIT* D816V mutation was positive in BM cells. The diagnosis of MCL associated with AML was assumed. The patient received corticosteroids, disodium cromoglycate, cladribine, idarubicin and cytosine arabinoside, high-dose cytosine arabinoside, and hematopoietic stem cell transplantation (HSCT). The outcome was favorable, with complete hematological remission two years after diagnosis and one year after HSCT. *Conclusions.* This case emphasizes the need of an exhaustive laboratory evaluation for the concomitant diagnosis of MCL and AML, and the therapeutic options.

1. Introduction

Mastocytoses are rare neoplasms defined by an abnormal expansion/accumulation of clonal mast cells (MC) in one or more organs or tissues [1, 2]. The 2016 revision to the "World Health Organization (WHO) Classification of Tumors of the Hematopoietic and Lymphoid Tissues" divides the disease into cutaneous mastocytosis (CM), systemic mastocytosis (SM), and localized mast cell tumors [1, 2]. Cutaneous mastocytosis includes maculopapular CM, also known as urticaria pigmentosa, diffuse CM, and mastocytoma of skin. Systemic mastocytosis is further divided into indolent SM (ISM), smoldering SM (SSM), and advanced SM variants; the latter includes aggressive SM (ASM), mast cell leukemia (MCL), and SM with associated hematological neoplasm (SM-AHN), previously known as SM with associated clonal hematological non-MC lineage disease (SM-AHNMD), and mast cell leukemia (MCL) [1, 2]. Associated hematological neoplasms may consist of myelodysplastic syndromes (MDS), myeloproliferative neoplasms (MPN), myelodysplastic/myeloproliferative neoplasms (MDS/MPN), and also acute myeloid leukemia (AML).

In the last years, serum tryptase levels [3], immunophenotypic characterization of BM mast cells by flow cytometry (FCM) [4, 5] and *KIT* mutation analysis [6], have proved to be useful for establishing the diagnosis, subclassifying and evaluating the prognosis of SM, adding important information to conventional cytomorphology and histopathology. Mast cells, and often other BM cells, from most patients with SM usually harbor the activating *KIT* D816V mutation. In addition, they regularly have abnormal morphology, from atypical MC type I, usually observed in ISM, to more immature atypical MC type II and metachromatic blasts, more frequently found in ASM and MCL, and they exhibit abnormal phenotypic features, from which the most frequent and more extensively studied are positivity for CD25 and/or CD2.

Mast cell leukemia accounts for <1% of all mastocytosis, it may appear de novo or secondary to a previously diagnosed MC disorder (usually ASM or SM-AHN), and it may associate with other hematological neoplasms (MCL-AHN) [7, 8]. Diagnosis is based on the presence of ≥20% atypical MC in the bone marrow (BM) and/or ≥10% in the peripheral blood (PB); an aleukemic variant with less than 10% of MC in the PB also exists. The European/American Consensus Group on Mastocytosis (EU/US-CGM) proposed a subclassification that distinguishes acute from chronic MCL based on the presence or absence of organ damage, respectively [9]. The neoplastic MC usually have an immature morphology and an abnormal immature and/or activated phenotype, although they often fail to have the abnormal CD2+CD25+ pattern encountered in most forms of SM; in addition, the *KIT* D816V mutation is detected in less than 50% of cases, and most patients have a normal karyotype. Symptoms of MC activation and involvement of the liver, spleen, peritoneum, digestive tract, and bones are relatively frequent, and skin lesions occur in only 1/3 of the cases. Treatment usually fails, and the median survival time is short. Due in part to the rarity, no standard therapy exists, and the role of hematopoietic stem cell transplantation (HSCT) needs further investigation.

Distinguishing MCL from SM associated with AML and from myelomastocytic leukemia (MML) is a challenge and requires a detailed laboratory investigation using cytology, cytochemistry, histopathology, immunohistochemistry, immunophenotypic, and genetic approaches [9–16]. The EU/US-CGM and the European Competence Network on Mastocytosis (ECNM) have recently proposed the criteria to establish the differential diagnosis between these entities [9].

We present a case of MCL diagnosed concomitantly to AML, given emphasis on the role of the laboratory exams, specially immunophenotyping and genetic testing, in establishing the differential diagnosis with MML. In addition, we compare the clinical and laboratory features of our patient with those described in previously published series of patients with MCL, ISM, ASM, and SM-ANH. Finally, we describe the success of the therapeutic strategy used in this patient, which included cladribine, anthracycline in combination with cytosine arabinoside, and HSCT.

2. Case Report

A 41-year-old Caucasian woman was admitted at the hospital with one-month history of asthenia, anorexia, fever, abdominal pain, early postprandial surfeit, and diarrhea. She had past history of an intermittent migratory pruritic maculopapular rash and mild episodes of flushing that had never been investigated, hypothyroidism, an anxiety disorder, and emotional instability, and she had smoked 20 cigarettes a day since the age of 13. There was no history of allergies or other pathologies.

When first observed at the hospital, she had a fever, a dark spot on the tongue, a slightly pruritic brownish erythematous maculopapular skin rash predominantly in the upper limbs, hepatomegaly (the left lobe of liver was enlarged and extended to epigastric region and the right lobe was four fingers below the right costal margin in the midclavicular line), and splenomegaly (5 fingers below the left costal margin). There was no peripheral lymphadenopathy.

Peripheral blood counts revealed pancytopenia: hemoglobin (Hg) 11.0 g/dl (normal range 12.0–15.0), platelets 16×10^9/L (normal range 150–400), and white blood cells (WBC) 4.25×10^9/L (normal range 4.0–11.0) with 7.0% neutrophils (0.3×10^9/L) (normal range 2.0–7.5), 6% blast cells (BC), and 20% of cells with metachromatic cytoplasmic granules that were initially classified as basophils by morphology (Figure 1), but whose immunophenotypic study subsequently revealed them to be an abnormal immature MC.

Serum biochemistry showed elevated lactate dehydrogenase (369 U/L, normal range 135–214 U/L) and abnormal hepatic tests with a cholestatic pattern: total bilirubin 1.2 mg/dl (normal range: 0.2–1.0), direct bilirubin 1.1 mg/dl (normal range: 0.0–0.2), indirect bilirubin 1.14 mg/dl (normal range: 0.0–1.0), alanine transaminase 90 U/L (normal range: 10–30), aspartate transaminase 36 U/L (normal range: 10–30), alkaline phosphatase 731 U/L (normal range: 32–104), and

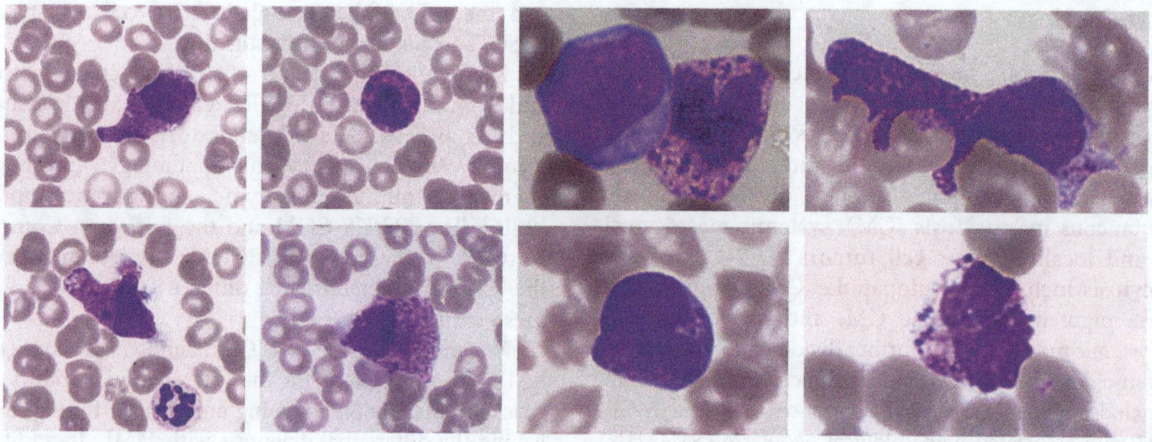

Figure 1: Peripheral blood smears showing different types of morphologically abnormal mast cells. Leishman's stain (a, 40x; b, 100x). Circulating mast cells (MC) had variable morphological features, from metachromatic blasts of medium to large cell size, round to oval shape, fine/immature nuclear chromatin, high nuclear : cytoplasmic ratio, and cytoplasmic metachromatic granules, to atypical MC type 2 with variable, sometimes spindle, cell shape, bilobated nucleus with fine to moderately condensed chromatin, variable nuclear : cytoplasmic ratio, and hypogranulated cytoplasm. Please note that in spite of these heterogeneous morphological features, all the MC present in the peripheral blood had an aberrant immature phenotype, corresponding to abnormal MC precursors (Figure 4).

gamma-glutamyl transferase 638 U/L (normal range: 6–39). There was also hypoalbuminemia (serum albumin 32 g/L, normal range: 35–50) and hypogammaglobulinemia (serum IgG 522 mg/dl, normal range: 793–1590; IgA 127 mg/dl, normal range: 114–457; IgM 170 mg/dl, normal range: 29–226). Serum tryptase levels were markedly increased (184 μg/L, normal range < 13 μg/L). Calcium and phosphate serum levels were normal, as did renal function tests. Coagulation tests, including prothrombin time, activated partial thromboplastin time, and fibrinogen levels, were within the normal range. Serological tests for hepatitis B and C viruses and human immunodeficiency virus type 1 and 2 were negative.

Bone marrow smears showed 24% myeloperoxidase (MPO) positive BC, 17% promyelocytes, 4% myelocytes, 3% metamyelocytes + neutrophils (AML-M2 classification by cytomorphology), 30% erythroid lineage, and 16% morphologically abnormal toluidine blue positive MC (Figure 2). These cells had variable morphological features, from atypical MC type I and II to metachromatic blasts. There was no BM eosinophilia, or evidence of myelodysplasia. Flow cytometry of the BM aspirate revealed 12% of CD45+ (low), CD117+, CD34+ myeloid precursor cells (MPC) also expressing CD123, HLA-DR (high), CD13, CD33, CD65 (low), and CD25 (low, in part of the cells) but lacking CD10, CD15, CD16, CD2, CD30, and FcεRI/IgE; 5% of CD45+ (low), CD117+, CD34− MC precursors (MCP), also being positive for CD123 (high), CD13, CD33, CD65 (low), CD25, CD30, FcεRI/IgE, and HLA-DR (high), and lacking CD10, CD15, CD16, and CD2; 34% promyelocytes with an aberrant phenotype (CD45+, CD34−, CD117+, CD13+low, CD33+, CD65+; CD15+, MPO+, and CD2, CD10, CD11b, CD16, CD25, CD30, FcεRI/IgE, and HLA-DR negative); a maturation blockage at the promyelocyte level, as revealed by an abnormal CD11b/CD13/CD16 maturation pattern, with <1% of CD16+CD10+ mature neutrophils; and 13% of abnormal CD45+, CD34−, CD117+high MC with a relatively immature (CD123+high, FcεRI/IgE+ low, and HLA-DR+high), activated (CD63+, CD69+), and aberrant (CD2−, CD25+, and CD30+) immunophenotype (Figure 3). Cytoplasmic carboxypeptidase and surface CD203 were also positive (data not shown). In addition, FCM performed in PB, showed 3% CD45+low, CD117+, CD34+ MPC, and 21% of CD45+low, CD117+, CD34− MCP, which were phenotypically similar to the correspondent BM cell populations, at least for the cell surface markers tested, but not CD45+, CD34−, and CD117+ high MC (Figure 4).

Bone marrow trephine biopsy revealed a hypercellular marrow with increased proportions of immature MPO+ myeloid cells and morphologically atypical CD117+ fusiform MC forming perivascular dense aggregates, and grade 2 fibrosis (Figure 5). Skin biopsy was not performed.

Cytogenetic analyses of at least 20 Giemsa-banded BM cell metaphases obtained from unstimulated 24 hour cultures disclosed a 46,XX karyotype, without numerical or structural abnormalities. Genetic studies using probes for relevant targets, including t(15;17) PML-RARA, t(8;21) RUNX1-RUNX1T1, inv(16) CBFB-MYH11, and t(9,22) BCR-ABL, gave negative results. Tests for *FLT3* (FMS-like tyrosine kinase 3) and *NPM-1* (Nucleophosmin-1) gene mutations were also negative. *KIT* mutation at the codon 816 (D816V) (A7176T) was detected in all sorted BM cell populations, except in T cells; BM cells harboring the *KIT* D816V mutation included MC, CD34+ cells, CD34-HLA-DR-, CD34-HLA-DR+, and CD34-HLA-DR++ cells.

Abdominopelvic computerized tomography scan affirmed hepatomegaly (18.5 cm) and mild splenomegaly (13 cm) with small hypodense nodules (maximum diameter 10 mm) and revealed retroperitoneal adenopathies forming a conglomerate extending from the lesser gastric curvature and involving the large vessels; the largest adenopathy was in the hepatic-duodenal ligament and had 2.4 cm of major diameter. There was also a lamina of peritoneal liquid in pelvic cavitation.

Digestive endoscopy revealed slight reduced distensibility of the gastric body, which had a congestive mucosa

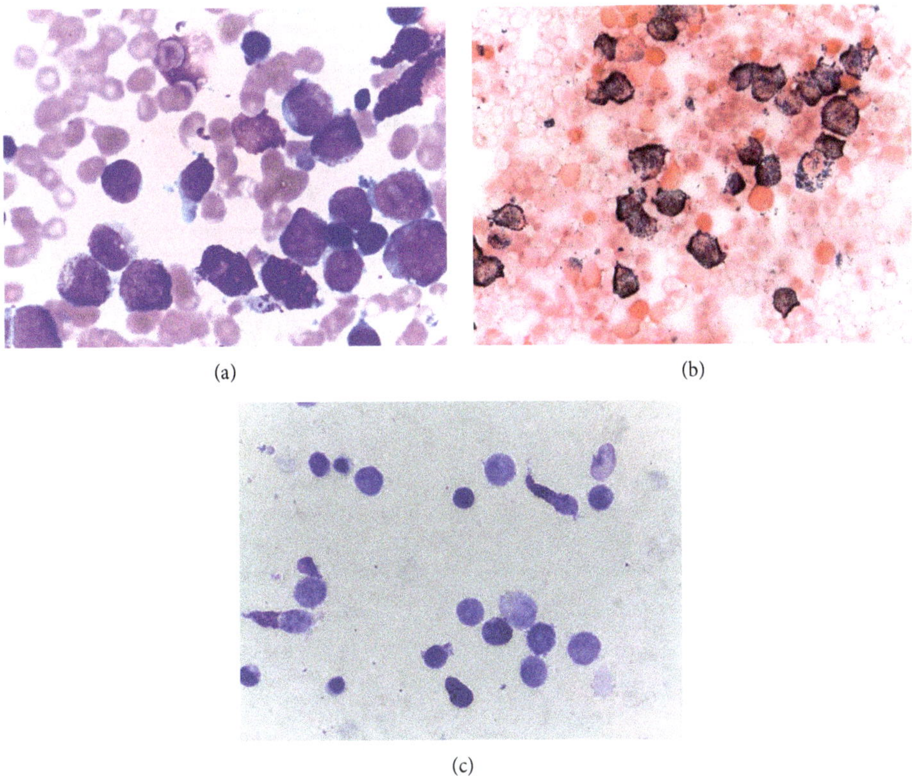

FIGURE 2: Bone marrow smears showing myeloperoxidase positive blast cells and promyelocytes, and morphologically abnormal toluidine blue positive mast cells. (a) Leishman. (b) Myeloperoxidase. (c) Toluidine blue staining.

with foci of erythema, and the duodenum had a congestive and micronodular mucosa. Biopsies were not performed due to severe thrombocytopenia. Skeleton radiography did not reveal osteolytic lesions. Thorax radiography had no evidence of mediastinal enlargement, lung consolidations, or pleural effusions.

According to the WHO criteria [1, 2], and to the consensus recommendations of the EU/US-CGM and the ECNM [9], the patient was diagnosed with *KIT* D816V+ MCL associated with AML with normal karyotype. She was immediately started with oral corticosteroids (prednisolone, 60 mg/day for one week, tapered to 20 mg/day over 1 month, and then maintaining 20 mg/day) and disodium cromoglycate (200 mg capsules, 4 times daily), and H1 (cetirizine, 10 mg/day, orally) and H2 (ranitidine, 150 mg twice a day, orally) antihistamines, which ameliorate the symptomatology. Then, she received two cycles of cladribine (0.14 mg/kg/day, administered over a 2-hour infusion for 5 days) with one month of interval, and the serum tryptase levels transiently decreased to 41 μg/L (Figure 6).

One month after, she maintained constitutional symptoms, hepatomegaly, and pancytopenia, and she developed cutaneous and mucosal hemorrhage (petechial rash, epistaxis, and spontaneous oral cavity bleeding), myalgia, and bone pain. By that time, the serum tryptase serum levels had increased to 123 μg/L (Figure 6), and the BM aspirate showed 47.0% myeloblasts, 8% promyelocytes, and 7.0% MC. Bone marrow FCM revealed 3% MPC (CD45+low, CD34+, CD117+, FcεRI/IgE−, CD2−, and CD25−/+), 7% MCP (CD45+ low, CD34−, CD117+, FcεRI/IgE+low, CD2−, and CD25+), 46% of immature granulocytic cells (almost complete maturational arrest at the promyelocyte stage), and 7% of CD45+, CD34−, CD117+ high, CD2−, and CD25+ MC. Peripheral blood counts were WBC 2.07×10^9/L, neutrophils 4.0% (0.08×10^9/L), MC 41.0%, BC 9.0%; Hg 8.8 g/dl; and platelets 28×10^9/L. Flow cytometry studies performed in the PB showed 48% CD45+ low, CD117+, CD34−, FcεRI/IgE+low, CD25+, CD2− MCP, 4% CD45+low, CD34+, CD117+, FcεRI/IgE−, CD25−/+, CD2− MPC; once again, circulating CD45+, CD34−, CD117+high, CD2−, CD25+ MC were not observed. By that time, she received induction therapy for AML consisting of two cycles of idarubicin (12 mg/m2/day, intravenous, for 3 days) and cytosine arabinoside (AraC) (100 mg/m2/day, intravenous, for 7 days), achieving hematological remission and normal tryptase levels after the second induction course (Figure 6). At that time, the BM smears were slightly hypocellular with 1.3% of BC and no MC. Bone marrow FCM studies detected 1.5% of CD117+ CD34+ MPC, 54% maturing granulocytic cells, from which 26% were promyelocytes, 53% were metamyelocytes and myelocytes, and 21% were mature neutrophils, and 0.03% were phenotypically abnormal MC (0.02% CD117+ CD34− CD2− CD25−/+low, FcεRI/IgE+ MCP, and 0.01% CD117+high CD34−, CD2−, CD25+, FcεRI/IgE+low MC). Consolidation therapy performed in the subsequent 2 months consisted of two courses of high-dose AraC (2 g/m2, intravenous).

As complication of treatment she had bartholinite, treated with piperacillin plus tazobactam, and

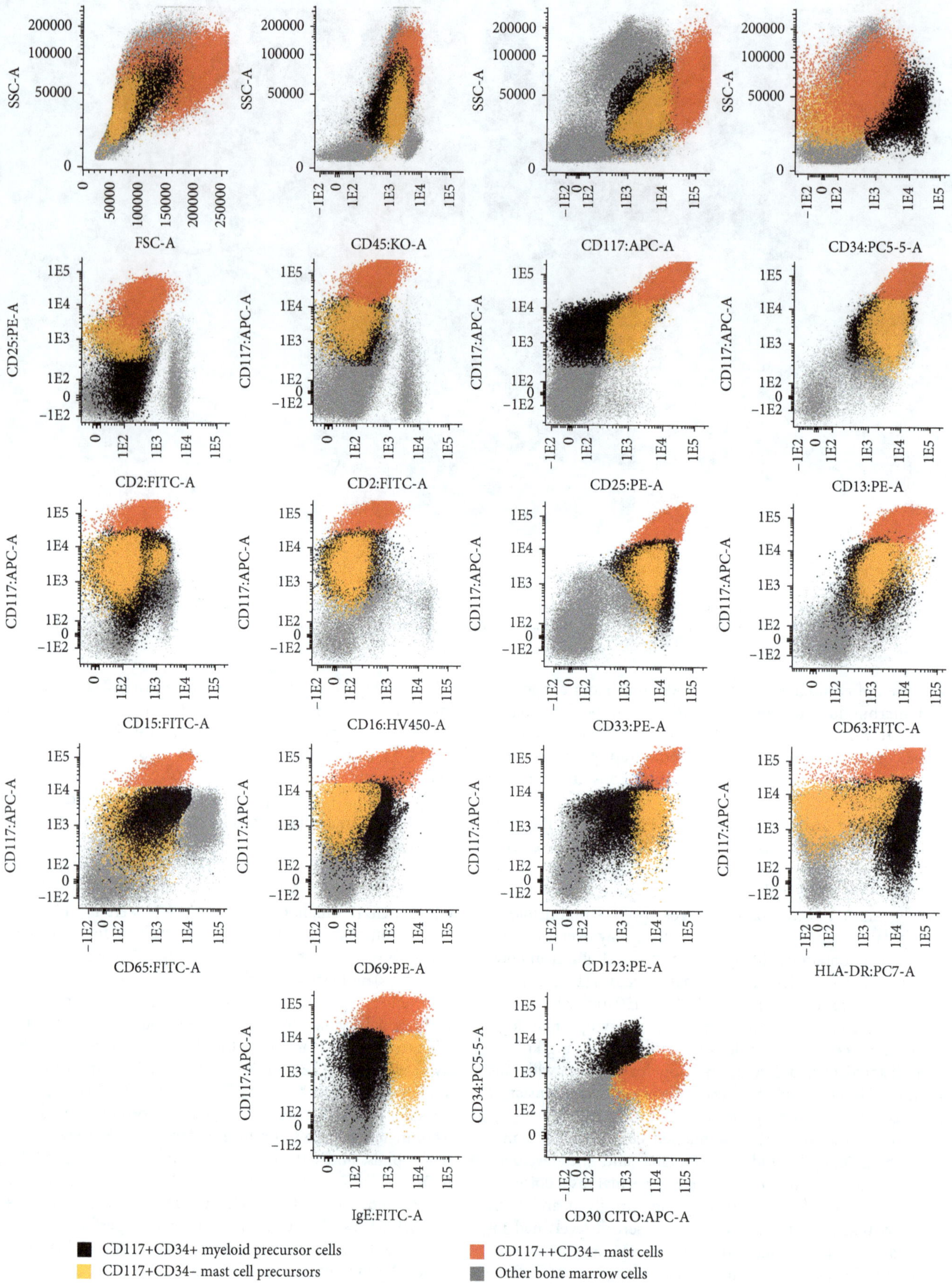

Figure 3: Continued.

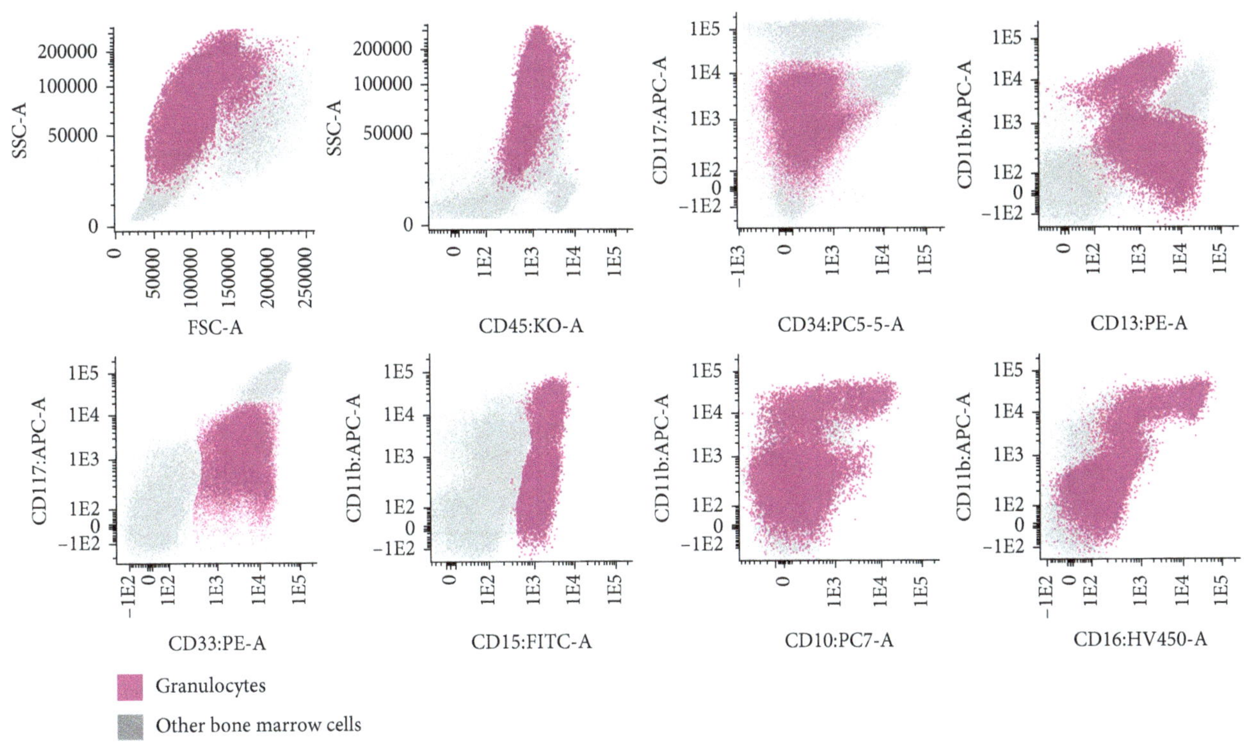

Figure 3: Bone marrow dot plots obtained by flow cytometry revealing 12% CD117+ CD34+ myeloid precursor cells (black dots), 5% CD117+CD34-mast cell precursors (orange dots), 13% of abnormal CD2− CD25+ mast cells (red dots), and 49% granulocytic cells with a maturation blockage at the promyelocyte level (purple dots). Myeloid precursor cells (black): CD117+, CD34+, CD2−, CD25−/+, CD13+, CD15−, CD16−, CD30−, CD33+, CD63+, CD65+low, CD69+low, CD123+, HLA-DR+high, and FcεRI/IgE−. Mast cell precursors (orange): CD117+, CD34−, CD2−, CD25+, CD13+, CD15−, CD16−, CD30+, CD33+, CD63+, CD65+low, CD69−, CD123+ high, HLA-DR−/+low, and FcεRI/IgE+. Mast cells (red): CD117+ high, CD34−, CD2−, CD25+ high, CD13+, CD15−, CD16−, CD30+, CD33+, CD63+, CD65+low, CD69+, CD123+ high, HLA-DR+high, and FcεRI/IgE+low.

metronidazole; oral mucositis grade II controlled with tramadol; febrile neutropenia with bacteremia by *Escherichia Coli* treated with piperacillin plus tazobactam; pneumonia without respiratory insufficiency, which was responsive to imipenem plus vancomycin, and pseudomembranous colitis by *Clostridium difficile*, treated with metronidazole.

Two months after the second course of consolidation chemotherapy, the patient received isogroup HLA-identical related allogeneic HSCT from her sister (10/10 match) (5.09×10^6/kg nonmanipulated peripheral blood CD34+ cells, totalizing 322×10^6 CD34+ cells). The reduced-intensity conditioning regimen included fludarabine (30 mg/m2/day for 5 days) and busulfan (4 mg/kg/day for 2 days). As acute complication, she had febrile neutropenia treated with meropenem. On day 30 after HSCT, she had recovery of the hematological counts, and no myeloblasts or MC were seen in the PB. Unfortunately, the BM aspirate was hypocellular and results from BM studies were unevaluable. Abdominal echography revealed stable hepatomegaly (17.5 cm), without splenomegaly, or adenomegalies. Three months after HSCT a complete chimerism was documented in PB and BM neutrophils, monocytes, and lymphocytes. She developed a chronic graft versus host disease with cutaneous manifestations, controlled with cyclosporine A and mycophenolate mofetil. By the time of this report (24 months after the diagnosis, 15 months after HSCT), she maintains normal serum tryptase levels, complete hematological remission, and complete chimerism in PB (Figure 6).

3. Discussion

According to the WHO classification, this complex case fulfils the criteria for the diagnosis of SM-AHN, more precisely, *KIT* D816V+ MCL associated with normal karyotype AML [1, 2]. Criteria for MCL include not only the conditions for SM, such as BM infiltration by morphologically and phenotypically abnormal MC forming dense aggregates (>15 MC), increased serum tryptase levels (>20 ng/ml), and the *KIT* (D816V) mutation in BM cells, but also 16% MC in the BM and 20% MC in the PB; criteria for AML were more than 20% MPO+ myeloblasts in the BM by cytomorphology. Curiously, FCM studies showed that the cells of the MC lineage were phenotypically heterogeneous, with both aberrant MCP and more mature MC being identified in the BM, and only the former being present in the PB. Interestingly, FCM studies also revealed that the granulocytic cells had an almost complete blockage at the promyelocyte stage, despite the fact that t(15;17) was negative. Thus, the MC and the granulocytic cell lineages were both compromised by the leukemic process. In accordance to this multilineage involvement, the *KIT*

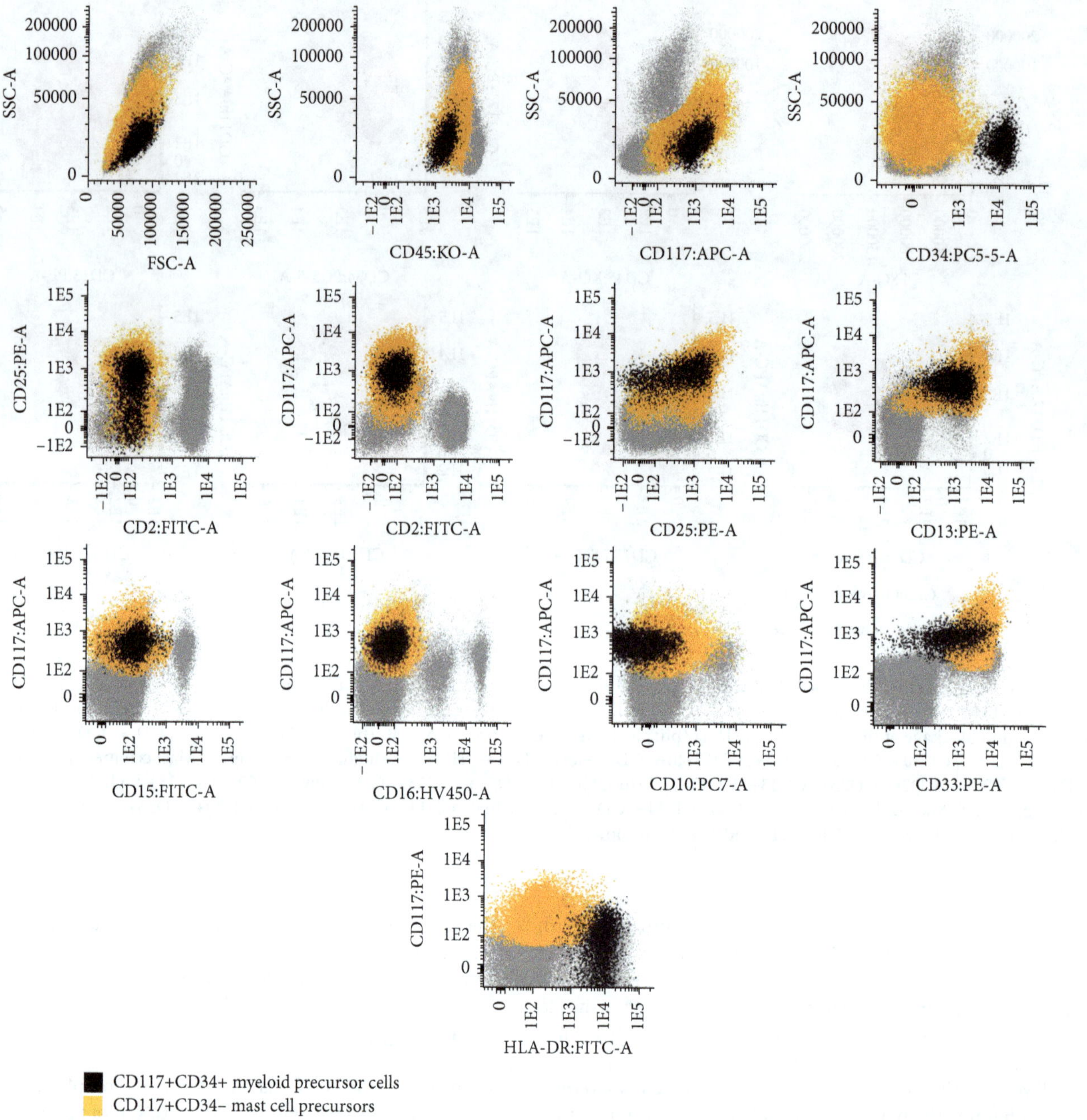

Figure 4: Peripheral blood dot plots obtained by flow cytometry showing 3% of CD117+ CD34+ myeloid precursor cells (black dots) and 49% of CD117+ CD34-mast cells precursors (orange dots). Please note that circulating myeloid precursor cells (black dots) and mast cells precursor (orange dots) had an immunophenotype like that observed in bone marrow (BM) myeloid precursor cells and BM mast cell precursors, respectively (please cf. Figure 3, same color code). Please also note that the relatively mature mast cells observed in BM (red dots, Figure 3) were not present in the peripheral blood.

D816V mutation was found in all BM cell populations tested, except in T cells. These findings are in line with previous studies, indicating that the occurrence of *KIT* mutations in an early progenitor cell results multilineage involvement, MC maturation blockade, immature MC phenotype, and aggressive disease [17–19]. The possibility of a secondary MCL arising in the context of a previously undiagnosed ISM is plausible, as the patient had a chronic maculopapular rash that had never been investigated. Unfortunately, skin biopsies were not performed, and thus, cutaneous infiltration by MC was not formally documented. It should however be mentioned, that secondary MCL usually occurs in patients with SM-AHN or ASM, and direct evolution from ISM to MCL is exceptionally rare [20–22].

The clinical and laboratory findings in patients with systemic MC neoplasms are diverse, depending on the disease subset and on the individual variability, and they are related to the release of MC mediators and/or to the infiltration of organs and tissues by the abnormal MC, which ultimately result in organ damage/failure (C-symptoms) [8, 20–22]. Except for

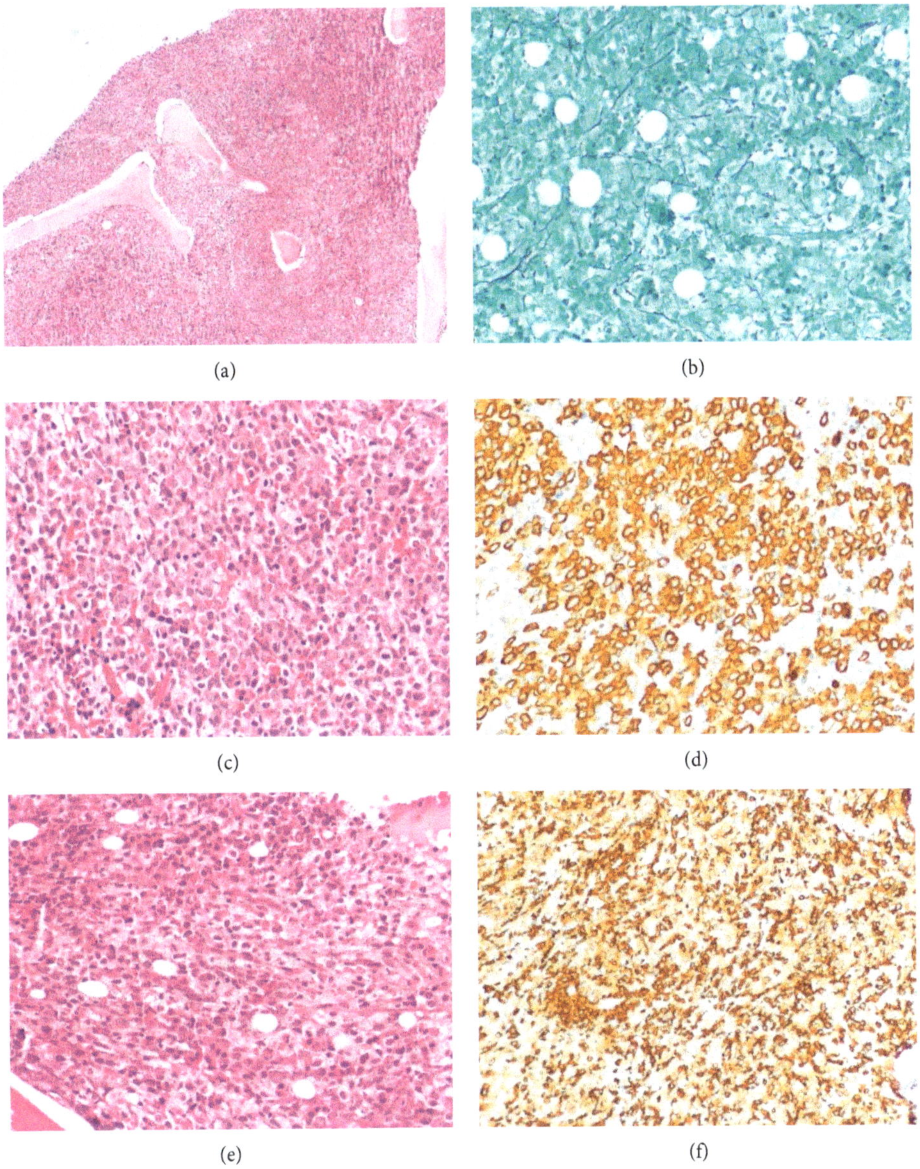

FIGURE 5: Bone marrow trephine biopsy showing a hypercellular marrow (a) with grade 2 fibrosis (b), and a preponderance of myeloid precursors with a diffuse proliferation of myeloperoxidase+ blast cells (c and d) and CD117+ mast cells (e and f). (a) Hematoxylin and eosin (H&E) stain, original amplification ×40. (b) Reticulin stain, original magnification ×100. (c) H&E stain, original amplification ×100. (d) MPO stain, original amplification ×100. (e) H&E stain, original amplification ×100. (f) CD117 stain, original amplification ×100.

a lower time from symptoms to diagnosis and a more severe neutropenia and thrombocytopenia, the clinical features observed in our patient with MCL + AML did not differ substantially from those usually found in patients with other advanced MC neoplasms, such as ASM and SM-AHN, as described in the largest series of patients with SM (342 cases), published by Lim et al. in 2009 (Table 1) [20]. In this series, ISM was the predominant SM subtype (46%), followed by SM-AHN (40%, subtype not specified) and ASM (12%), and only 4 cases were MCL (1%).

The clinical and laboratory features of our patient were those expected to occur in cases of MCL, as previously described in the literature (Table 2). In 2013, Georgin-Lavialle et al. revised all the MCL cases that had been published in scientific journals indexed in the MedLine [8]. In total, they provided data from 51 cases, including a series of 10 cases of MCL, published by Valentini et al. in 2008 [21], several cases reported individually from 1950 to 2012, and 4 personal unpublished cases; in 41 cases, they had enough data to classify them as de novo MCL ($n = 30$) or as secondary MCL ($n = 11$), and to compare the clinical and biological features of these entities (Table 2) [8]. Very recently, in 2017, Jawhar et al. reported on the clinical and laboratorial characteristics of 28 patients with MCL, from which 12 (43%) had secondary MCL and 20 (71%) had associated hematological neoplasms (MCL-AHN), other than AML [22] (Table 2). To the best of our knowledge, data available in the literature are not enough to establish if MCL-AHN has worse outcome

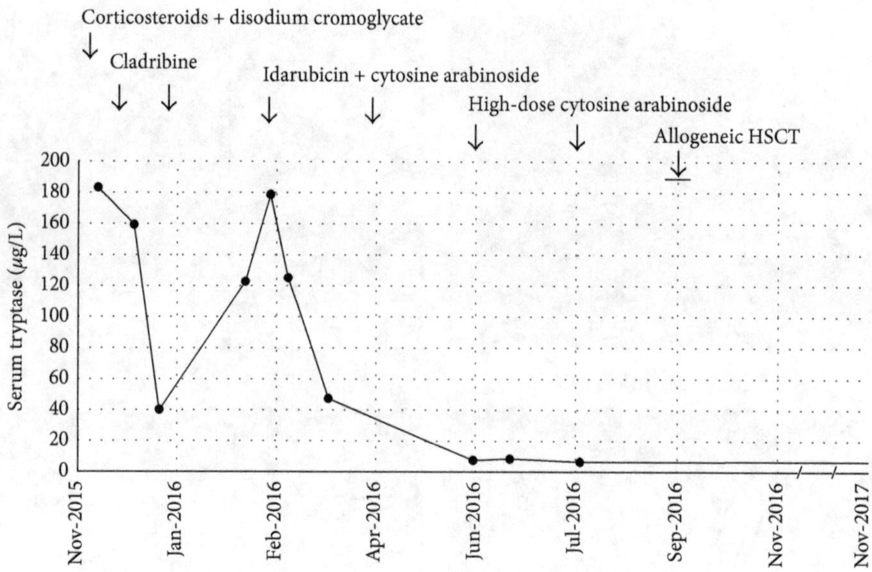

FIGURE 6: Serum tryptase levels from diagnosis of MCL-AML to date. Serum tryptase levels were markedly increased at the diagnosis (184 μg/L, October 2015) and decreased transiently to 41 μg/L after two cycles of cladribine (5 days, with one month of interval: December 2015; January 2016). However, one month later (February 2016), the serum tryptase levels increased again to 123 μg/L, and the BM aspirate showed 47% myeloblasts. At that time, the patient received two cycles of combined therapy with idarubicin and cytosine arabinoside (3 + 7 days) (February 2016; April 2016) followed by two cycles of high-dose cytosine arabinoside (June 2016; July 2016). At day +32 of reinduction chemotherapy (May 2016), the patient achieved complete hematological remission, and the serum tryptase levels decreased to 8 mg/L, remaining normal to date. At the end of August 2016, the patient received allogeneic hematopoietic stem cell transplantation (HSCT) from her sister. By the time of this report (November 2017, 24 months after the diagnosis, 15 months after HSCT), she maintains a complete hematological remission and a complete chimerism in peripheral blood.

than SM- (other than MCL) AHN, or if the type of AHN is more important for prognosis.

Rare cases of MCL have been diagnosed previously, subsequently or concomitantly to AML, as occurring in this patient [23–25]. Mast cell leukemia-AML cases exhibit a substantial increase (>20%) in myeloblasts in the BM, and they must be distinguished from MML where an AML may also be diagnosed, but criteria for SM are not met (Table 3).

Myelomastocytic leukemia is a very rare type of leukemia that is not yet incorporated in the WHO classification of the tumors of lymphoid and hematopoietic tissues [9, 16]. It is characterized by an expansion (>10%) of atypical MC together with BC with metachromatic granules (identified as MC precursors by immunophenotyping) in the BM and/or PB, concomitantly with criteria for an advanced myeloid neoplasm, which may have features of AML, MDS with excess of blast cells, or accelerated/blast phase of a MPN or a MDS/MPN. By definition, MML carries no specific (recurrent) molecular and immunophenotypic markers for SM. Specifically, activating point mutations at codon 816 of *KIT* are not found, and the aberrant CD2+/CD25+ MC immunophenotype, which is typically found in the majority of SM cases, is rare in MML. In addition, in patients with MML, the karyotype usually reflects the underlying disease (e.g., MDS, MPN, MDS/MPN, and AML) and chromosomal aberrations are frequently complex; in contrast, no recurrent chromosome abnormalities are known for patients with MCL [9, 16]. In addition, the neoplastic MC in MCL usually express CD117, low tryptase, and low FcεRI, and are often CD25+, whereas in MML, MC also express CD117 and tryptase, but they habitually stain negative for CD25. CD2 is usually negative in both cases, being frequently detected in MC from patients with indolent or smoldering SM (Table 4). Some other markers, including HLA-DR, CD30, and CD123, may also be positive in MCL cells, as observed in our patient. Thus, the clinical and laboratory findings observed in this case would favor the diagnosis of MCL associated to AML, instead of MML.

Management of patients with AML relies on genetic tests that allows for the diagnosis, informs about prognosis, and predicts response to therapy, and the value of genetics is reinforced in the WHO classification scheme for AML. For instance, cytogenetic aberrations have long been recognized as important prognostic variables in AML patients [26]. However, patients with AML and normal karyotype have had a very heterogeneous outcome, and previous studies have indicated that many other molecular aberrations do influence the response to treatment as well as in the risk of relapse [27]. For example, AML with normal cytogenetics may carry poor prognostic genetic lesions, such as *FLT3* mutations, overexpression of *BAALC* (brain and acute leukemia cytoplasmic), *ERG* (ETS/E26 transformation-specific-related gene), or *MN1* (meningioma 1) genes, or they may have aberrations that predict better prognosis as are cases with isolated *NPM-1* or *CEBPA* (CCAAT/enhancer binding protein alpha) mutations [27]. Among them, *FLT3* and *NPM-1* mutations were found to be absent in this patient. Also negative were studies for other relevant targets including t(15;17) PML-RARA, t(8;21) RUNX1-RUNX1T1, inv(16) CBFB-MYH11, and t(9,22) BCR-ABL. As mentioned before, *SRSF2*, *ASXL1*,

Table 1: Clinical and laboratory features observed in our patient with MCL + AML, as compared to those described in a series of 342 patients with SM, including ISM, ASM, and SM-AHN, published by Lim et al. in 2009 [20].

	Lim et al. series [20]			This case (MCL-AML)
	ISM ($n = 159$)	ASM ($n = 41$)	SM-AHN ($n = 138$)	
Demographic data				
Age, years	49 (19–84)	65 (32–85)	65 (20–87)	41
Gender, males/females	69 (43)/90 (57)	19 (46)/22 (54)	97 (70)/41 (30)	Female
Clinical features				
Time from symptoms to diagnosis, months	72 (0–516)	18 (1–372)	15 (1–360)	1 month
Maculopapular skin lesions	100 (63)	15 (37)	25 (18)	Yes
Cutaneous symptoms	20 (71)	16 (62)	10 (83)	Yes
Constitutional symptoms	3 (19)	24 (59)	85 (62)	Yes
MC mediators-related symptoms	110 (69)	9 (22)	39 (28)	Yes
Anaphylactoid reactions	53 (33)	2 (5)	2 (1)	No
Musculoskeletal symptoms	48 (30)	17 (41)	41 (30)	No
Gastrointestinal symptoms	113 (71)	26 (63)	79 (57)	Yes
Hepatomegaly	22 (14)	16 (39)	53 (38)	Yes
Splenomegaly	26 (17)	18 (44)	76 (57)	Yes
Lymphadenopathy	22 (14)	11 (27)	40 (29)	Yes
C-findings	NA	41 (100)	36 (26)	Yes
BM dysfunction with cytopenia(s)	NA	13 (32)	NA	Yes
Hepatomegaly with functional impairment	NA	11 (27)	20 (14)	Yes
Splenomegaly with hypersplenism	NA	9 (22)	16 (12)	Yes
Osteolysis/pathological fractures	NA	18 (44)	5 (4)	No
Malabsorption with weight loss	NA	2 (5)	1 (1)	No
Peripheral blood findings				
Hemoglobin, g/dl	13.9 (8.1–16.7)	11.3 (5.1–16.5)	10.9 (6.4–17.4)	11.0
Hemoglobin, <10.0 g/dl	4 (3)	10 (24)	48 (45)	No
Platelets, $\times 10^9$/L	260 (39–570)	179 (20–561)	129 (2–1625)	16
Platelets, $<100 \times 10^9$/L	2 (1)	11 (27)	50 (37)	Yes
Neutrophils, $\times 10^9$/L	4.2 (0.6–12.4)	4.2 (0.9–17.8)	4.8 (0.2–42.5)	0.3
Neutrophils, $<100 \times 10^9$/L	2 (1)	2 (5)	11 (8)	Yes
Serum tryptase, μg/L	53.6 (11.4–1410)	145 (10–2000)	75.4 (3.7–1360)	184
Increased tryptase: >11.5/>200 μg/L	89 (99)/11 (12)	14 (93)/6 (40)	49 (92)/15 (28)	>11.5/<200
Decreased albumin (<35 g/L)	10 (9)	10 (26)	29 (27)	Yes
Increased AP (>115 U/L)	36 (25)	24 (60)	65 (50)	Yes
Increased AST (>48)/ALT (>55 U/L)	10 (7)/4 (7)	5 (13)/1 (9)	22 (17)/5 (16)	Yes
Increased total bilirubin	3 (11)	10 (28)	42 (32)	Yes
Increased LDH (>222 U/L)	2 (4)	1 (9)	25 (25)	Yes
Bone marrow findings				
BM cellularity: increased/decreased	49 (32)/15 (10)	24 (67)/3 (8)	123 (91)/1 (1)	Increased
MC in BM biopsy: <10%	58 (41)	9 (26)	42 (35)	NA
MC in BM biopsy: 10–30%/>30%	68 (48)/15 (11)	17 (50)/8 (24)	66 (55)/12 (10)	NA
Fibrosis grade 2 or more	5 (14)	8 (47)	31 (46)	Grade 2
MC phenotype, FCM: CD2+/CD25+	27 (66)/39 (95)	4 (50)/8 (100)	7 (33)/18 (86)	No/Yes
MC nuclear morphology: oval/elongated	87 (78)/24 (22)	21 (66)/7 (22)	82 (73)/17 (15)	Mixed
MC nuclear morphology: indented/round	0 (0)/0 (0)	3 (9)/1 (3)	10 (9)/3 (3)	
Blasts in BM smears: 5–10%/>10%	0 (0)/0 (0)	0 (0)/0 (0)	16 (12)/11 (8)	24%
Molecular and chromosomal aberrancies				
KIT D816V mutation	(78)	(82)	(60)	Yes
FIP1L1-PDGFRA rearrangement	(52)	NA	NA	No

Table 1: Continued.

	Lim et al. series [20]			This case (MCL-AML)
	ISM ($n = 159$)	ASM ($n = 41$)	SM-AHN ($n = 138$)	
JAK2 V617F mutation	(4)	NA	NA	NA
Abnormal karyotype	(5)	(20)	(31)	No
Survival and leukemic transformation				
Transformation into AML or MCL	1 (<1)	2 (5)	18 (13)	MCL + AML
Median survival time from diagnosis, mo	198	41	24	Alive, 24 mo
Deaths after median follow-up of 21 mo	26 (16)	25 (61)	99 (72)	NA

AHN, associated hematological neoplasm; ALT, alanine transaminase; AML: acute myeloid leukemia; AP, alkaline phosphatase; AST, aspartate transaminase; BM: bone marrow; FCM, flow cytometry; LDH, lactate dehydrogenase; MC, mast cells; MCL, mast cell leukemia; mo, months; NA, not available, not evaluated or not applicable. Not all parameters were evaluated in all patients. Results are presented as median (range) values or as number (percentage) of patients with the mentioned characteristic.

Table 2: Clinical and laboratory features observed in our patient with MCL + AML, as compared to those described in a review of 51 cases of MCL performed by Georgin-Lavialle et al. in 2013 [8], and in a series of 28 patients with MCL published by Jawhar et al. in 2017 [22].

	Georgin-Lavialle et al. review [8]			Jawhar et al. series [22]			This case (MCL-AML)
	MCL ($n = 51$)	De novo MCL ($n = 30$)	Secondary MCL ($n = 11$)	MCL ($n = 28$)	De novo MCL ($n = 16$)	Secondary MCL ($n = 12$)	
Demographic data							
Age, years	52 (5–76)	52 (18–76)	35 (5–75)	67 (45–82)	69 (47–82)	65 (45–73)	41
Gender, males/females	20 (40)/30 (60)	11 (38)/18 (62)	6 (55)/5 (45)	16 (57)/12 (43)	10 (63)/6 (37)	6 (50)/6 (50)	Female
Diagnosis							
MCL (without AHN)	36/40 (90)	27 (89)	11 (100)	8 (29)	6 (38)	2 (17)	No
MCL-AHN (other than AML)*	4/40 (10)	3 (11)	0 (0)	20 (71)	10 (62)	10 (83)	No
MC disorder prior to MCL**	11 (40)	0 (0)	11 (100)	12 (43)	0 (0)	12 (100)	Probably yes
ASM	NA	NA	NA	2 (7)	0 (0)	2 (17)	No
SM-AHN	NA	NA	NA	10 (36)	0 (0)	10 (83)	No
Leukemic MCL (MC in the PB ≥ 10%)	18/47 (38)	15 (50)	3 (30)	2 (7)	NA	NA	Yes (20)
Peripheral blood findings							
Tryptase, μg/L	433 (21–2357)	433 (21–742)	250 (173–2357)	520 (157–1854)	520 (157–1854)	544 (160–1250)	184 μg/L
Tryptase > 200 μg/L	NA	NA	NA	26 (93)	15 (94)	11 (92)	No
Cytopenias	NA	NA	NA	26 (93)	15 (94)	11 (92)	Yes
Hemoglobin, gr/dl	9.9 (5.4–14.0)	9.0 (5.4–13.7)	11.0 (8.1–13.3)	8.9 (7.9–14.3)	9.2 (7.9–13.3)	8.7 (7.9–14.3)	11.0
Neutrophils, $\times 10^9$/L	3.7 (1.0–15.3)	6.0 (1.0–14)	NA	NA	NA	NA	0.3
Platelets, $\times 10^9$/L	110 (5–318)	82 (5–202)	111 (30–150)	69 (21–795)	64 (21–795)	86 (26–331)	16
Hypoalbuminemia < 35 g/L	NA	NA	NA	11 (39)	5 (31)	6 (50)	Yes (32 g/L)
Alkaline phosphatase > 150 U/L	NA	NA	NA	20 (71)	10 (62)	10 (62)	Yes (731 U/L)
% Mast cells	6 (0–72)	7 (0–72)	0 (0–12)	NA	NA	NA	21%
Other relevant findings							
Splenomegaly	38/49 (65)	23 (82)	9 (82)	28 (100)	16 (100)	12 (100)	Yes
Hepatomegaly	32/47 (68)	21 (78)	6 (60)	NA	NA	NA	Yes
Skin lesions	15/50 (30)	4 (14)	5 (45)	NA	NA	NA	Yes
Ascites	9/50 (18)	5 (17)	1 (9)	13 (46)	7 (44)	6 (50)	Yes

Table 2: Continued.

	Georgin-Lavialle et al. review [8]			Jawhar et al. series [22]			This case (MCL-AML)
	MCL ($n = 51$)	De novo MCL ($n = 30$)	Secondary MCL ($n = 11$)	MCL ($n = 28$)	De novo MCL ($n = 16$)	Secondary MCL ($n = 12$)	
Asthenia	NA (78)	NA	NA	NA	NA	NA	Yes
Weight loss > 10% in 6 months	NA (38)	NA	NA	12 (43)	8 (50)	4 (33)	NA
Anorexia	NA (20)	NA	NA	NA	NA	NA	Yes
Flushing and other MCAS	39/50 (78)	24 (83)	8 (73)	NA	NA	NA	Yes
Bone marrow findings							
% MC in BM smears	NA	NA	NA	25 (20–95)	25 (20–95)	20 (20–95)	16
% MC in BM biopsy	50 (20–100)	60 (20–100)	60 (25–90)	65 (20–95)	60 (20–95)	65 (30–95)	NA
Phenotypic aberrancies							
CD2+	15/29 (52)	6 (46)	1	NA	NA	NA	No
CD25+	18/24 (75)	6 (50)	3	NA	NA	NA	Yes
Molecular and chromosomal aberrancies							
KIT D816V mutation	13/28 (46)	6 (40)	1 (20)	16 (68)	10 (63)	9 (75)	Yes
Other *KIT* mutations	6/28 (22)	3 (19)	3 (60)	6 (21)	4 (25)	2 (17)	NA
SRSF2, ASXL1, or *RUNX1* mutations	NA	NA	NA	13 (52)	7 (50)	6 (55)	NA
Normal karyotype***	20/23 (83)	8 (73)	NA	19 (79)	11 (79)	8 (10)	Normal
Survival and leukemic transformation							
Survival, months	6 (0.5–98)	4 (0.5–24)	5 (1–18)	17 (1–86)	NA	NA	>24
Progression into secondary AML****	NA	NA	NA	3 (11)	2 (13)	1 (8)	MCL + AML
Deaths	33/48 (69)	24 (83)	5 (62)	18 (64)	10 (63)	8 (67)	Alive

AHN, associated hematological neoplasm; AML, acute myeloid leukemia; BM, bone marrow; CEL, chronic eosinophilic leukemia; CM, cytomorphology; CMML, chronic myelomonocytic leukemia; MC, mast cells; MCAS, mast cell activation-related symptoms; MCL, mast cell leukemia; MCL-AHN, mast cell leukemia with associated hematological neoplasm; MDS, myelodysplastic syndrome; MDS/MPN, myelodysplastic myeloproliferative neoplasm; NA, not available or not evaluated. Results are presented as median (range) values or as number (percentage) of patients with the mentioned characteristic. Not all parameters were evaluated in all patients. *AHN included MDS ($n = 3$) and CMML ($n = 1$) in the Georgin-Lavialle review, and CMML ($n = 8$), MDS/MPN unclassifiable ($n = 5$), MDS ($n = 5$) or CEL ($n = 2$) in the Jawhar series. **Our patient had past history of uninvestigated maculopapular skin lesions and flushing episodes, and a maculopapular rash at the diagnosis (skin biopsy not performed). ***In the Jawhar series, karyotype was available in 24 patients with MCL (14 patients with de novo MCL and 10 patients with secondary MCL); 5 patients (21%) had an aberrant karyotype (3 patients with de novo MCL, 21%; 2 patients with secondary MCL, 20%), with 3 patients having a complex karyotype (≥3 aberrations) and 2 patients having del(5q) or del(12p), respectively. Cytogenetic studies were available for 23 of 51 cases reviewed by Georgin-Lavialle et al., and a normal karyotype was found in 83% cases (83%). Two patients (9%) had a 5q deletion and were diagnosed as having MCL-MDS, and 2 patients with de novo MCL had t(10;16)(q22;q13q22) and t(8;21)(q22;q22). Thus, there are no recurrent cytogenetic abnormalities in MCL. ****Three patients from the Jawhar series progressed into secondary AML 18, 28, and 34 months, respectively, after the diagnosis of MCL had been established.

and *RUNX1* mutations, described to be present in around 50% of MCL patients and found to affect adversely response to treatment and to predict lower OS [22], were not examined in this case.

Due fundamentally to the extreme rarity of MCL, no standard treatment exists, and therapies frequently consist on those commonly used in aggressive SM, such as cladribine (2-chloro-deoxy-adenosine, 2-CDA), interferon alpha 2a (IFN-α2a), and tyrosine kinase (TK) inhibitors (TKI). As MCL is presumably a clonal disorder of hematopoietic myeloid stem cells, chemotherapy with drugs proven successful in AML, such as anthracyclines in combination with AraC, have also been used to treat patients with MCL. If hematological remission is achieved, additional therapy with curative intent involving HSCT might be attempted, as in this patient [7, 8].

The rationale behind the use of cladribine, which was the first therapy tried in our patient, is based on the value of this drug in the treatment of aggressive SM, which has been confirmed in several studies [28, 29]. However, 2-CDA had no or little activity in this case, as in most previously reported cases of MCL treated with this purine analogue [22, 30], although in rare cases transient or prolonged partial response has been observed [21, 31, 32]. Reports on the use of IFN-α2a in MCL are scarce, and the results obtained were also not encouraging [21, 31].

Tyrosine kinase inhibitors have been actively investigated for the treatment of patients with mastocytosis because *KIT* mutations often cause constitutive activation of TK activity of the *KIT* receptor [33]. Imatinib is effective in patients with increased mast cells and eosinophils associated

TABLE 3: Clinical and laboratory features in our patient as compared to those observed in patients with MCL or MML, as schematized by Valent et al. in 2014 [9].

	Mast cell leukemia (MCL)	Myelomastocytic leukemia (MML)	This case (MCL-AML)
Clinical features			
Skin lesions	Present in a subset of patients	Absent	Yes (maculopapular rash)
Spleen involvement/splenomegaly	Found in a subset of patients	Usually present at diagnosis	Yes (13 cm; splenic nodules)
Liver involvement/ hepatomegaly, ascites	Often found	Usually not found	Yes (18.5 cm; cholestasis; ascites)
MC mediators-related symptoms	Frequent	Frequent	Yes (flushing; diarrhea)
Peripheral blood findings			
Serum tryptase (μg/L)	Markedly elevated (usually >200; often >500)	Moderately elevated (usually <100; often <50)	184 μg/L
Circulating MC	Present in a subset of patients	Present in a subset of patients	Yes (CM: 20%); FCM: 21% MCP
Circulating myeloblasts	No (except MCL-AHN)	Present in a subset of patients	Yes (CM: 6%); FCM: 3% MPC
Bone marrow findings			
Underlying non-MC myeloid neoplasms	No (except MCL-AHN)	Yes	AML (concomitant diagnosis)
Increased myeloblasts	No (except MCL-AHN)	Almost always seen	Yes (CM: 24% myeloblasts + 17% promyelocytes); FCM: 12% MPC + 34% promyelocytes
MC clusters and sheets in BM biopsy	Yes	No	Yes
Diffuse MC infiltrate in the BM biopsy	Yes	Yes	Yes
MC in BM smears	≥20%	≥10%	Yes (CM: 16%); FCM: 5% MCP + 13% MC
Karyotype	Normal or abnormal with a few lesions (except MCL-AHN)**	Usually complex**	Normal
CD25+ MC	Yes	No	Yes
KIT D816V or other codon 816 mutation	Present	Not found	Yes (BM mast cells, CD34+ precursors and other myeloid cells)
KIT mutations in non-816-codons	Found in a subset of patients	Found in a subset of patients	Not investigated

AHN, associated hematological neoplasm; AML, acute myeloid leukemia; BM, bone marrow; CM, cytomorphology; FCM, flow cytometry; MC, mast cells; MCL, mast cell leukemia; MCL-AHN, mast cell leukemia with associated hematological neoplasm; MCP, mast cell precursors; MML, myelomastocytic leukemia; MPC, myeloid precursor cells. *Past history of uninvestigated maculopapular skin lesions and flushing episodes; maculopapular rash at the diagnosis (skin biopsy not performed). **In MML, the karyotype usually reflects the nature of the underlying disease, whereas no recurrent chromosome abnormalities are known for patients with MCL.

with *FIP1L1/PDGFRA* (Factor Interacting with PAPOLA and CPSF/Platelet-derived growth factor receptor A) fusion gene (e.g., myeloid neoplasm with eosinophilia and rearrangement of PDGFRA) [34] or rare patients with SM associated with *KIT* mutations outside of exon 17 [30]. However, the results from imatinib and other TKI, such as masitinib and dasatinib, in MCL and other D816V+ SM have been disappointing [21, 35–37].

Midostaurin (PKC412), a multitarget TKI, is a promising agent for patients with advanced SM, as it inhibits the growth of neoplastic MC exhibiting various mutant forms of *KIT*, including *KIT* D816V [38]. In contrast to other *KIT*-targeting drugs, midostaurin also impedes IgE-dependent release of histamine [39, 40]. Midostaurin has been reported to be efficacious in patients with advanced SM, including ASM and MCL [22, 41, 42]. Data from a Phase 2 single-arm open-label trial (CPKC412D2201), which included 89 with mastocytosis-related organ damage (16 with aggressive SM, 57 with SM-AHN, and 16 MCL), revealed that treatment with midostaurin 100 mg twice daily resulted in an overall response rate of 60% with a median duration of response of 24 months and a median overall survival of 29 months [42]. Unfortunately, midostaurin was not yet approved for patients with advanced SM, including MCL, and the drug was not available for compassionate use at the time the MCL was diagnosed in our patient. Brentuximab vedotin has also been considered for the treatment of patients with advanced SM. The results obtained in a small series of 4 patients with SM have suggested that this anti-CD30 monoclonal antibody-drug conjugate can induce durable responses with

TABLE 4: Cell molecules expressed in MC from our patient as compared to those usually expressed in the MC from patients with MCL or MML, as schematized by Valent et al. in 2014 [9].

Markers	Normal MC	ISM	SSM	ASM	MCL	MML	This case
CD34 (HPCA-1)	–	–	–	–	–	–	–
CD117 (*KIT*)	+	+	+	+	+	+	+
Tryptase	+	+	+	+	+	+	NA
CD33 (Siglec-3)	+	+	+	+	+	+	+
CD123 (IL-3RA)	–	–	–	+/–	+/–	–	+
CD2 (LFA-2)	–	+/–	+/–	–/+	–/+	–	–
CD25 (IL-2RA)	–	+	+	+	+	–	+
CD30 (Ki1)	–	–/+	+	+	+	NA	+
FcεRI	+	+	+	+	–/+ (low)	–	+ (low)

HPCA-1, human precursor cell antigen-1; IL-2RA, interleukin-2 receptor alpha chain; IL-3RA, interleukin-3 receptor alpha chain; ISM, indolent systemic mastocytosis; SSM, smoldering SM; ASM, aggressive SM; MCL, mast cell leukemia; MML, myelomastocytic leukemia; NA, not available. +, expressed in MCs in almost all (>90% of) cases; +/–, expressed in a majority of MC in a considerable proportion of cases; –/+, expressed in a minority of MC in a smaller subset of cases; –, not expressed. In a few cases, one of the two markers, either CD2 or CD25, may be expressed in neoplastic MCs in MML.

a manageable toxicity profile [43], and a clinical trial in patients with CD30 positive ASM and MCL is currently going on in the United States (NCT01807598). Thus, midostaurin and brentuximab vedotin may be considered alternative adjuvant therapies in case of disease relapse in our patient.

Induction chemotherapy has been used in some patients with MCL. According to the review performed by Georgin-Lavialle et al., AML-type chemotherapy was used in 6 of 51 MCL patients reported till 2013; the median survival time was 7 months, and all patients died between 2 and 29 months, because of disease progression or multiorgan failure [8]. A few cases of patients with MCL who received HSCT have also been reported, but sustained remission was not achieved in any of them [21, 44–46]. Ustun et al. have reported on a retrospective series of 57 patients with SM, including SM-AHN ($n = 38$), ASM ($n = 7$) and MCL ($n = 12$), who received allogeneic HSCT either after myeloablative ($n = 36$) or nonmyeloablative reduced-intensity ($n = 21$) conditioning regimens [47]. Responses were observed in 70% of the patients, with complete remission in 28%. Twenty-one percent of patients had stable disease, and 9% had primary refractory disease. The best responses were obtained in SM-AHN (AML/MDS), and the worst were obtained in MCL patients. Overall survival at 3 years was 57% for all patients, 74% for patients with SM-AHN, 43% for those with ASM, and 17% for those with MCL, and the strongest risk factor for poor overall survival was MCL. Survival was also lower in patients receiving nonmyeloablative compared with myeloablative conditioning regimens and in patients having progression compared with patients having stable disease or response. Although allogeneic HSCT may be considered a potentially curative treatment for advanced SM, including MCL, its definitive role needs to be determined by prospective clinical trials. Our patient maintains hematological remission of both diseases (MCL and AML) with complete chimerism, 15 months after HLA-identical HSCT.

In summary, we described an extremely rare case of an adult female with *KIT* D816V+ MCL associated with normal karyotype AML without *FLT3* and *NPM-1* mutations, who was refractive to cladribine and who achieved complete hematological remission after receiving induction chemotherapy with idarubicin and AraC, followed by allogeneic HLA-identical sibling HSCT preceded by a reduced-intensity conditioning regimen.

Conflicts of Interest

The authors declare that they have no conflicts of interest.

Authors' Contributions

Marta Lopes collected data and contributed to manuscript writing. Patrícia Seabra, Vanessa Mesquita, Cláudia Casais, Renata Cabral, and Jorge Coutinho provided clinical support and were responsible for the therapeutic decisions. José-Palla Garcia and José Ramón Vizcaíno performed analysis of bone marrow trephine biopsy and immunohistochemical staining. Maria dos Anjos Teixeira contributed to flow cytometry data analysis and interpretation, and case discussion. Catarina Lau participated in flow cytometry data interpretation. Inês Freitas performed analysis of the bone marrow smears, cytomorphology, and cytochemical staining. João Rodrigues performed cytogenetic and molecular genetic studies. Maria Jara-Acevedo performed cell sorting and *KIT* mutation analysis. Luís Escribano was involved in data interpretation and case discussion. Alberto Orfao was involved in flow cytometry data analysis and interpretation, and in case discussion. Margarida Lima participated in flow cytometry data analysis, data interpretation and case discussion, and gave major contributions to manuscript writing. All authors read, discussed, and approved the final version of the manuscript.

References

[1] H. Horny, C. Akin, D. Arber et al., "Mastocytosis," in in *World Health Organization Classification of Tumours Pathology & Genetics Tumours of Haematopoietic and Lymphoid Tissues*, S. Swerdlow, E. Campo, N. Harris et al, Eds., International Agency for Research on Cancer (IARC) Press, Lyon, France, 2016.

[2] P. Valent, C. Akin, K. Hartmann et al., "Advances in the classification and treatment of mastocytosis: current status and outlook toward the future," *Cancer Research*, vol. 77, no. 6, pp. 1261–1270, 2017.

[3] A. Matito, J. M. Morgado, I. Álvarez-Twose et al., "Serum tryptase monitoring in indolent systemic mastocytosis: association with disease features and patient outcome," *PLoS One*, vol. 8, no. 10, article e76116, 2013.

[4] J. M. Morgado, L. Sánchez-Muñoz, C. Teodósio, and L. Escribano, "Identification and immunophenotypic characterization of normal and pathological mast cells," *Methods in Molecular Biology*, vol. 1192, pp. 205–226, 2014.

[5] C. Teodosio, A. Mayado, L. Sánchez-Muñoz et al., "The immunophenotype of mast cells and its utility in the diagnostic work-up of systemic mastocytosis," *Journal of Leukocyte Biology*, vol. 97, no. 1, pp. 49–59, 2015.

[6] M. Arock, K. Sotlar, C. Akin et al., "*KIT* mutation analysis in mast cell neoplasms: recommendations of the European Competence Network on Mastocytosis," *Leukemia*, vol. 29, no. 6, pp. 1223–1232, 2015.

[7] R. Stone and S. Bernstein, "Mast cell leukemia and other mast cell neoplasms," in *Holland-Frei Cancer Medicine*, D. Kufe, R. Pollock, R. Weichselbaum et al, Eds., BC Decker, Hamilton, Ontario, Canada, 6th edition, 2003, http://www.ncbi.nlm.nih.gov/books/NBK12354/.

[8] S. Georgin-Lavialle, L. Lhermitte, P. Dubreuil, M.-O. Chandesris, O. Hermine, and G. Damaj, "Mast cell leukemia," *Blood*, vol. 121, no. 8, pp. 1285–1295, 2013.

[9] P. Valent, K. Sotlar, W. R. Sperr et al., "Refined diagnostic criteria and classification of mast cell leukemia (MCL) and myelomastocytic leukemia (MML): a consensus proposal," *Annals of Oncology*, vol. 25, no. 9, pp. 1691–1700, 2014.

[10] P. Valent, W. R. Sperr, P. Samorapoompichit et al., "Myelomastocytic overlap syndromes: biology, criteria, and relationship to mastocytosis," *Leukemia Research*, vol. 25, no. 7, pp. 595–602, 2001.

[11] P. Valent, P. Samorapoompichit, W. R. Sperr, H.-P. Horny, and K. Lechner, "Myelomastocytic leukemia: myeloid neoplasm characterized by partial differentiation of mast cell-lineage cells," *Hematology*, vol. 3, no. 2, pp. 90–94, 2002.

[12] W. R. Sperr, J. Drach, A. W. Hauswirth et al., "Myelomastocytic leukemia: evidence for the origin of mast cells from the leukemic clone and eradication by allogeneic stem cell transplantation," *Clinical Cancer Research*, vol. 11, no. 19, pp. 6787–6792, 2005.

[13] A. R. Arredondo, J. Gotlib, L. Shier et al., "Myelomastocytic leukemia versus mast cell leukemia versus systemic mastocytosis associated with acute myeloid leukemia: a diagnostic challenge," *American Journal of Hematology*, vol. 85, no. 8, pp. 600–606, 2010.

[14] S. Intzes, S. Wiersma, and H. J. Meyerson, "Myelomastocytic leukemia with t(8;21) in a 3-year-old child," *Journal of Pediatric Hematology/Oncology*, vol. 33, no. 8, pp. e372–e375, 2011.

[15] A. Rich, J. Sun, A. S. Aldayel et al., "Myelomastocytic leukemia with aberrant CD25 expression: case report and review of the literature," *Clinical Lymphoma Myeloma and Leukemia*, vol. 14, no. 5, pp. e173–e177, 2014.

[16] H.-P. Horny, K. Sotlar, A. Reiter et al., "Myelomastocytic leukemia: histopathological features, diagnostic criteria and differential diagnosis," *Expert Review of Hematology*, vol. 7, no. 4, pp. 431–437, 2014.

[17] A. C. Garcia-Montero, M. Jara-Acevedo, C. Teodosio et al., "*KIT* mutation in mast cells and other bone marrow hematopoietic cell lineages in systemic mast cell disorders: a prospective study of the Spanish Network on Mastocytosis (REMA) in a series of 113 patients," *Blood*, vol. 108, no. 7, pp. 2366–2372, 2006.

[18] C. Teodosio, A. C. Garcia-Montero, M. Jara-Acevedo et al., "Mast cells from different molecular and prognostic subtypes of systemic mastocytosis display distinct immunophenotypes," *Journal of Allergy and Clinical Immunology*, vol. 125, no. 3, pp. 719.e4–726.e4, 2010.

[19] C. Teodosio, A. C. Garcia-Montero, M. Jara-Acevedo et al., "An immature immunophenotype of bone marrow mast cells predicts for multilineage D816V *KIT* mutation in systemic mastocytosis," *Leukemia*, vol. 26, no. 5, pp. 951–958, 2012.

[20] K. H. Lim, A. Tefferi, T. L. Lasho et al., "Systemic mastocytosis in 342 consecutive adults: survival studies and prognostic factors," *Blood*, vol. 113, no. 23, pp. 5727–5736, 2009.

[21] C. G. Valentini, M. Rondoni, E. M. Pogliani et al., "Mast cell leukemia: a report of ten cases," *Annals of Hematology*, vol. 87, no. 6, pp. 505–508, 2008.

[22] M. Jawhar, J. Schwaab, M. Meggendorfer et al., "The clinical and molecular diversity of mast cell leukemia with or without associated hematologic neoplasm," *Haematologica*, vol. 102, no. 6, pp. 1035–1043, 2017.

[23] A. Beghini, R. Cairoli, E. Morra, and L. Larizza, "In vivo differentiation of mast cells from acute myeloid leukemia blasts carrying a novel activating ligand-independent C-kit mutation," *Blood Cells Molecules and Diseases*, vol. 24, no. 2, pp. 262–270, 1998.

[24] J. Gotlib, C. Berubé, J. D. Growney et al., "Activity of the tyrosine kinase inhibitor PKC412 in a patient with mast cell leukemia with the D816V *KIT* mutation," *Blood*, vol. 106, no. 8, pp. 2865–2870, 2005.

[25] M. H. Bae, H.-K. Kim, C.-J. Park et al., "A case of systemic mastocytosis associated with acute myeloid leukemia terminating as aleukemic mast cell leukemia after allogeneic hematopoietic stem cell transplantation," *Annals of Laboratory Medicine*, vol. 33, no. 2, pp. 125–129, 2013.

[26] M. L. Gulley, T. C. Shea, and Y. Fedoriw, "Genetic tests to evaluate prognosis and predict therapeutic response in acute myeloid leukemia," *Journal of Molecular Diagnostics*, vol. 12, no. 1, pp. 3–16, 2010.

[27] S. Z. Zaidi, T. Owaidah, F. Al Sharif, S. Y. Ahmed, N. Chaudhri, and M. Aljurf, "The challenge of risk stratification in acute myeloid leukemia with normal karyotype," *Hematology/Oncology and Stem Cell Therapy*, vol. 1, no. 3, pp. 141–158, 2008.

[28] H. C. Kluin-Nelemans, J. M. Oldhoff, J. J. van Doormaal et al., "Cladribine therapy for systemic mastocytosis," *Blood*, vol. 102, no. 13, pp. 4270–4276, 2003.

[29] A. Pardanani, A. V. Hoffbrand, J. H. Butterfield et al., "Treatment of systemic mast cell disease with 2-chlorodeoxyadenosine," *Leukemia Research*, vol. 28, no. 2, pp. 127–131, 2004.

[30] A. Mital, A. Piskorz, K. Lewandowski et al., "A case of mast cell leukaemia with exon 9 *KIT* mutation and good response to imatinib," *European Journal of Haematology*, vol. 86, no. 6, pp. 531–535, 2011.

[31] O. Penack, K. Sotlar, F. Noack et al., "Cladribine therapy in a patient with an aleukemic subvariant of mast cell leukemia," *Annals of Hematology*, vol. 84, no. 10, pp. 692-693, 2005.

[32] F. Noack, K. Sotlar, M. Notter, E. Thiel, P. Valent, and H.-P. Horny, "Aleukemic mast cell leukemia with abnormal immunophenotype and c-kit mutation D816V," *Leukemia and Lymphoma*, vol. 45, no. 11, pp. 2295–2302, 2004.

[33] C. Ustun, D. L. DeRemer, and C. Akin, "Tyrosine kinase inhibitors in the treatment of systemic mastocytosis," *Leukemia Research*, vol. 35, no. 9, pp. 1143–1152, 2011.

[34] Y. Yamada and J. A. Cancelas, "FIP1L1/PDGFR alpha-associated systemic mastocytosis," *International Archives of Allergy and Immunology*, vol. 152, no. 1, pp. 101–105, 2010.

[35] S. Georgin-Lavialle, L. Lhermitte, F. Suarez et al., "Mast cell leukemia: identification of a new c-Kit mutation, dup(501-502), and response to masitinib, a c-Kit tyrosine kinase inhibitor," *European Journal of Haematology*, vol. 89, no. 1, pp. 47–52, 2012.

[36] K. J. Aichberger, W. R. Sperr, K. V. Gleixner et al., "Treatment responses to cladribine and dasatinib in rapidly progressing aggressive mastocytosis," *European Journal of Clinical Investigation*, vol. 38, no. 11, pp. 869–873, 2008.

[37] M. S. Spector, I. Iossifov, A. Kritharis et al., "Mast-cell leukemia exome sequencing reveals a mutation in the IgE mast-cell receptor β chain and *KIT* V654A," *Leukemia*, vol. 26, no. 6, pp. 1422–1425, 2012.

[38] K. V. Gleixner, M. Mayerhofer, K. J. Aichberger et al., "PKC412 inhibits in vitro growth of neoplastic human mast cells expressing the D816V-mutated variant of *KIT*: comparison with AMN107, imatinib, and cladribine (2CdA) and evaluation of cooperative drug effects," *Blood*, vol. 107, no. 2, pp. 752–759, 2006.

[39] M.-T. Krauth, I. Mirkina, H. Herrmann et al., "Midostaurin (PKC412) inhibits immunoglobulin E-dependent activation and mediator release in human blood basophils and mast cells," *Clinical and Experimental Allergy*, vol. 39, no. 11, pp. 1711–1720, 2009.

[40] B. Peter, G. E. Winter, K. Blatt et al., "Target interaction profiling of midostaurin and its metabolites in neoplastic mast cells predicts distinct effects on activation and growth," *Leukemia*, vol. 30, no. 2, pp. 464–472, 2016.

[41] M. O. Chandesris, G. Damaj, D. Canioni et al., "Midostaurin in advanced systemic mastocytosis," *New England Journal of Medicine*, vol. 374, no. 26, pp. 2605–2607, 2016.

[42] J. Gotlib, H. C. Kluin-Nelemans, T. I. George et al., "Efficacy and safety of midostaurin in advanced systemic mastocytosis," *New England Journal of Medicine*, vol. 374, no. 26, pp. 2530–2541, 2016.

[43] U. Borate, A. Mehta, V. Reddy, M. Tsai, N. Josephson, and I. Schnadig, "Treatment of CD30-positive systemic mastocytosis with brentuximab vedotin," *Leukemia Research*, vol. 44, pp. 25–31, 2016.

[44] T.-Y. Chen, J.-S. Chen, W.-T. Huang, W.-C. Su, and C.-J. Tsao, "Rapid engraftment of mast cells of donor origin in a case of acute myeloid leukemia with mast cell leukemia after allogeneic stem cell transplantation," *Bone Marrow Transplantation*, vol. 32, no. 1, pp. 111–114, 2003.

[45] R. Nakamura, S. Chakrabarti, C. Akin et al., "A pilot study of nonmyeloablative allogeneic hematopoietic stem cell transplant for advanced systemic mastocytosis," *Bone Marrow Transplantation*, vol. 37, no. 4, pp. 353–358, 2006.

[46] R. Chantorn and T. Shwayder, "Death from mast cell leukemia: a young patient with longstanding cutaneous mastocytosis evolving into fatal mast cell leukemia," *Pediatric Dermatology*, vol. 29, no. 5, pp. 605–609, 2012.

[47] C. Ustun, A. Reiter, B. L. Scott et al., "Hematopoietic stem-cell transplantation for advanced systemic mastocytosis," *Journal of Clinical Oncology*, vol. 32, no. 29, pp. 3264–3274, 2014.

Dasatinib and Prednisolone Induction Therapy for a Case of Philadelphia Chromosome-Positive Acute Lymphoblastic Leukemia with Dilated Cardiomyopathy Accompanied by Life-Threatening Ventricular Tachycardia

Mitsutaka Nishimoto,[1] Hirohisa Nakamae,[1] Kana Matsumoto,[2] Kunihiko Morita,[2] Yuki Koga,[3] Dai Momose,[4] and Masayuki Hino[1]

[1]*Hematology, Graduate School of Medicine, Osaka City University, 1-4-3 Asahi-machi, Abeno, Osaka, Japan*

[2]*Department of Clinical Pharmaceutics, Faculty of Pharmaceutical Sciences, Doshisha Women's College of Liberal Arts, Kodo, Kyotanabe, Kyoto, Japan*

[3]*Department of Cardiovascular Medicine, Graduate School of Medicine, Osaka City University, 1-4-3 Asahi-machi, Abeno, Osaka, Japan*

[4]*Department of Hematology, Osaka General Hospital, West Japan Railway Company, 1-2-22 Matsuzaki-cho, Abeno, Osaka, Japan*

Correspondence should be addressed to Mitsutaka Nishimoto; nishimo@med.osaka-cu.ac.jp

Academic Editor: Ramon Tiu

A 56-year-old man being treated for dilated cardiomyopathy presented with epigastralgia. He was diagnosed with ventricular tachycardia and Philadelphia chromosome-positive acute lymphoblastic leukemia. After treating incessant ventricular tachycardia, we commenced induction therapy for leukemia with dasatinib and prednisolone to minimize toxicity towards cardiomyocytes and the cardiac conduction system. Although dasatinib was temporarily withheld because of a recurrence of ventricular tachycardia, we rechallenged dasatinib while using bisoprolol and amiodarone and achieved a complete hematological response three weeks later. Although drug interactions between dasatinib and amiodarone were of concern, the blood concentration of each drug remained within the safe range after concomitant use, and there were no adverse cardiac effects such as QT prolongation after rechallenging dasatinib. Induction therapy with dasatinib and prednisolone may be an acceptable therapeutic option for Philadelphia chromosome-positive acute lymphoblastic leukemia with severe cardiac complications.

1. Introduction

Dasatinib, a second-generation tyrosine kinase inhibitor (TKI), has profoundly improved the prognosis for Philadelphia chromosome-positive leukemia [1]. Combined with steroids, dasatinib has been used to effectively treat Philadelphia chromosome-positive acute lymphoblastic leukemia (Ph^+ ALL) [2]. It is well known that TKIs have cardiovascular toxicity and can cause ventricular tachycardia (VT) because of QT prolongation [3–5]. In a randomized phase-3 trial, drug-related adverse cardiac effects occurred in 17 of 258 leukemia patients treated with dasatinib [6]. Dasatinib was also discontinued after QT prolongation in one patient among 26 Japanese leukemia patients [7]. In patients with advanced solid tumors, a high dasatinib blood concentration has been associated with prolongation of the QTc interval [8]. We should be aware of adverse cardiac effects when using TKIs. However, there are few data regarding treatments for Ph^+ ALL patients with cardiomyopathy or life-threatening ventricular arrhythmias. Although it has been reported that drug interactions between dasatinib and amiodarone can occur [9], there has not yet been much clinical data. Herein, we describe induction therapy with dasatinib plus prednisolone with concomitant use of bisoprolol and amiodarone

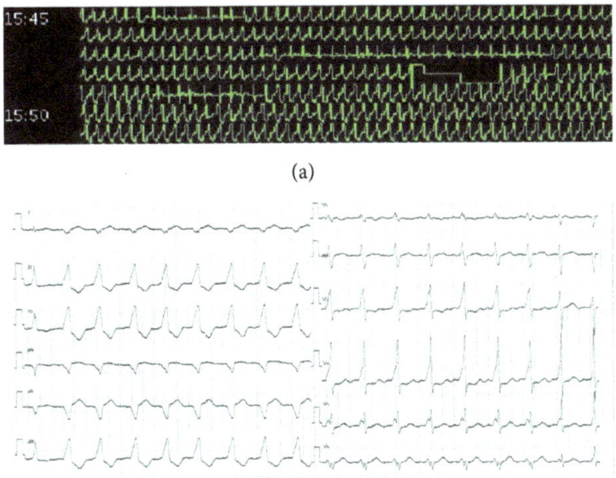

(a)

(b)

Figure 1: The 24-hour and twelve-lead electrocardiograms on admission. The 24-hour electrocardiogram shows a ventricular arrhythmia persisting for more than five minutes, and the twelve-lead electrocardiogram on admission shows incessant ventricular tachycardia.

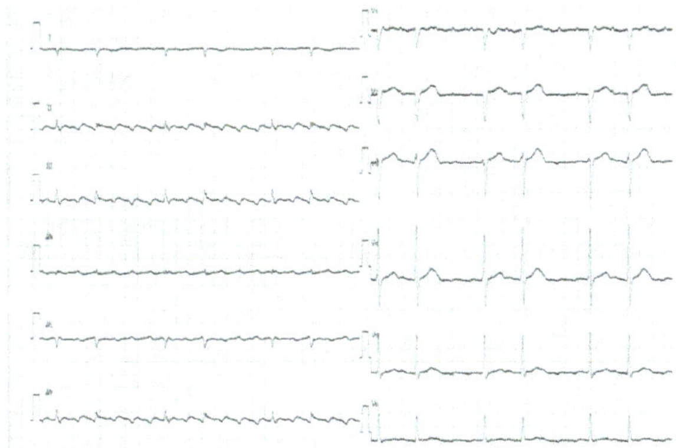

Figure 2: Electrocardiogram on the 22nd day after dasatinib retreatment. Potentially fatal ventricular arrhythmias have been replaced by atrial flutter.

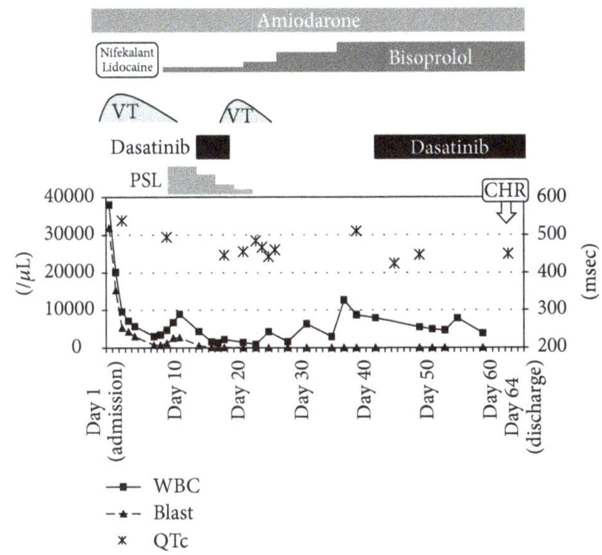

Figure 3: Clinical course before and after dasatinib treatment. VT, ventricular tachycardia; PSL, prednisolone; CHR, complete hematological response.

for a patient with Ph^+ ALL who had dilated cardiomyopathy and incessant VT.

2. Case

A 56-year-old man who had been treated for dilated cardiomyopathy and atrial fibrillation presented at the hospital with epigastralgia. His electrocardiogram showed nonsustained VT, which developed into VT storms even after starting amiodarone (Figure 1). Nifekalant hydrochloride and lidocaine were also administered, and the ventricular arrhythmias then decreased, and atrial flutter was seen. After the hemodynamics had been stabilized, we started bisoprolol with a dose of 0.625 mg daily. While treating the cardiac complications, we assessed the patient's blood sample. Severe anemia and blastoid cells were observed in the peripheral blood. The bone marrow contained 96% lymphoid blast cells with a 46, XY, t(9;22)(q34;q11.2) karyotype, and minor bcr-abl mRNA transcripts were detected at 7.0×10^5 copies/μg RNA. The patient was diagnosed with Ph^+ ALL and received induction therapy with dasatinib 50 mg twice daily and prednisolone 100 mg daily to minimize toxicity towards cardiomyocytes and the cardiac conduction system. We started dasatinib at a lower dose because of concerns about cardiotoxicity. Five days after initiating dasatinib and prednisolone, dasatinib was discontinued because of increments in nonsustained VT although the QTc interval had not become significantly prolonged (455 ms). We gradually increased the dose of bisoprolol to 3.75 mg daily. After being withdrawn for 22 days, dasatinib was rechallenged, and we could continue without the appearance of nonsustained VT or the prolongation of QTc intervals (Figures 2 and 3). The serum concentration of dasatinib one hour after oral administration ($C_{1\,\mathrm{hr}}$) and the plasma concentrations of amiodarone and desethylamiodarone approximately 12 hours after oral administration on the 10th day of concomitant use were 45.7 ng/mL, 660.6 ng/mL, and 449.0 ng/mL, respectively. Three weeks after retreatment with dasatinib, we confirmed a complete hematological response and a 2-log reduction in minor bcr-abl mRNA transcripts in the patient's bone marrow (Table 1). He wished to be discharged from hospital and refused a dose-escalation of dasatinib or chemotherapy. On the 88th day after his admission, blastoid cells appeared in the peripheral blood. We discontinued dasatinib at that time because of the refractoriness of his leukemia. Although VT recurred and lasted for five days, it disappeared following the initiation of steroid pulse therapy and furosemide. After that, VT did not recur. We did not add any other TKIs or chemotherapy except for dexamethasone and the short-term use of mercaptopurine. Eventually, he died from leukemia on the 183rd day after his admission.

TABLE 1: Laboratory data.

	Admission to hospital	Before retreatment with dasatinib	22 days after retreatment
Peripheral blood samples			
Leukocytes ($\times 10^2/\mu L$)	380	79	78
Neutrophils (%)	4	67	65
Lymphocytes (%)	7	28	15
Monocytes (%)	0	2	7
Blastoid cells (%)	84	0	0
Hemoglobin (g/dL)	7.6	9.4	8.2
Platelet ($\times 10^4/\mu L$)	5.4	19.8	6.8
Bone marrow samples			
Total nucleated cells ($/\mu L$)	74500		11000
Blastoid cells (%)	96		0.4
Minor bcr-abl mRNA (copy/μg RNA)	7.0×10^5		7.9×10^3
Karyotype by G-banding	46XY, t(9;22)(q34;q11.2) [17/20]		46XY [20/20]

3. Discussion

We encountered a Ph$^+$ ALL patient with dilated cardiomyopathy accompanied by incessant VT and achieved a complete hematological response with dasatinib and prednisolone treatment without worsening the cardiomyopathy and ventricular arrhythmias.

Since chemotherapy including anthracycline confers a high risk of congestive heart failure [10], we avoided cardiotoxic antitumor agents and used dasatinib plus prednisolone instead. Dasatinib may also induce congestive heart failure because of fluid retention, pulmonary arterial hypertension, and ventricular arrhythmias [11]. In particular, we should be aware of adverse cardiac effects in a patient who has cardiac complications prior to therapy. In our case, we achieved a complete hematological response without fluid retention, pulmonary arterial hypertension, or ventricular arrhythmias, although this might have been affected by the short duration of dasatinib therapy.

We also continued dasatinib without exacerbating the VT. Spechbach et al. described a case of ventricular arrhythmia induced by dasatinib and the successful continuation of dasatinib with concomitant use of antiarrhythmic agents [12]. In the current case, we used bisoprolol and amiodarone to control VT during dasatinib therapy. Bisoprolol restrains excessive myocyte activity by inhibiting the myocardial beta 1 receptor [13], and amiodarone prolongs phase 3 cardiac action potential [14]. Dasatinib is not thought to directly harm cardiac mitochondrial function but to affect Purkinje-fiber assays and human ether-a-go-go-related gene potassium ion channels (HERG K$^+$) [5, 15], which is why we might have been able to continue dasatinib without increments in VT during treatment with bisoprolol and amiodarone.

Dasatinib and amiodarone are both thought to be metabolized mainly by CYP3A4, and the concurrent use of these two drugs can elevate the concentration of each drug [9]. The actual dasatinib $C_{1\,\mathrm{hr}}$ was not particularly high, and the plasma concentration of amiodarone stayed within the safe range. It was speculated that the drug concentrations might have not reached a high enough range to inhibit CYP3A4 [16, 17].

Since a low plasma concentration of dasatinib can cause the bcr-abl T315I point mutation, we should use a substantial dose of dasatinib, if possible [18]. In the present case, there was a possibility that T315I mutations had occurred at the time of relapse, though this could not be assessed. The pharmacokinetics of dasatinib vary widely in individuals [8, 18]. Thus, we could consider a dose-escalation of dasatinib to prevent the occurrence of bcr-abl point mutations while monitoring the dasatinib blood concentration. We should have increased the dose of dasatinib to 140 or 180 mg daily and tried to maintain the dasatinib Cmax above 50 ng/mL [18, 19].

In conclusion, induction therapy with dasatinib and prednisolone may be an acceptable therapeutic option for Ph$^+$ ALL patients with dilated cardiomyopathy and life-threatening ventricular arrhythmias. We can consider escalating the dose of dasatinib while monitoring its blood concentration. More cases should be accumulated to establish the optimal therapy for Ph$^+$ ALL with severe cardiac complications.

Competing Interests

Masayuki Hino received a research grant from Bristol-Myers Squibb and Astellas. Hirohisa Nakamae received a research grant from Bristol-Myers Squibb. All other authors have declared no financial interests/relationships relating to the topic of this article.

Acknowledgments

The authors would like to thank T. Katayama for managing and processing the stored samples.

References

[1] M. Talpaz, N. P. Shah, H. Kantarjian et al., "Dasatinib in imatinib-resistant Philadelphia chromosome-positive leukemias," *New England Journal of Medicine*, vol. 354, no. 24, pp. 2531–2541, 2006.

[2] R. Foà, A. Vitale, M. Vignetti et al., "Dasatinib as first-line treatment for adult patients with Philadelphia chromosome-positive acute lymphoblastic leukemia," *Blood*, vol. 118, no. 25, pp. 6521–6528, 2011.

[3] M. H. Chen, R. Kerkelä, and T. Force, "Mechanisms of cardiac dysfunction associated with tyrosine kinase inhibitor cancer therapeutics," *Circulation*, vol. 118, no. 1, pp. 84–95, 2008.

[4] T. Force, D. S. Krause, and R. A. Van Etten, "Molecular mechanisms of cardiotoxicity of tyrosine kinase inhibition," *Nature Reviews Cancer*, vol. 7, no. 5, pp. 332–344, 2007.

[5] E. L. Strevel, D. J. Ing, and L. L. Siu, "Molecularly targeted oncology therapeutics and prolongation of the QT interval," *Journal of Clinical Oncology*, vol. 25, no. 22, pp. 3362–3371, 2007.

[6] H. M. Kantarjian, N. P. Shah, J. E. Cortes et al., "Dasatinib or imatinib in newly diagnosed chronic-phase chronic myeloid leukemia: 2-year follow-up from a randomized phase 3 trial (DASISION)," *Blood*, vol. 119, no. 5, pp. 1123–1129, 2012.

[7] S. Fujisawa, H. Nakamae, M. Ogura et al., "Efficacy and safety of dasatinib versus imatinib in Japanese patients with newly diagnosed chronic-phase chronic myeloid leukemia (CML-CP): subset analysis of the DASISION trial with 2-year follow-up," *International Journal of Hematology*, vol. 99, no. 2, pp. 141–153, 2014.

[8] F. M. Johnson, S. Agrawal, H. Burris et al., "Phase 1 pharmacokinetic and drug-interaction study of dasatinib in patients with advanced solid tumors," *Cancer*, vol. 116, no. 6, pp. 1582–1591, 2010.

[9] A. Haouala, N. Widmer, M. A. Duchosal, M. Montemurro, T. Buclin, and L. A. Decosterd, "Drug interactions with the tyrosine kinase inhibitors imatinib, dasatinib, and nilotinib," *Blood*, vol. 117, no. 8, pp. e75–e87, 2011.

[10] K. Shan, A. M. Lincoff, and J. B. Young, "Anthracycline-induced cardiotoxicity," *Annals of Internal Medicine*, vol. 125, no. 1, pp. 47–58, 1996.

[11] Dasatinib Prescribing Information, http://www.sprycel.com.

[12] H. Spechbach, P. Morel, K. I. Lorenzini et al., "Reversible ventricular arrythmia induced by dasatinib," *Clinical Case Reports*, vol. 1, no. 1, pp. 20–25, 2013.

[13] P. Lechat, K. W. Brunhuber, R. Hofmann et al., "The Cardiac Insufficiency Bisoprolol Study II (CIBIS-II): a randomised trial," *The Lancet*, vol. 353, no. 9146, pp. 9–13, 1999.

[14] S. M. Yabek, R. Kato, and B. N. Singh, "Effects of amiodarone and its metabolite, desethylamiodarone, on the electrophysiologic properties of isolated cardiac muscle," *Journal of Cardiovascular Pharmacology*, vol. 8, no. 1, pp. 197–207, 1986.

[15] Y. Will, J. A. Dykens, S. Nadanaciva et al., "Effect of the multitargeted tyrosine kinase inhibitors imatinib, dasatinib, sunitinib, and sorafenib on mitochondrial function in isolated rat heart mitochondria and H9c2 cells," *Toxicological Sciences*, vol. 106, no. 1, pp. 153–161, 2008.

[16] K. Ohyama, M. Nakajima, M. Suzuki, N. Shimada, H. Yamazaki, and T. Yokoi, "Inhibitory effects of amiodarone and its N-deethylated metabolite on human cytochrome P450 activities: prediction of in vivo drug interactions," *British Journal of Clinical Pharmacology*, vol. 49, no. 3, pp. 244–253, 2000.

[17] X. Li, Y. He, C. H. Ruiz, M. Koenig, and M. D. Cameron, "Characterization of dasatinib and its structural analogs as CYP3A4 mechanism-based inactivators and the proposed bioactivation pathways," *Drug Metabolism and Disposition*, vol. 37, no. 6, pp. 1242–1250, 2009.

[18] N. Takahashi, M. Miura, S. A. Scott, T. Niioka, and K. Sawada, "Pharmacokinetics of dasatinib for Philadelphia-positive acute lymphocytic leukemia with acquired T315I mutation," *Journal of Hematology & Oncology*, vol. 5, article 23, 2012.

[19] M. Miura, "Therapeutic drug monitoring of imatinib, nilotinib, and dasatinib for patients with chronic myeloid leukemia," *Biological and Pharmaceutical Bulletin*, vol. 38, no. 5, pp. 645–654, 2015.

Composite t(14;18)-Negative Follicular Lymphoma and Nodular Lymphocyte-Predominant Hodgkin Lymphoma

John Patrick O'Neill,[1] Fiona Quinn,[1] Anita Dowling,[1] Jan Walker,[1] Triona Hayes,[2] Brian Bird,[2] and Richard Flavin[1]

[1]*St. James's Hospital, Dublin, Ireland*
[2]*Bons Secours Hospital, Cork, Ireland*

Correspondence should be addressed to John Patrick O'Neill; oneilljp@tcd.ie

Academic Editor: Takashi Sonoki

A composite lymphoma is the rare simultaneous occurrence of two or more distinct lymphomas within a single tissue or organ. Herein, we describe a case of a 51-year-old man presenting with a history of lower limb rash, fatigue, and bulky abdominopelvic lymphadenopathy. An excisional left iliac lymph node biopsy was notable for the composite presence of two distinct lymphoid neoplasms, nodular lymphocyte-predominant Hodgkin lymphoma (NLPHL), and follicular lymphoma (FL). Multiplex PCR and FISH analyses failed to demonstrate a t(14;18)(q32;q21) translocation in either composite lymphoma component. A clonal light-chain kappa (V/JC intron-kde) gene rearrangement was detected in the FL component only.

1. Introduction

Composite lymphomas (CLs) are defined by the rare simultaneous occurrence of two or more distinct lymphomas within one tissue or organ and were first described as an entity in 1954 [1]. It is estimated that CL accounts for approximately 1–4% of all lymphoma diagnoses [2]. CL has been typically found to comprise a classical Hodgkin lymphoma (cHL) and a non-Hodgkin lymphoma (NHL) such as follicular lymphoma (FL) [3], chronic lymphocytic leukaemia (CLL) [4], mantle cell lymphoma (ML) [5], or diffuse large B-cell lymphoma (DLBCL) [6]. Combinations of two NHL subtypes have also been described [7].

A rare occurrence is that of a CL including nodular lymphocyte-predominant Hodgkin lymphoma (NLPHL). Herein, we describe a case of composite FL and NLPHL diagnosed concurrently within the same lymph node.

2. Clinical History

A 51-year-old man with a background history of lower limb rash and unexplained fatigue had an incidental finding of bulky abdominopelvic lymphadenopathy during investigation for prostatitis. Skin punch biopsy of the flank and medial left calf noted features of papular urticaria in both specimens. In addition, the left calf biopsy showed features of a mixed septal and lobular panniculitis. Retroperitoneal lymph node core biopsy and open intra-abdominal nodal biopsy at minilaparotomy in another institution failed to yield sufficiently the diagnostic material, and a PET-directed laparoscopic left iliac lymph node excisional biopsy was performed. Following diagnosis, he was treated with bendamustine and rituximab with a complete metabolic response. He has completed 1 of 2-year maintenance rituximab with no clinical evidence of relapse.

3. Pathological Findings

Haematoxylin and eosin (H&E) staining of the lymph node showed one discrete block of the biopsy nodular areas composed of small lymphocytes, epithelioid histiocytes, immunoblasts, and lymphocyte-predominant (LP) cells (Figure 1). There was background progressive transformation of germinal centres (PTGC). The LP cells were

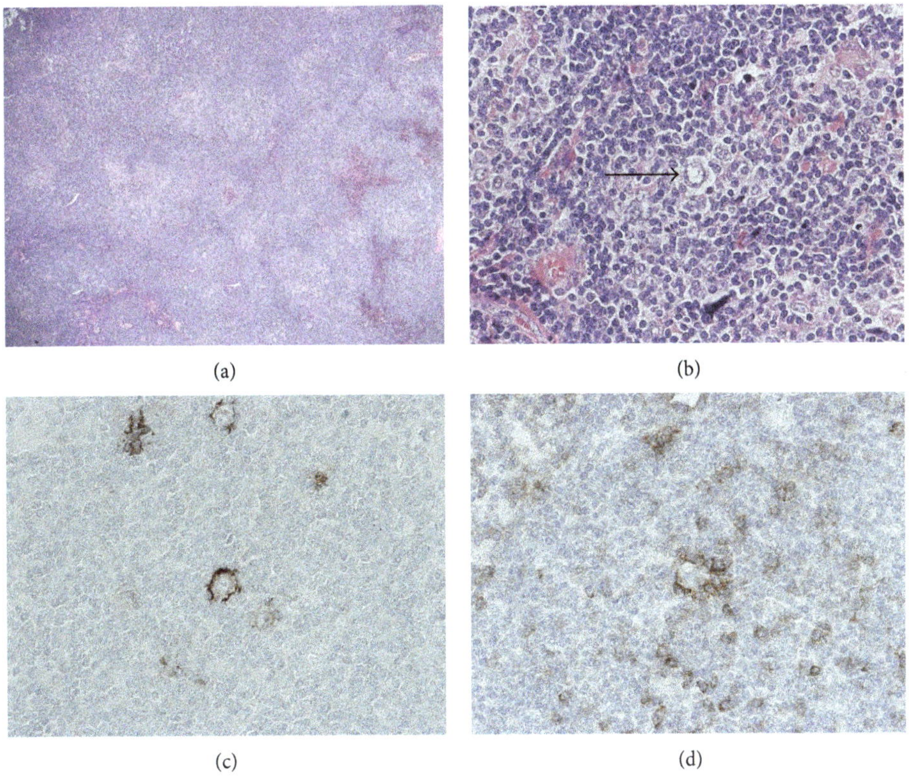

FIGURE 1: NLPHL. (a) H&E staining, low power, showing vague nodular effacement. (b) H&E staining, high power, showing large LP cells (centre arrow) in a background population of small lymphocytes and histiocytes. (c) Immunostaining for EMA showing membrane positivity in LP cells. (d) Immunostaining for PD-1 showing positive membrane staining of T-cell rosettes surrounding LP cells.

positive for immunohistochemical stains CD45, CD20, CD79a, PAX-5, OCT-2, BOB-1, BCL-6, EMA, and MUM-1 and were negative for CD30 and CD15. The background T-cell population was CD4 predominant without aberrant T-cell antigen loss (CD2, CD5, and CD7 positive). PD-1-positive T-cell rosettes were seen around LP cells [8]. The follicular dendritic meshwork was highlighted by CD21 and CD23 staining. EBV-encoded small RNAs in situ hybridization (EBER-ISH) was negative. Overall, the above morphology and immunoprofile were felt to be in keeping with NLPHL. Multiplex polymerase chain reaction (PCR) analysis was performed on a whole discrete section of NLPHL, and a polyclonal immunoglobulin (Ig) gene rearrangement profile was detected. In addition, the t(14;18) BCL2-JH translocation was not detected. Insufficient material was available for FISH analysis and for laser capture microdissection for downstream PCR analysis.

In a separate block section of the same lymph node biopsy, there were neoplastic follicles present containing centroblasts (numbering >15 per high-power field) and admixed centrocytes (Figure 2). Immunohistochemistry showed that the neoplastic follicles were positive for CD20, CD79a, CD10, BCL-6, and BCL-2 (weak) with equivocal staining for MUM-1. The Ki-67 proliferation index within follicles was 50%. The morphology and immunoprofile were in keeping with a follicular lymphoma (FL), grade 3a, follicular pattern. Multiplex PCR performed on FFPE tissue from a distinct area of FL detected a clonal Ig light-chain kappa (V/JC intron-kde) gene rearrangement. Multiplex PCR did not detect a t(14;18) BCL2-JH translocation. Fluorescence in situ hybridization (FISH) did not detect either the t(14;18)(q32;q21) translocation or a BCL-2 rearrangement (Figure 3).

4. Materials and Methods

The lymph node was fixed in 10% neutral-buffered formalin followed by paraffin embedding. Immunohistochemistry and in situ hybridization were performed routinely following standardized protocols. Antibodies used were CD3, CD4, CD5, CD7, CD8, CD10, CD15, CD20, CD23, CD30, EMA, Ki-67, Pax-5, and Bcl-2 (Ventana); CD21, CD79a, MUM-1, Bcl-6, and PD-1 (Cell Marque); and Oct-2 and Bob-1 (Leica). EBV-encoded small RNAs in situ hybridization (EBER-ISH) was performed on FFPE sections using the fluorescein-conjugated PNA probe (Roche). Fluorescence in situ hybridization analyses for t(14;18) and BCL-2 rearrangements were performed on FFPE samples according to standardized protocols using probe sets LSI IGH/BCL2 t (14;18)(q32;q21) and LSI BCL2 (dual colour) (Abbott Vysis Inc, Downers Grove, IL). t(14;18)(q32;q21) and LSI BCL2 were deemed positive if >10% of nonoverlapped lymphoma nuclei had a demonstrable translocation or break-apart signals, respectively. DNA was extracted from FFPE using Qiagen DNAse kits. Multiplex polymerase chain reaction (PCR) analysis was performed using BioMED primers and

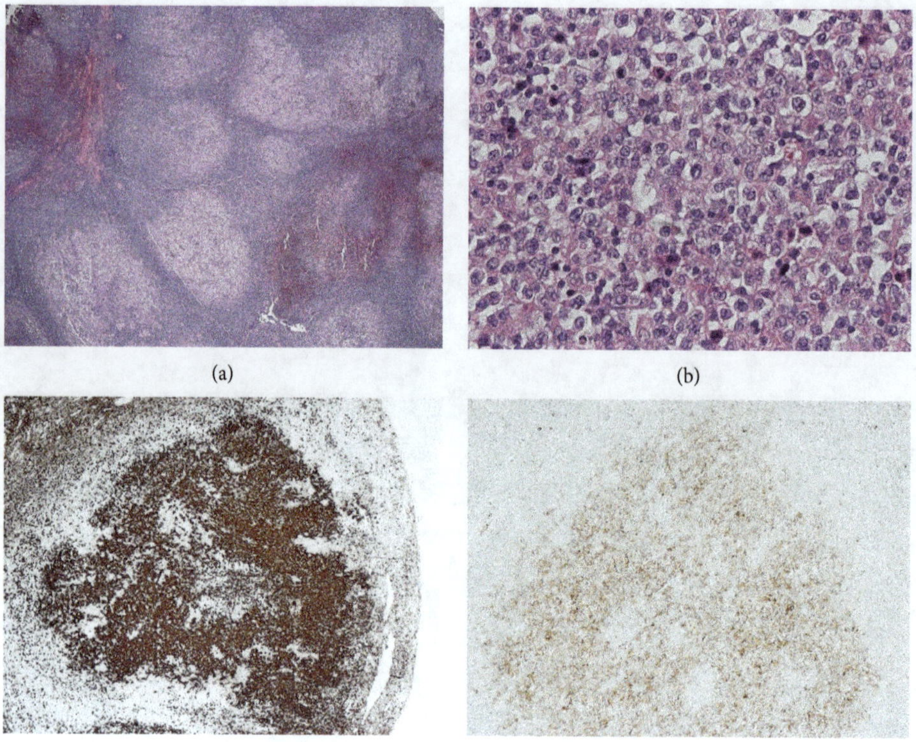

(a) (b) (c) (d)

FIGURE 2: Follicular lymphoma. (a) H&E staining, low power, showing pronounced nodular effacement by closely packed nodules lacking mantle zones. (b) H&E staining, high power, showing neoplastic follicle containing centroblasts (>15 per HPF). Immunostaining for (c) CD20 and (d) CD10 showing follicle positivity.

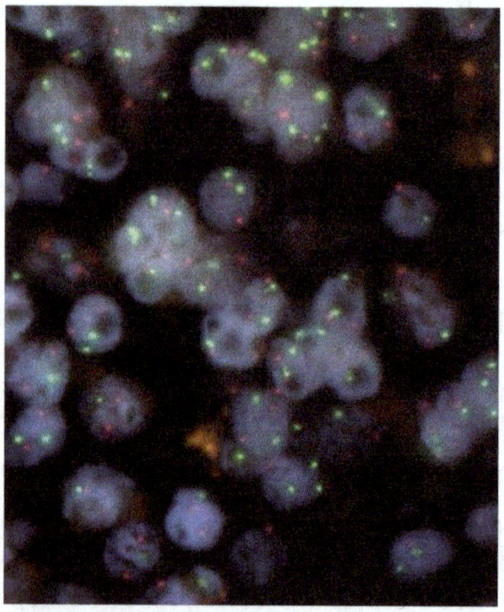

FIGURE 3: Fluorescence in situ hybridization photomicrograph of the follicular lymphoma component using LSI IGH/BCL2 t(14;18) (q32;q21) dual colour probes showing no evidence of t(14;18) translocation in nonoverlapped nuclei.

probes with PCR products visualized using GeneScan as previously described [9]. Extracted DNA from FFPE was also tested for the presence of the t(14;18) BCL2-JH translocation using multiplex PCR.

5. Discussion

This report outlines a second documented case of a composite lymphoma comprising NLPHL and FL. In the previously published case of composite NLPHL and FL, the t(14; 18) translocation was detected by FISH, but interestingly, no clonal immunoglobulin gene rearrangements were detected in the FL component, which is in direct contrast to our case.

Cases of composite cHL and FL have been previously described [10–12]. In two of these cases, the cHL and FL components were shown to be clonally related, with shared and distinct Ig V mutations in each instance [10, 11]. This suggests a common origin of the cHL and FL components. Indeed, in an extended series of 19 composite cases involving cHL and other non-Hodgkin lymphomas, where clonality was examined, shared clonality was demonstrated in 12/19 (63%) cases [13]. Furthermore, in four composite cases involving NLPHL, shared clonality has been shown in cases involving DLBCL [14], T-cell-rich large B-cell lymphoma [15], and cHL [16, 17]. The common finding of shared clonality in cases described as composite lymphomas raises the question of whether these lymphomas are in fact "distinct" entities by Custer's 1954 definition [1, 18]. Composite lymphomas where common clonality is present may just represent differing phenotypes of an identical progenitor clone. In our case, we were unable to determine whether shared clonality was present due to insufficient tissue available for laser capture microdissection. In the single other reported instance of composite NLPHL and FL, the authors were also unable to determine the clonal relationship [19].

Finally, composite lymphomas may be more common than previously thought. A 2015 Japanese study examined 154 cHL cases and found a 20% incidence of composite lymphoma in patients ≥40 years [12]. Interestingly, they also noted that marrow involvement by the cHL component and the presence of a high-grade component were adverse prognostic factors.

Conflicts of Interest

The authors declare that they have no conflicts of interest.

References

[1] R. Custer, "Pitfalls in the diagnosis of lymphoma and leukemia from the pathologist's point of view," in *Proceedings of Second National Cancer Conference*, pp. 554–557, New York City, NY, USA, 1954.

[2] S. Thirumala, M. Esposito, and A. Fuchs, "An unusual variant of composite lymphoma: a short case report and review of the literature," *Archives of Pathology and Laboratory Medicine*, vol. 124, no. 9, pp. 1376–1378, 2000.

[3] T. Marafioti, M. Hummel, I. Anagnostopoulos et al., "Classical Hodgkin's disease and follicular lymphoma originating from the same germinal center B cell," *Journal of Clinical Oncology*, vol. 17, no. 12, pp. 3804–3809, 1999.

[4] L. de Leval, M. Vivario, B. De Prijck et al., "Distinct clonal origin in two cases of Hodgkin's lymphoma variant of Richter's syndrome associated with EBV infection," *American Journal of Surgical Pathology*, vol. 28, no. 5, pp. 679–686, 2004.

[5] A. Caleo, A. Sánchez-Aguilera, S. Rodríguez et al., "Composite Hodgkin lymphoma and mantle cell lymphoma: two clonally unrelated tumors," *American Journal of Surgical Pathology*, vol. 27, no. 12, pp. 1577–1580, 2003.

[6] R. K. Thomas, C. Wickenhauser, D. Kube et al., "Repeated clonal relapses in classical Hodgkin's lymphoma and the occurrence of a clonally unrelated diffuse large B-cell non-Hodgkin lymphoma in the same patient," *Leukemia and Lymphoma*, vol. 45, no. 5, pp. 1065–1069, 2004.

[7] D. F. Boyer, N. I. Lindeman, N. L. Harris, and J. A. Ferry, "Peripheral T-cell lymphomas with cytotoxic phenotype in patients with chronic lymphocytic leukemia/small lymphocytic lymphoma," *American Journal of Surgical Pathology*, vol. 38, no. 2, pp. 279–288, 2014.

[8] S. H. Nam-Cha, G. Roncador, M. A. Piris et al., "PD-1 a follicular T-cell marker useful for recognising nodular lymphocyte predominant Hodgkin lymphoma," *American Journal of Surgical Pathology*, vol. 32, no. 8, pp. 1252–1257, 2008.

[9] J. J. Van Dongen, A. W. Langerak, M. Brüggemann et al., "Design and standardization of PCR primers and protocols for detection of clonal immunoglobulin and T-cell receptor gene recombinations in suspect lymphoproliferations: report of the BIOMED-2 Concerted Action BMH4-CT98-3936," *Leukemia*, vol. 17, no. 12, pp. 2257–2317, 2003.

[10] A. Bräuninger, M. L. Hansmann, J. G. Strickler et al., "Identification of common germinal-center B-cell precursors in two patients with both Hodgkin's disease and non-Hodgkin's lymphoma," *New England Journal of Medicine*, vol. 340, no. 16, pp. 1239–1247, 1999.

[11] R. Küppers, A. B. Sousa, A. S. Baur, J. G. Strickler, K. Rajewsky, and M. L. Hansmann, "Common germinal-center B-cell origin of the malignant cells in two composite lymphomas, involving classical Hodgkin's disease and either follicular lymphoma or B-CLL," *Molecular Medicine*, vol. 7, no. 5, pp. 285–292, 2001.

[12] A. M. Maeshima, H. Taniguchi, J. Nomoto et al., "Clinicopathological features of classical Hodgkin lymphoma in patients ≥ 40 years old, with special reference to composite cases," *Japanese Journal of Clinical Oncology*, vol. 45, no. 10, pp. 921–928, 2015.

[13] R. Küppers, U. Dührsen, and M. L. Hansmann, "Pathogenesis, diagnosis, and treatment of composite lymphomas," *Lancet Oncology*, vol. 15, no. 10, pp. e435–e446, 2014.

[14] T. Ohno, J. Z. Huang, G. Wu, K. H. Park, D. D. Weisenburger, and W. C. Chan, "The tumor cells in nodular lymphocyte-predominant Hodgkin disease are clonally related to the large cell lymphoma occurring in the same individual. Direct demonstration by single cell analysis," *American Journal of Clinical Pathology*, vol. 116, no. 4, pp. 506–511, 2001.

[15] S. Shimodaira, E. Hidaka, and T. Katsuyama, "Clonal identity of nodular lymphocyte-predominant Hodgkin's disease and T-cell-rich B-cell lymphoma," *New England Journal of Medicine*, vol. 343, no. 15, pp. 1124-1125, 2000.

[16] J. Y. Song, F. C. Eberle, L. Xi et al., "Coexisting and clonally identical classic Hodgkin lymphoma and nodular lymphocyte predominant Hodgkin lymphoma," *American Journal of Surgical Pathology*, vol. 35, no. 5, pp. 767–772, 2011.

[17] M. Szczepanowski, N. Masqué-Soler, I. Oschlies et al., "Composite lymphoma of nodular lymphocyte-predominant and classical Hodgkin lymphoma-Epstein-Barr virus association suggests divergent pathogenesis despite clonal relatedness," *Human Pathology*, vol. 44, no. 7, pp. 1434–1439, 2013.

[18] M. Steinhoff, M. Hummel, C. Assaf et al., "Cutaneous T cell lymphoma and classic Hodgkin lymphoma of the B cell type within a single lymph node: composite lymphoma," *Journal of Clinical Pathology*, vol. 57, no. 3, pp. 329–331, 2004.

[19] J. L. Dargent, L. Lespagnard, I. Meiers, C. Bradstreet, P. Heimann, and C. De Wolf-Peeters, "Composite follicular lymphoma and nodular lymphocyte predominance Hodgkin's disease," *Virchows Archiv*, vol. 447, no. 4, pp. 778–780, 2005.

11

Myelodysplastic Syndrome/Acute Myeloid Leukemia Arising in Idiopathic Erythrocytosis

Stephen E. Langabeer,[1] Eibhlin Conneally,[2] and Catherine M. Flynn[2]

[1]*Cancer Molecular Diagnostics, St. James's Hospital, Dublin 8, Ireland*
[2]*Department of Haematology, St. James's Hospital, Dublin 8, Ireland*

Correspondence should be addressed to Stephen E. Langabeer; slangabeer@stjames.ie

Academic Editor: Sergio Storti

The term "idiopathic erythrocytosis (IE)" is applied to those cases where a causal clinical or pathological event cannot be elucidated and likely reflects a spectrum of underlying medical and molecular abnormalities. The clinical course of a patient with IE is described manifesting as a persistent erythrocytosis with a low serum erythropoietin level, mild eosinophilia, and with evidence of a thrombotic event. The patient subsequently developed a myelodysplasic syndrome (MDS) and acute myeloid leukemia (AML), an event not observed in erythrocytosis patients other than those with polycythemia vera (PV). Application of a next-generation sequencing (NGS) approach targeted for myeloid malignancies confirmed wild-type *JAK2* exons 12–15 and identified a common *SH2B3* W262R single-nucleotide polymorphism associated with the development of hematological features of myeloproliferative neoplasms (MPNs). Further NGS analysis detected a *CBL* L380P mutated clone expanding in parallel with the development of MDS and subsequent AML. Despite the absence of *JAK2, MPL* exon 10, or *CALR* exon 9 mutations, a similarity with the disease course of PV/MPN was evident. A clonal link between the erythrocytosis and AML could be neither confirmed nor excluded. Future molecular identification of the mechanisms underlying IE is likely to provide a more refined therapeutic approach.

1. Introduction

The causes of erythrocytosis are many and can be broadly divided into either primary or secondary forms. Primary causes are due to a defect intrinsic to the erythroid compartment of the bone marrow which leads to increased red cell generation, whereas secondary causes are due to factors external to the bone marrow that are produced in excess and drive red cell production [1]. The most common cause of acquired primary erythrocytosis is the myeloproliferative neoplasm (MPN) of polycythemia vera (PV) that is molecularly characterized by the *JAK2* p.V617F and exon 12 mutations [2]. Mutations of other genes in the erythropoiesis, oxygen sensing, and oxygen transport pathways are known to result in erythrocytosis; however, the underlying causes are unknown in a large number of cases, particularly those recognized as congenital erythrocytosis, and remain classified as idiopathic erythrocytosis (IE) [3]. Several clinical and biological differences exist between IE and PV, including a considerably lower risk of thrombotic events in IE patients compared to PV patients [4] with transformation to acute myeloid leukemia (AML) exceedingly rare in individuals with IE or other molecularly annotated forms of erythrocytosis [5]. A case is described in which application of the myeloid malignancy-targeted, next-generation sequencing (NGS) approach retrospectively provided insights into the molecular appearance of myelodysplastic syndrome (MDS)/AML in a patient with IE.

2. Case Report

An overweight 62-year-old male with hypertension and hyperlipidemia presented with a hemoglobin level of 20.4 g/dL, hematocrit of 0.59, normal white cell and platelet counts, and a mild eosinophilia (Table 1). The patient had no clinical signs of PV, normal spleen size, normal oxygen

Table 1: Hematological indices and molecular analysis throughout the patient's clinical course.

Time (months)	Hb	HCT	RCC	PLT	WCC	Eos	BM blasts (IP/morphology)	Mutations detected (variant allele frequency)	
Dx	20.4	0.59	6.20	140	5.8	1.0	—	—	
41	16.2	0.49	6.29	158	6.8	0.9	—	*SH2B3* p.W262R (52.4%)	
149	19.7	0.58	6.78	75	8.1	1.9	—	*SH2B3* p.W262R (45.9%)	*CBL* p.L380P (3.6%)
157	8.9	0.26	2.62	112	4.0	0.2	4%/0%	—	
159	10.1	0.30	3.00	106	3.3	0.1	8%/6%	—	
161	10.1	0.29	3.19	35	6.1	0.4	15%/22%	*SH2B3* p.W262R (56.8%)	*CBL* p.L380P (37.2%)

Hb: hemoglobin (g/dL); HCT: hematocrit; RCC: red cell count ($\times 10^{12}$/L); PLT: platelet count ($\times 10^9$/L); WCC: white cell count ($\times 10^9$/L); Eos: eosinophil count ($\times 10^9$/L); BM blasts: bone marrow myeloblasts; IP: immunophenotyping; Dx: diagnosis.

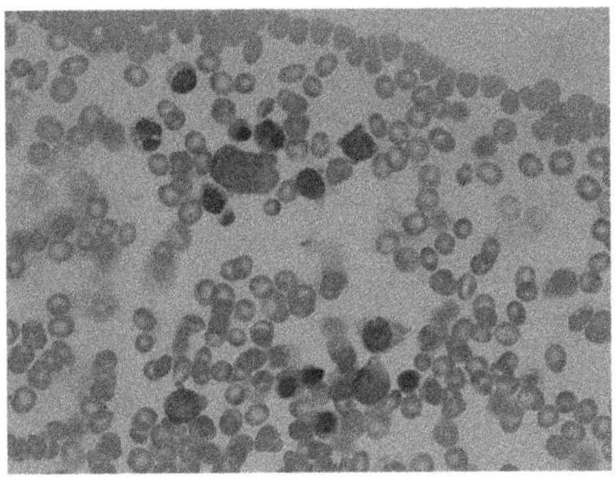

Figure 1: Bone marrow morphology at development of myelodysplasia/acute myeloid leukemia showing myeloblasts and dysplastic red blood cell precursors.

saturation, no endogenous erythrocyte colony formation, no evidence of abnormal hemoglobin, and no family history of a hematological abnormality. The patient was managed with intermittent venesection alone for nine years with no evidence of the *JAK2* p.V617F mutations by allele-specific PCR or the *JAK2* exon 12 mutations by high-resolution melt curve analysis, excluding a diagnosis of PV [2]. At 149 months after diagnosis, thrombocytopenia (75×10^9/L) and increasing eosinophilia (1.9×10^9/L) were noted with a low serum erythropoietin (EPO) level of 0.6 IU/L (normal range 2.6–18.5 IU/L). At 154 months after diagnosis, the patient had temporoparietal stroke. Worsening pancytopenia at 157 months prompted bone marrow biopsy which demonstrated 4% myeloblasts (Table 1). Subsequent bone marrow investigations showed progressively increasing myeloblast cell numbers by both morphological and immunophenotypic evaluation with reduced dysplastic megakaryocytes, dyserythropoiesis with basophilic stippling, and binuclear red cell forms, all consistent with MDS progressing to AML (Figure 1). The karyotype at 159 months was normal. The patient was not fit for intensive treatment and was given best supportive care with EPO, intermittent red cell transfusions, and low-dose steroids but died of infection at 161 months.

A targeted NGS approach panel was retrospectively employed to detect mutations possibly contributing to the erythrocytosis and subsequent development of MDS/AML in archival peripheral blood or bone marrow DNA samples from 41, 149, and 161 months. Amplicon libraries covering thirty commonly mutated genes implicated in myeloid malignancies, either covering the entire coding region (*CALR, CEBPA, ETV6, EZH2, RUNX1, SH2B3, TET2, TP53,* and *ZRSR2*) or mutational hotspots (*ABL1, ASXL1, BRAF, CBL, CSF3R, DNMT3A, FLT3, GATA2, IDH1, IDH2, JAK2, KIT, KRAS, MPL, NPM1, NRAS, PTPN11, SETBP1, SF3B1, SRSF2,* and *U2AF1*), were generated. Sequencing was performed with Ion AmpliSeq™ methodology (Thermo Fisher Scientific, Paisley, UK). Calling of somatic mutations was achieved using an algorithm that excluded synonymous mutations, variants located within intronic or untranslated regions, and those present at a variant allele frequency (VAF) of <5%. A minimum target depth of coverage for variant calls was set at 500x as previously described [6, 7]. The nonsynonymous *SH2B3* exon 2, single-nucleotide polymorphism (SNP) W262R (c.784T>C, NP_005466.1, rs3184504) was present at all three time points analyzed at VAFs of approximately 50% (Table 1). No mutations were detected in *MPL* exon 10 or *CALR* exon 9. A single *CBL* L380P mutation (c.1139T>C, NP_005179.2) was detected in the bone marrow sample at 161 months. Reinterrogation of sequencing data revealed this *CBL* mutation to be present a year previously at a VAF of 3.6% (Table 1).

3. Discussion

Despite the absence of either the *JAK2* V617F or exon 12 mutations in the patient, a high degree of suspicion remained throughout the clinical course for a diagnosis of PV or "PV-like" MPN given the persistently raised hematocrit, the low serum EPO, a mild eosinophilia, and clinically a thrombotic episode (stroke). While NGS confirmed the absence of the *JAK2* V617F and exon 12 mutations, several alternative mutations of *JAK2* have been identified in sporadic cases of "PV-like" MPN and hereditary erythrocytosis [8–13], yet none were identified by NGS in exons 12–15 in the patient.

Of interest is the presence of the *SH2B3* W262R SNP. *SH2B3* (formerly *LNK*) encodes the *LNK* inhibitory adaptor protein that modulates thrombopoietin and erythropoietin signalling by interacting with *JAK2* and inhibiting downstream STAT activation. Disruption of this function by a mutant protein results in aberrant JAK-STAT signalling and cytokine responsiveness. Low frequency but recurrent, acquired, and germ line mutations of *SH2B3* have been reported in both sporadic and familial MPN, respectively, particularly in those cases and kindred identified with IE [14, 15]. While no somatic mutations were identified within the entire coding region of *SH2B3*, this patient was heterozygous (T/C) for the common W262R SNP [16]. This SNP and others within *SH2B3* have been shown to be associated with an increase in platelets, eosinophils, and elevated hemoglobin and hematocrit levels [17–22]. Furthermore, some recent evidence exists for the T allele of this SNP to be associated with the development of MPN and *JAK2* V617F-positive hematopoiesis [16, 21, 22]. Despite *in vitro* functional analysis of another nonsynonymous *SH2B3* SNP (E400K) in a patient with IE indicating no impairment of *SH2B3* inhibiting *JAK2*-STAT5 activation, subtle loss of function induced by *SH2B3* SNPs cannot be excluded [23]. While tempting to speculate a causal role for this *SH2B3* SNP in the development of erythrocytosis in this patient, no specific evidence exists for such an association, suggesting involvement of additional genetic and/or epigenetic events.

Transformation to AML is a recurrent event in PV with reported risks of 2.3–14.4% at ten years [24]. However, transformation to or development of MDS/AML in other forms of molecularly annotated erythrocytosis or IE is exceedingly rare [25]. A true transformation of the erythrocytosis could neither be confirmed nor excluded in this case due to the absence of a pre-MDS/AML marker of clonality with the possibility that the erythrocytosis and MDS/AML represent two unrelated pathologies. Activating mutations of *CBL*, a negative regulator of receptor tyrosine kinases, including the p.L380P detected in this case, is recurrent in myeloid malignancies and is associated with progression of MDS to AML [26].

In conclusion, we describe a patient with IE possessing a clinical similarity to PV in which there are persistent erythrocytosis, a thrombotic event, and the acquisition of somatic mutations that resulted in MDS/AML. Employment of an NGS gene panel specifically targeted for investigation of IE has recently demonstrated the benefits of this type of approach [27]. The potential exists for identifying those patients at increased risk of developing a myeloid malignancy, enabling refined counseling and therapeutic decision-making throughout the disease course.

Conflicts of Interest

The authors declare that there are no conflicts of interest regarding the publication of this paper.

References

[1] G. Lee and M. O. Arcasoy, "The clinical and laboratory evaluation of the patient with erythrocytosis," *European Journal of Internal Medicine*, vol. 26, no. 5, pp. 297–302, 2015.

[2] D. A. Arber, A. Orazi, R. Hasserjian et al., "The 2016 revision to the World Health Organization classification of myeloid neoplasms and acute leukemia," *Blood*, vol. 127, no. 20, pp. 2391–2405, 2016.

[3] C. Bento, H. Almeida, T. M. Maia et al., "Molecular study of congenital erythrocytosis in 70 unrelated patients revealed a potential causal mutation in less than half of the cases (where is/are the missing gene(s)?)," *European Journal of Haematology*, vol. 91, no. 4, pp. 361–368, 2013.

[4] I. Bertozzi, M. Ruggeri, I. Nichele, G. Biagetti, E. Cosi, and M. L. Randi, "Thrombotic and hemorrhagic complications in idiopathic erythrocytosis," *American Journal of Hematology*, vol. 92, no. 11, pp. E639–E641, 2017.

[5] M. F. McMullin, "Investigation and management of erythrocytosis," *Current Hematologic Malignancy Reports*, vol. 11, no. 5, pp. 342–347, 2016.

[6] K. Haslam, M. A. Catherwood, E. Dobbin, A. Sproul, S. E. Langabeer, and K. I. Mills, "Inter-laboratory evaluation of a next-generation sequencing panel for acute myeloid leukemia," *Molecular Diagnosis & Therapy*, vol. 20, no. 5, pp. 457–461, 2016.

[7] S. E. Langabeer, K. Haslam, and C. M. Flynn, "Isolated erythrocytosis associated with a *CALR* mutation," *Blood Cells, Molecules & Diseases*, vol. 66, pp. 6-7, 2017.

[8] S. Schnittger, U. Bacher, W. Kern, M. Schröder, T. Haferlach, and C. Schoch, "Report on two novel nucleotide exchanges in the *JAK2* pseudo-kinase domain: D620E and E627E," *Leukemia*, vol. 20, no. 12, pp. 2195–2197, 2006.

[9] F. Grünebach, U. Bross-Bach, L. Kanz, and P. Brossart, "Detection of a new D620E mutation in addition to V617F in a patient with polycythemia vera," *Leukemia*, vol. 20, no. 12, pp. 2210-2211, 2006.

[10] B. Bahar, K. Barton, and A. R. Kini, "The role of exon 13 G571S *JAK2* mutation in myeloproliferative neoplasms," *Leukemia Research Reports*, vol. 6, pp. 27-28, 2016.

[11] C. Cleyrat, J. Jelinek, F. Girodon et al., "*JAK2* mutation and disease phenotype: a double L611/V617F in cis mutation of *JAK2* is associated with isolated erythrocytosis and increased activation of AKT and ERK1/2 rather than STAT5," *Leukemia*, vol. 34, no. 5, pp. 1069–1073, 2010.

[12] I. S. Tiong, D. A. Casolari, S. Moore et al., "Apparent *JAK2*-negative polycythaemia vera due to compound mutations in exon 14," *British Journal of Haematology*, vol. 178, no. 2, pp. 333–336, 2017.

[13] K. Kapralova, H. Horvathova, C. Pecquet et al., "Cooperation of germ line *JAK2* mutations E845D and R1063H in hereditary erythrocytosis with megakaryocytic atypia," *Blood*, vol. 128, no. 10, pp. 1418–1423, 2016.

[14] M. F. McMullin and H. Cario, "*LNK* mutations and myeloproliferative disorders," *American Journal of Hematology*, vol. 91, no. 2, pp. 248–251, 2016.

[15] N. Maslah, B. Cassinat, E. Verger, J. J. Kiladjian, and L. Velazquez, "The role of *LNK/SH2B3* genetic alterations in myeloproliferative neoplasms and other hematological disorders," *Leukemia*, vol. 31, no. 8, pp. 1661–1670, 2017.

[16] E. Lesteven, M. Picque, C. Conejero Tonetti et al., "Association of a single-nucleotide polymorphism in the *SH2B3* gene with *JAK2* V617F-positive myeloproliferative neoplasms," *Blood*, vol. 123, no. 5, pp. 794–796, 2014.

[17] M. K. Christiansen, S. B. Larsen, M. Nyegaard et al., "The *SH2B3* and KCNK5 loci may be implicated in regulation of platelet count, volume, and maturity," *Thrombosis Research*, vol. 158, pp. 86–92, 2017.

[18] D. F. Gudbjartsson, U. S. Bjomsdottir, E. Halapi et al., "Sequence variants affecting eosinophil numbers associate with asthma and myocardial infarction," *Nature Genetics*, vol. 41, no. 3, pp. 342–347, 2009.

[19] M. E. Daly, "Determinants of platelet count in humans," *Haematologica*, vol. 96, no. 1, pp. 10–13, 2011.

[20] S. K. Ganesh, N. A. Zakai, F. J. A. van Rooiij et al., "Multiple loci influence erythrocyte phenotypes in the CHARGE consortium," *Nature Genetics*, vol. 41, no. 11, pp. 1191–1198, 2009.

[21] Y. Chen, F. Fang, Y. Hu et al., "The polymorphisms in *LNK* gene correlated to the clinical type of myeloproliferative neoplasms," *PLoS One*, vol. 11, no. 4, article e0154183, 2016.
[22] D. A. Hinds, K. E. Barnholt, R. A. Mesa et al., "Germ line variants predispose to both *JAK2* V617F clonal hematopoiesis and myeloproliferative neoplasms," *Blood*, vol. 128, no. 8, pp. 1121–1128, 2016.
[23] M. F. McMullin, C. Wu, M. J. Percy, and W. Tong, "A nonsynonymous *LNK* polymorphism associated with idiopathic erythrocytosis," *American Journal of Hematology*, vol. 86, no. 11, pp. 962–964, 2011.
[24] S. Cerquozzi and A. Tefferi, "Blast transformation and fibrotic progression in polycythemia vera and essential thrombocythemia: a literature review of incidence and risk factors," *Blood Cancer Journal*, vol. 5, no. 11, p. e366, 2015.
[25] K. Labno-Kirszniok, T. Niesporek, A. Wiecek, G. Helbig, and J. Lubinski, "Acute myeloid leukemia in a 38-year-old hemodialyzed patient with von Hippel-Lindau disease," *Hereditary Cancer in Clinical Practice*, vol. 11, no. 1, p. 11, 2013.
[26] C. Reindl, H. Quentmeier, K. Petropoulos et al., "*CBL* exon 8/9 mutants activate the FLT3 pathway and cluster in core binding factor/11q deletion acute myeloid leukemia/myelodysplastic syndrome subtypes," *Clinical Cancer Research*, vol. 15, no. 7, pp. 2238–2247, 2009.
[27] C. Camps, N. Petousi, C. Bento et al., "Gene panel sequencing improves the diagnostic work-up of patients with idiopathic erythrocytosis and identifies new mutations," *Haematologica*, vol. 101, no. 11, pp. 1306–1318, 2016.

12

Incidental Discovery of Multiorgan Extramedullary Plasmacytomas in the Setting of Newly Diagnosed Multiple Myeloma and Delayed Hemolytic Transfusion Reaction

Joselle Cook,[1] Steven Song,[1] Anthony Ventimiglia,[2] and Carol Luhrs[3]

[1]*Department of Medicine, SUNY Downstate Medical Center, Brooklyn, NY 11203, USA*
[2]*College of Medicine, SUNY Downstate Medical Center, Brooklyn, NY 11203, USA*
[3]*Division of Hematology and Oncology, SUNY Downstate Medical Center, Brooklyn, NY 11203, USA*

Correspondence should be addressed to Joselle Cook; joselle.cook@downstate.edu

Academic Editor: Marie-Christine Kyrtsonis

Extramedullary plasmacytomas (EMPs) are defined by the presence of clonal plasma cell proliferation outside of the bone marrow, portending an overall poor prognosis. This case highlights extramedullary plasmacytomas as an unusual presenting manifestation of multiple myeloma. Through incidental discovery during a delayed hemolytic transfusion reaction workup, EMPs were found in the liver, spleen, and possibly the lung. Though rare at presentation, this case emphasizes that the presence of EMPs should be considered at the outset as it not only impacts the treatment regimen for such patients but also considerably affects prognosis.

1. Introduction

Multiple myeloma (MM) is the malignant proliferation of plasma cells. It usually occurs in the seventh or eighth decade of life. Newly diagnosed cases often present with symptoms of anemia (fatigue, shortness of breath, and decreased exercise tolerance) and may require RBC transfusions. Through incidental discovery during evaluation of a delayed hemolytic transfusion reaction, multiorgan extramedullary plasmacytomas were found in the liver and spleen, with possible involvement of the lung. This case report reinforces the need for increased awareness of the varied presentations of advanced multiple myeloma.

2. Case Presentation

A 58-year-old woman, who recently arrived from Guyana, presented to the primary care clinic with complaints of generalized fatigue, hip pain, and low back pain for the preceding 8 months. She denied fever, chills, unintentional weight loss, abdominal pain, diarrhea, constipation, and cardiopulmonary or neurological symptoms. Routine lab work demonstrated anemia (hemoglobin: 8 mg/dL), hypercalcemia (13.8 mg/dL), and renal impairment (creatinine: 2.83 mg/dL). Remaining labs including liver function tests were remarkable for total protein of 13.4 g/dL. A metastatic bone survey revealed diffuse lytic lesions consistent with multiple myeloma. The patient was admitted to the hospital for management of symptomatic anemia and hypercalcemia and to complete myeloma evaluation.

Intravenous (IV) fluids and dexamethasone were initiated. Further evaluation of the myeloma revealed a monoclonal IgG lambda of 7600 mg/dL and a kappa/lambda ratio of 0.01. Bone marrow biopsy demonstrated 58% plasma cell infiltration. Flow cytometry, immunohistochemistry, and FISH of the biopsy showed a monoclonal IgG-λ plasma cell population, with trisomy 11 and 17p del. Spine MRI demonstrated multifocal areas of pathologic marrow replacement of the entire axial spine without signs of cord compression.

The patient received one cycle of bortezomib and RBC transfusion for symptomatic anemia. Because of her high risk for pathologic fracture, the patient underwent prophylactic intramedullary nailing of the left humerus and femur. While awaiting right lower extremity intramedullary nailing, there was an acute and unexpected increase in total bilirubin to 4.5 mg/dL, with an indirect predominance and an acute drop in hemoglobin from 8 mg/dL to 6 mg/dL. Other labs were

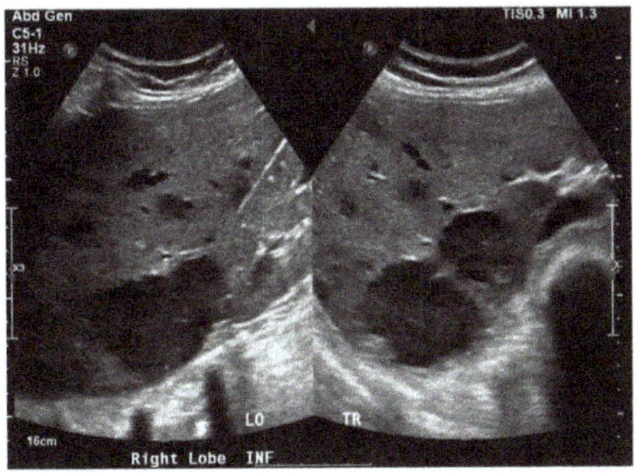

FIGURE 1: Right lobe liver ultrasound (inferior view) showing innumerable hypoechoic heterogeneous masses, the largest of which was located inferiorly and measured 6.0 × 4.3 × 5.4 cm.

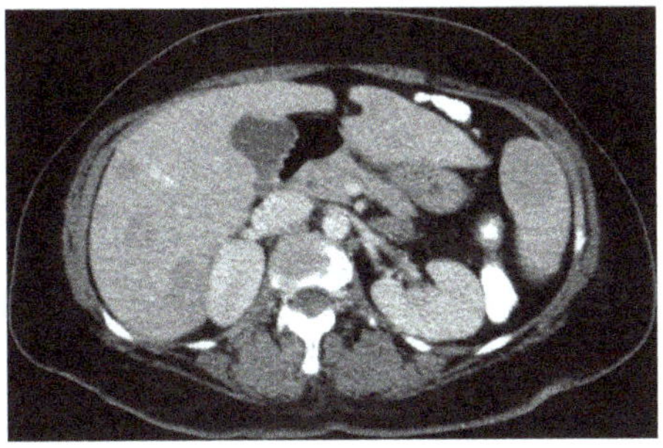

FIGURE 2: CT of the abdomen showing numerous low attenuation lesions in the liver and spleen suspicious for metastatic disease along with soft tissue nodules in the anterior abdominal wall and numerous lytic lesions in the axial skeleton.

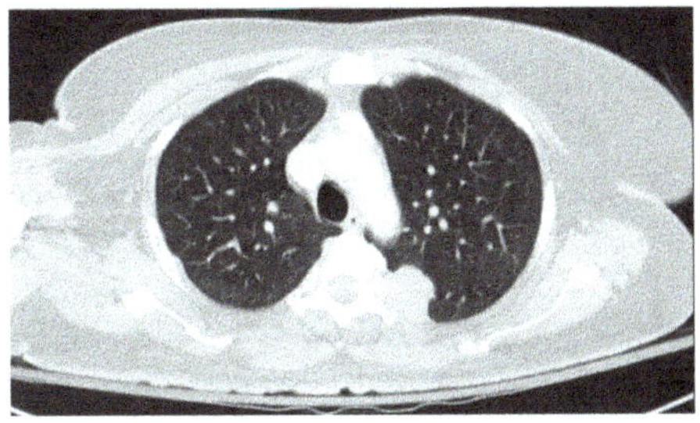

FIGURE 3: CT of the chest showing a subpleural mass in the upper left lobe that measured 3.3 × 3.0 × 2.7 cm concerning for metastasis.

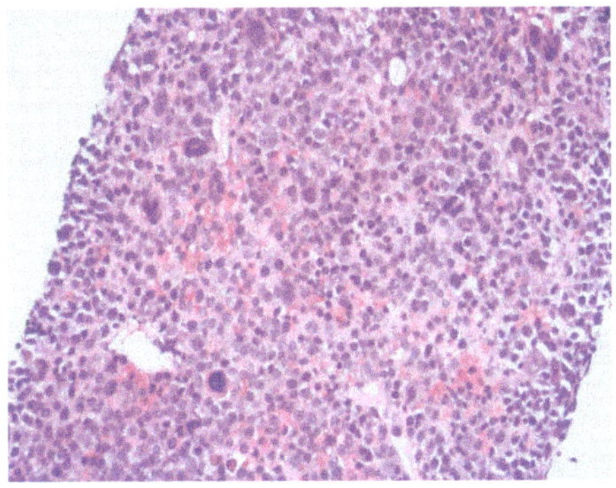

FIGURE 4: Liver biopsy H&E stain demonstrating compact sheets of atypical plasma cells, consistent with extramedullary hepatic plasmacytoma.

remarkable for elevated LDH (2009 mg/dL), reticulocytosis (absolute reticulocyte count: 354,576 cells/mm^3), and a positive direct antiglobulin test suggesting a delayed hemolytic transfusion reaction. Right upper quadrant ultrasound performed revealed innumerable hypoechoic hepatic masses (Figure 1). CT of the chest and abdomen showed numerous low attenuation lesions in the liver and spleen suspicious for metastatic disease, along with soft tissue nodules in the anterior abdominal wall and a subpleural mass in the left upper lobe (Figures 2 and 3). Biopsy of one of the hepatic lesions was consistent with extramedullary plasmacytoma (Figures 4–7). After 4 days of supportive care, the hemolysis resolved. Prophylactic right humerus and femur intramedullary nailing was performed, with subsequent initiation of VD-PACE chemotherapy.

3. Discussion

Multiple myeloma (MM) is the clonal proliferation of plasma cells originating in the bone marrow that predominantly affects the axial skeleton [1]. Extramedullary plasmacytoma (EMP) is defined by the presence of clonal plasma cell proliferation outside of the bone marrow. Formerly thought to be an uncommon manifestation, EMPs are increasingly being recognized as part of the clinical constellation of MM [2]. The utilization of more sensitive imaging modalities has resulted in earlier recognition of EMPs [3]. The incidence of EMP on diagnosis ranges from 7 to 18%, with a notable association with IgD myeloma [2–4]. EMP is associated with a more aggressive albeit heterogenous natural history, dictated by biologics and genetic mutations unique to this disease subtype [2, 3, 5]. Isolated case reports detail the presence of EMP with an uncharacteristically asymptomatic systemic myelomatous disease [5].

A complexity of high risk cytogenetics and altered tumor biologics within the bone microenvironment signal the aberrant spread of the myeloma cells into the extramedullary realm [2, 5, 6]. Increased expression of CD44, together with low CD56 expression and low p-selectin levels, is a proposed mechanism for EMPs, resulting in decreased adhesion molecule expression and the potential for extramedullary spread [6, 7]. CXCR4 and its ligand CXCL12, thought to mediate the homing of bone marrow progenitor cells, are found to have increased expression with EMPs through induction of an epithelial-mesenchymal transition-like pattern [6, 8]. Increased genetic instability and aberrant cell proliferation have been demonstrated by a high level of mutations in tumor protein p53, high MIB-1 antibody proliferation indices [2, 5, 6]. A demonstrable association has been made between EMPs and poor prognostic cytogenetics such as t[4;14] translocation, 17p deletion, and t[14;16] translocation [2, 6, 9]. As a result of these genetic and cellular irregularities, together with hypoxia and increased angiogenesis, a "bone marrow escape" mechanism is proposed, through extension

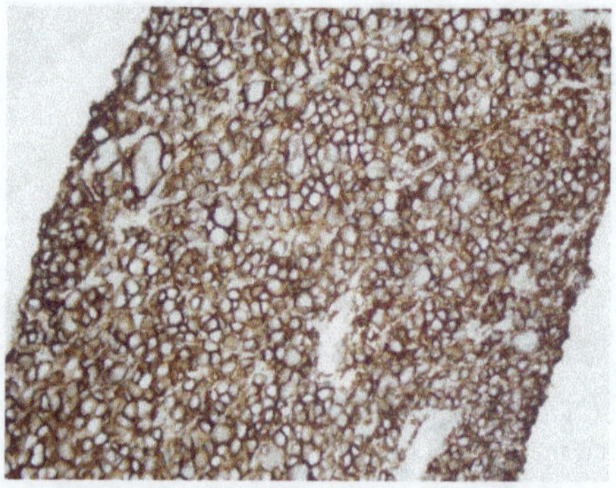

FIGURE 5: Liver biopsy CD138 marker confirming neoplastic extramedullary plasma cell infiltration from multiple myeloma.

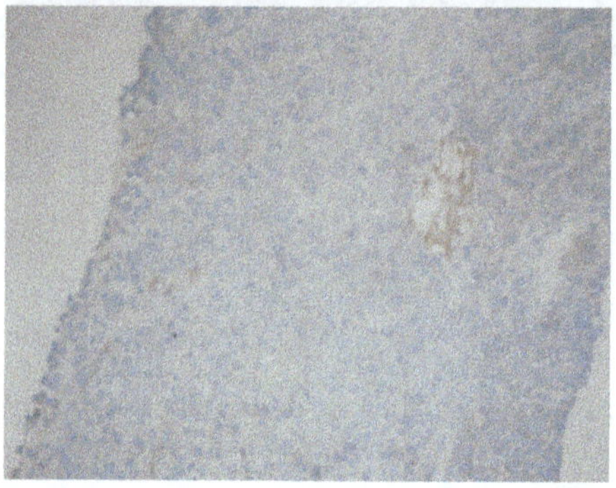

FIGURE 6: Liver biopsy stained for kappa light chain immunoglobulin confirming neoplastic extramedullary plasma cell infiltration from multiple myeloma.

from skeletal plasmacytomas, or by hematogenous spread to various organs, most commonly lymph nodes, the liver, lung, muscles, the mesentery, and also the skin [2, 5, 7]. Alternatively proposed is the release of plasma cells incited by any surgical intervention during the course of disease [2, 5, 9]. The resultant plasma cells of EMPs are notably less differentiated, with production of predominantly light chains instead of intact immunoglobulins [2, 6]. Patients usually present with more severe manifestations of the myeloma spectrum and high LDH levels [6, 9].

In the diagnostic workup, PET-CT scan would best determine the presence of extramedullary disease and should be performed early as part of initial staging in determined high risk patients [7, 10]. Once the presence of EMPs is established, after the initial PET-CT, it should be repeated to assess response 2 cycles after treatment and at treatment completion to ensure complete remission [2]. It is noteworthy to add that the International Myeloma Working Group recently published a consensus statement recommending the use of PET-CT in the initial workup of all newly diagnosed patients with multiple myeloma, as well as patients with refractory or relapsed myeloma, given its high sensitivity in detecting extramedullary disease as well as its superiority in determining metabolically active disease and early determination of treatment response [11].

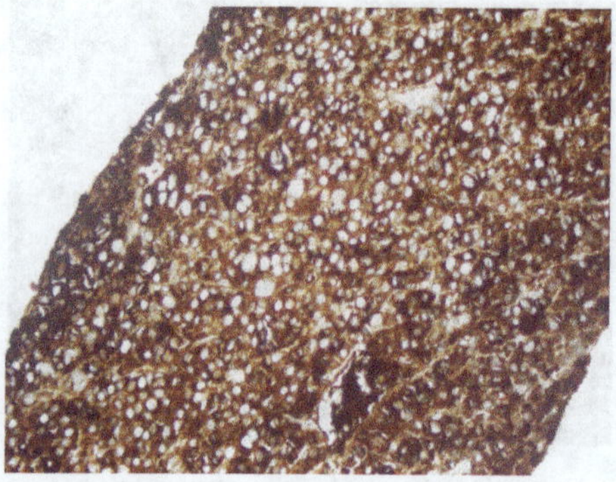

FIGURE 7: Liver biopsy stained for lambda light chain immunoglobulin confirming neoplastic extramedullary plasma cell infiltration from multiple myeloma.

With currently evolving practice patterns for MM presenting with EMPs, a favorable response has been seen with the use of high dose combination regimens with lenalidomide, glucocorticoids, chemotherapy with bortezomib, heralded as an "antimyeloma agent," and cyclophosphamide [2–4, 12]. Improved sustained responses may be seen with high dose therapy and autologous stem cell transplantation after induction therapy in eligible candidates [2–4, 7, 12]. Contrary to previous concerns, several meta-analyses have demonstrated no association between the use of novel agents and targeted treatments such as bortezomib and thalidomide and relapse of extramedullary disease [2, 3, 6, 13].

Outcomes for patients with EMPs at diagnosis continue to emerge through reports of various case series and clinical trials. Varettoni et al. established shorter progression-free survival (PFS) with no significant difference in median overall survival (OS) in patients with EMPs compared to patients without EMPs [3, 6, 7]. Alternatively, outcomes from an autologous stem cell transplant (ASCT) trial by PETHEMA group showed decreased OS, but no difference in PFS [7, 12]. Notably, should relapse of extramedullary disease occur posttreatment, the prognosis for overall survival is significantly worse compared to myeloma without EMPs [6].

In summary, the presence of EMPs is a poor prognosticator, demonstrating decreased overall patient survival, increased rates of disease progression, associated with more severe cytopenias, increased cytogenetic abnormalities, and poorer response to traditional chemotherapeutic regimens [1–3, 9]. This unusual case describes the incidental discovery of extensive EMPs during evaluation of a hemolytic transfusion reaction on the grounds of newly diagnosed multiple myeloma. Myeloma with extramedullary disease proves at this time to be an enigmatic condition with an ominous clinical course, for which definitive treatment and practice patterns are still evolving [5, 6]. High risk genomics and tumor biologics potentially may predict those patients at higher risk of extramedullary disease and should be considered in such patients with newly diagnosed MM [6, 9, 10]. The judicious use of imaging modalities such as PET-CT scan in high risk patients at the initial diagnostic evaluation may facilitate an earlier diagnosis of EMPs.

Conflicts of Interest

The authors declare that there are no conflicts of interest regarding the publication of this article.

References

[1] S. F. Low, N. H. M. Tap, T. Y. Kew, C. S. Ngiu, and R. Sridharan, "Non secretory multiple myeloma with extensive extramedullary plasmacytoma: A diagnostic dilemma," *Iranian Journal of Radiology*, vol. 12, no. 3, Article ID e11760, 2015.

[2] J. Bladé, C. Fernández de Larrea, L. Rosiñol, M. T. Cibeira, R. Jiménez, and R. Powles, "Soft-tissue plasmacytomas in multiple myeloma: incidence, mechanisms of extramedullary spread, and treatment approach," *Journal of Clinical Oncology*, vol. 29, no. 28, pp. 3805–3812, 2011.

[3] M. Varettoni, A. Corso, G. Pica, S. Mangiacavalli, C. Pascutto, and M. Lazzarino, "Incidence, presenting features and outcome of extramedullary disease in multiple myeloma: a longitudinal study on 1003 consecutive patients," *Annals of Oncology*, vol. 21, no. 2, pp. 325–330, 2010.

[4] P. Wu, F. E. Davies, K. Boyd et al., "The impact of extramedullary disease at presentation on the outcome of myeloma," *Leukemia and Lymphoma*, vol. 50, no. 2, pp. 230–235, 2009.

[5] S. E. Schols and L. L. Tick, "Recurrent extramedullary plasmacytoma in asymptomatic multiple myeloma: A case report," *Journal of Medical Case Reports*, vol. 9, no. 37, 2015.

[6] C. Touzeau and P. Moreau, "How i treat extramedullary myeloma," *Blood*, vol. 127, no. 8, pp. 971–976, 2016.

[7] J. Bladé, C. F. de Larrea, and L. Rosiñol, "Extramedullary involvement in multiple myeloma," *Haematologica*, vol. 97, no. 11, pp. 1618-1619, 2012.

[8] A. M. Roccaro, Y. Mishima, A. Sacco et al., "CXCR4 regulates extra-medullary myeloma through epithelial-mesenchymal-transition-like transcriptional activation," *Cell Reports*, vol. 12, no. 4, pp. 622–635, 2015.

[9] S. Z. Usmani, C. Heuck, A. Mitchell et al., "Extramedullary disease portends poor prognosis in multiple myeloma and is over-represented in high-risk disease even in the era of novel agents," *Haematologica*, vol. 97, no. 11, pp. 1761–1767, 2012.

[10] D. Ajay and C. Abhinav, "A multiple myeloma patient presenting with multiple hepatic masses," *Journal of Medical Cases*, pp. 673–675, 2013.

[11] M. Cavo, E. Terpos, C. Nanni et al., "Role of 18 F-FDG PET/CT in the diagnosis and management of multiple myeloma and other plasma cell disorders: a consensus statement by the International Myeloma Working Group," *The Lancet Oncology*, vol. 18, no. 4, pp. e206–e217, 2017.

[12] L. Rosiñol, A. Oriol, A. I. Teruel et al., "Superiority of bortezomib, thalidomide, and dexamethasone (VTD) as induction pretransplantation therapy in multiple myeloma: a randomized phase 3 PETHEMA/GEM study," *Blood*, vol. 120, no. 8, pp. 1589–1596, 2012.

[13] P. Raanani, O. Shpilberg, and I. Ben-Bassat, "Extramedullary disease and targeted therapies for hematological malignancies—Is the association real?" *Annals of Oncology*, vol. 18, no. 1, pp. 7–12, 2007.

13

Prevention of High-Dose Cytosine Arabinoside-Induced Acute Pericarditis with Preemptive Dexamethasone Administration

Weerapat Owattanapanich and Theera Ruchutrakool

Division of Hematology, Department of Medicine, Faculty of Medicine, Siriraj Hospital, Mahidol University, Bangkok, Thailand

Correspondence should be addressed to Theera Ruchutrakool; sitrc@mahidol.ac.th

Academic Editor: Chihaya Imai

Pericarditis/pericardial effusion (PC/PEEF) is a rare but fatal complication of cytosine arabinoside (Ara-C). We report an acute myeloid leukemia (AML) patient who developed massive pericardial effusion after a second Ara-C exposure. As Ara-C was most beneficial in controlling the leukemia, she was treated with a further cycle of Ara-C along with dexamethasone to prevent the complication from reoccurring. No PC/PEEF was subsequently detected.

1. Introduction

AML is the most common acute leukemia in adults. Its annual incidence in Thailand is 1.4 per 100,000 population, with 5-year disease-free survival and overall-survival rates of 41.0% and 22.2%, respectively [1]. The most efficient chemotherapeutic agents are anthracyclin and Ara-C. Ara-C is administered as a standard dose during induction and a high dose during consolidation. Besides bone marrow suppression, nausea, vomiting, fatigue, and mouth sores, the side effects of high-dose Ara-C (HIDAC) include conjunctivitis and cerebellar toxicity. PC/PEEF, a rare but often lethal complication of standard and high-dose Ara-C, was first reported in 1984 [2]. No management guidelines exist for PC/PEEF. Based on a literature review and our experience with an AML patient with this rare complication after Ara-C treatment, we propose a strategy to manage it and rechallenge with Ara-C without the complication.

2. Case Report

A 38-year-old female presented with fatigue for 2 months. On examination, pale skin and petechiae along both legs were observed; others were unremarkable. The initial blood count showed a hemoglobin of 7.8 g/dL, WBC of 242.7×10^9/L (myeloblasts and monoblasts constituted over 90%), and platelet count of 21×10^9/L. By flow cytometry, the malignant cells (86%) were positive for CD13, CD33, CD11b, CD11c, CD14, CD64, CD117, and MPO which were compatible with AML-M4 according to FAB classification. By G-banding karyotyping, no abnormalities were observed. After establishing the diagnosis of AML, the patient received standard remission induction therapy with Ara-C (100 mg/M^2/day; 12-hour continuous infusion once daily for 7 consecutive days) and idarubicin (12 mg/M^2/day; intravenous infusion for 3 consecutive days). She regenerated at day 24 and entered complete remission without grade 4 complications except cytopenia. It was planned that she would receive allogeneic stem cell transplantation. While awaiting approval of this treatment from her covered medical expenses, we decided to control her disease with consolidation therapy, HIDAC regimen for 3 cycles.

A week after complete remission, Ara-C (1,000 mg/M^2/day; 2-hour continuous infusion every 12 hours for 6 doses) commenced. On day 3 of this regimen, during administration of the fourth Ara-C dose, she complained of a sudden onset of dyspnea and sharp, persistent pain in the substernal and epigastric areas. She had no fever, sweating, cough, or palpitation. Her temperature was 36.8°C and pulse rate was

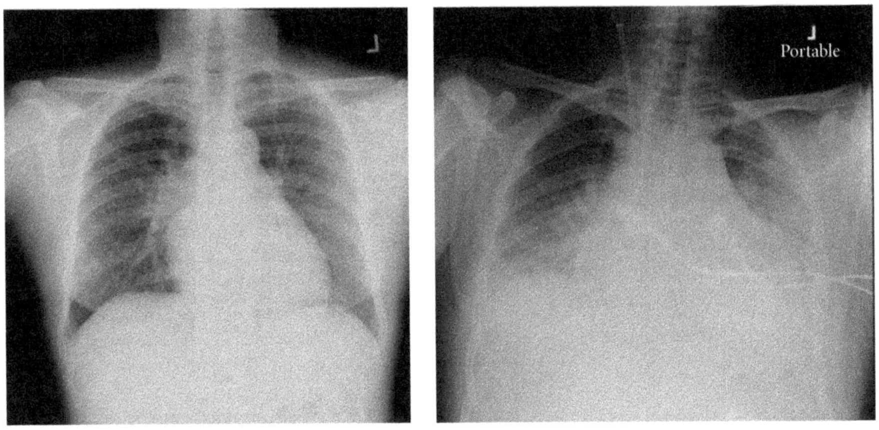

(a) (b)

Figure 1: Chest X-rays: (a) prior to cytosine arabinoside; (b) day 3 of the first cycle of HIDAC.

80/min and regular, but her blood pressure, measured repeatedly at all extremities, was 80/40 mmHg. A chest X-ray revealed massive cardiomegaly (Figure 1(b)) relative to the baseline cardiac size on the admission day (Figure 1(a)). Electrocardiography showed normal sinus rhythm and no low voltage, electrical alternans, or ST-T abnormality.

An echocardiography disclosed massive PEEF without cardiac tamponade. The left ventricular ejection fraction was 71% without either an abnormal wall motion or significant valve dysfunction. Computed tomography of the chest and abdomen was unremarkable except revealing massive PEEF. Troponin-T was under 0.003 ng/mL (<0.01 ng/mL), and CK-MB was 0.67 IU/L (5–25 IU/L). Viral serologic studies (herpes simplex virus, cytomegalovirus, Epstein–Barr virus, and hepatitis B virus) detected by IgM and IgG were all negative. Antinuclear antibody was also negative.

Given no other apparent causes of PC/PEEF, Ara-C-induced PC/PEEF was highly suspected. After 2,000 mL of normal saline infusion within 15 minutes, hypotension was unimproved. The initial central venous pressure revealed 24 cm H_2O. Dopamine (10 μg/kg/minute) was started. Besides ceasing Ara-C, 10 mg/day of intravenous dexamethasone was initiated. The substernal and epigastric pain subsequently disappeared within six hours, with BP stabilized at 110/80 mmHg. The inotropic drug was discontinued within 26 hours. The cardiac shadow was markedly decreased three days after commencement of the dexamethasone treatment. At day 7, an echocardiography revealed only small pericardial effusion, so a planned pericardiocentesis was canceled. The dexamethasone was tapered and stopped by day 11. She was discharged on day 23, still without evidence of effusion.

As Ara-C was deemed essential for the AML treatment, it was decided to repeat the HIDAC consolidation therapy but with preemptive, high-dose dexamethasone. Ten mg/day intravenous dexamethasone was therefore initiated the day before cytoreduction and continued for 6 days of each cycle. The HIDAC regimen administration went without complications. The patient successfully underwent a matched-sibling stem cell transplantation in July 2012. As of January 2017, she remains in remission.

3. Discussion

PC/PEEF is an uncommon, but potentially fatal, AML complication. Its pathogenesis is multifactorial, possibly resulting from the underlying disease, the concomitant infection, accompanying bleeding complications arising from thrombocytopenia or DIC, the chemotherapy, or radiation. Thus, Ara-C-induced PC/PEEF should always be an exclusion diagnosis. In our case, we excluded both virological and autoimmune pathogenesis. Despite the lack of cytology of the pericardial effusion, we deemed that leukemic involvement and hemorrhagic complications in this patient, who was in remission and without any complaints, could be ruled out. Thus, this severe episode should be described to the cytoreductive regimen. Chemotherapeutic agents which have been reported to induce PC/PEEF include daunorubicin, doxorubicin, cyclophosphamide, bleomycin, and actinomycin D. Our patient received anthracycline six weeks before the development of PC/PEEF; the longest duration of anthracycline-induced PC/PEEF onset ever reported was 29 days. Therefore, Ara-C is the most likely cause of PC/PEEF in our patient, rather than doxorubicin.

Ara-C-induced PC/PEEF was first described by Vaickus in 1984 [2]; a literature review revealed that only 10 patients (including our patient) have been reported. Interestingly, two patients developed two episodes of this complication [3, 4]. The pathogenesis of these severe complications is unclear, but type IV delayed hypersensitivity [4–9], anaphylaxis [10], and direct toxicity to the endothelium [11] have been suggested.

Table 1 tabulates previously published series of PC/PEEF. The onset of PC/PEEF varied between 2 and 29 days (median: 3 days) after receiving repeated doses of Ara-C. Most patients received the HIDAC regimen. Our patient developed PC/PEEF three days after HIDAC; we hypothesize that there was a type IV delayed hypersensitivity, compatible with such reactions developing within 10 days of the last exposure. To prove this, a cardiac muscle biopsy showing infiltration of T-lymphocytes would be required.

Table 1: Reported cases of Ara-C-induced pericarditis/pericardial effusion.

Author	Year	Patients/disease	Site of complication	Chemotherapy regimen and onset of event (day after receiving chemotherapy)	Treatment of pericarditis or pericardial effusion	Results
Vaickus and Letendre	1984	25-year-old man with relapsed ALL	PC/PEEF with cardiac tamponade	Day 2 after the fourth dose of the second cycle of high-dose Ara-C ($3\,g/M^2$ for 10 doses/cycle) (consolidation)	Prednisolone 10 mg twice daily and salicylate 500 mg twice daily for 2 days, but no response; pericardiocentesis was performed	Full recovery after pericardiocentesis
Gillis et al.	1992	51-year-old woman	PC with minimal PEEF	Day 3 after the fifth dose of the first cycle of high-dose Ara-C ($3\,g/M^2$ for 12 doses/cycle) (consolidation)	Hydrocortisone 200 mg once daily intravenously	Full recovery within a week without pericardiocentesis
Reykdal et al.	1995	47-year-old man with AML-M4	PC, no PEEF	Day 11 after the last dose of the first cycle of high-dose Ara-C ($2\,g/M^2$ every 12 hours for 6 days) (consolidation)	Supportive treatment with NSAIDs	Pain relieved by NSAIDs within a day
Hermans et al.	1997	37-year-old man with AML-M2	PC/PEEF	Day 4 after the 5th dose of 3rd cycle of high-dose Ara-C ($3\,g/M^2$ every 12 hours for 4 days) (consolidation)	Methylprednisolone 0.5 mg/kg orally for 8 days, and tapered off at day 11	Complete recovery by day 7 of methylprednisolone
Yamada et al.	1998	61-year-old man with AML-M2 and 65-year-old man with MDS-related AML-M2	PEEF	Relapsed AML, low-dose Ara-C (induction remission) AML-M2 low-dose Ara-C (consolidation)	Pulse methylprednisolone plus pericardiocentesis	Not reported
Woods et al.	1999	47-year-old man with AML-M2	Large PEEF	Day 9 after the first induction remission with daunorubicin and Ara-C ($100\,mg/M^2$ D1-7); then, high-dose Ara-C ($2\,g/M^2$ on D8-10) (induction remission)	Pericardiocentesis	Recovery by 6 weeks
Gähler et al.	2003	64-year-old man with AML-M4	1st: PC/small PEEF	1st episode: day 29 after 7 + 3 regimen ($200\,mg/M^2$ Ara-C) (induction remission)	1st: NSAIDs	Recovery in 48 hours
			2nd: PC with PEEF and cardiac tamponade	2nd episode: day 3 after high-dose Ara-C ($1\,g/M^2$ every 12 hours for 6 days) (consolidation)	2nd: Pericardiocentesis	Immediately improved after pericardiocentesis
Lee et al.	2011	25-year-old woman with AML-M4	Recurrent PC	1st episode: day 6 after the sixth dose of high-dose Ara-C (second cycle of induction remission)	1st: high-dose ibuprofen (1,200 mg/day)	Responded well
				2nd episode: day 2 after the sixth dose of high-dose Ara-C (first consolidation)	2nd: high-dose ibuprofen (1,200 mg/day) + colchicine (0.6 mg/day)	Responded well within 10 days
This study	2017	38-year-old woman with AML-M4	PC/PEEF	Day 3 after the fourth dose of high-dose Ara-C (first consolidation)	Dexamethasone 10 mg intravenously once daily	Complete recovery within 3 days

These considerations leave us with the question of how to treat PC/PEEF, either prophylactically or upon occurrence. PEEF management depends on the degree of cardiac tamponade; if clinical cardiac tamponade is detected, pericardiocentesis is the treatment of choice. Systemic corticosteroids were first introduced in treating this complication in 1984 [2] with the hypothesis of a delayed hypersensitivity or anaphylaxis, but the response was undesirable. This could be due to an insufficient amount of steroid being used (prednisolone 20 mg/day). Subsequently, Gillis introduced higher dose of steroid (hydrocortisone 200 mg/day), and the results were promising [5], similar to our patient. Successful results with various types and dosage of corticosteroids, such as intravenous hydrocortisone (200 mg/day) and oral methylprednisolone (0.5 mg/kg/day), have been reported [6–8]. Furthermore, we insisted on using the HIDAC regimen for the second course of consolidation chemotherapy with prophylactic dexamethasone. As PC/PEEF did not reappear, we suggest that patients with Ara-C-induced PC/PEEF may be treated with the same regimen combined with a systemic high-dose corticosteroid. From our experience, the optimal dexamethasone dosage to prevent this complication is at least 8–10 mg/day, which is equivalent to hydrocortisone dose of 200–250 mg/day or prednisolone dose of 40–50 mg/day.

Conflicts of Interest

The authors have no conflicts of interest regarding the publication of this manuscript.

Acknowledgments

The authors would like to thank Professor Peter Hokland for his comments and wonderful suggestions about this manuscript.

References

[1] P. Niparuck, S. Chuncharunee, A. Ungkanont et al., "Long-term outcomes of de novo acute myeloid leukemia in Thai patients," *Journal of the Medical Association of Thailand*, vol. 92, no. 9, pp. 1143–1149, 2009.

[2] L. Vaickus and L. Letendre, "Pericarditis induced by high-dose cytarabine therapy," *Archives of Internal Medicine*, vol. 144, no. 9, pp. 1868-1869, 1984.

[3] A. Gähler, F. Hitz, U. Hess, and T. Cerny, "Acute pericarditis and pleural effusion complicating cytarabine chemotherapy," *Oncology Research and Treatment*, vol. 26, no. 4, pp. 348–350, 2003.

[4] G. Y. Lee, K. T. Ahn, C. W. Jung et al., "Recurrent pericarditis after chemotherapy for acute myeloid leukemia: a case report and a modern approach to chemotherapy-induced pericarditis," *Cardiology*, vol. 120, no. 3, pp. 130–134, 2011.

[5] S. Gillis, E. J. Dann, Y. Ilan et al., "Pericarditis associated with high-dose cytarabine therapy for acute myeloblasts leukemia: a rare complication of therapy," *Leukemia & Lymphoma*, vol. 6, no. 6, pp. 525-526, 1992.

[6] S. Reykdal, R. Sham, and P. Kouides, "Cytarabine-induced pericarditis: a case report and review of the literature of the cardio-pulmonary complications of cytarabine therapy," *Leukemia Research*, vol. 19, no. 2, pp. 141–144, 1995.

[7] C. Hermans, N. Straetmans, J. L. Michaux et al., "Pericarditis induced by high-dose cytosine arabinoside chemotherapy," *Annals of Hematology*, vol. 75, no. 1-2, pp. 55–57, 1997.

[8] T. Yamada, H. Tsurumi, T. Hara, M. Sawada, M. Oyama, and H. Moriwaki, "Cytarabine-induced pericarditis," *Rinsho Ketsueki*, vol. 39, no. 11, pp. 1115–1120, 1998.

[9] T. Woods, B. Vidarsson, D. Mosher et al., "Transient effusive-constrictive pericarditis due to chemotherapy," *Clinical Cardiology*, vol. 22, no. 4, pp. 316–318, 1999.

[10] B. L. Powell, P. J. Zekan, H. B. Muss et al., "Ara-C syndrome during low-dose continuous infusion therapy," *Medical and Pediatric Oncology*, vol. 14, no. 6, pp. 310–312, 1986.

[11] M. A. Boogaerts, S. Malbrain, and R. L. Verwilghen, "The Ara-C syndrome: direct endothelial cytotoxicity," *British Journal of Haematology*, vol. 66, p. 423, 1987.

14

Two Cases of γ-Heavy Chain Disease and a Review of the Literature

I. Ramasamy[1] and Z. Rudzki[2]

[1]*Department of Biochemistry, Worcester Royal Hospital, Worcester, UK*
[2]*Heart of England NHS Trust, Birmingham, UK*

Correspondence should be addressed to I. Ramasamy; indrar@ozemail.com.au

Academic Editor: Marie-Christine Kyrtsonis

Gamma heavy chain disease (γ-HCD) is a rare lymphoproliferative disorder characterised by the production of a truncated immunoglobulin heavy chain. Fewer than 200 cases have been reported in the literature. In some cases, γ-HCD occurs with other lymphoid neoplasms. This study reports clinical, biochemical, haematological, and histological findings in two cases of γ-HCD. We describe newer biochemical diagnostic tools (HevyLite measurement, capillary electrophoresis, and immunotyping) that can aid in the characterisation of γ-HCD. The first case is an 88-year-old woman with γ-HCD. The second case is an 81-year-old woman who developed γ-HCD during treatment for Waldenstrom's macroglobulinemia. In the second patient, histopathology identified a separate clone responsible for the secretion of the gamma heavy chain. Studies on the clonal evolution of the disease may provide insight into therapeutic implications and the genomic complexity of the disease.

1. Introduction

Gamma heavy chain disease (γ-HCD) is also called Franklin's disease, named after the author of the first report in 1964. The disease is defined as a neoplasm of lymphocytes, plasmacytoid lymphocytes, and plasma cells characterised by the production of an abnormally truncated gamma heavy chain protein that lacks associated light chains. Since Franklin first reported the case, fewer than 200 cases have been described in the literature. A wide variety of disorders have been associated with γ-HCD. In some cases, γ-HCD occurs with other lymphoid neoplasms or with a history of autoimmune disorder. γ-HCD shows a wide clinical spectrum ranging from completely asymptomatic to progressively malignant forms.

Normal heavy chains not associated with light chains have not been detected in serum of healthy individuals. In γ-HCD abnormally short truncated heavy chains can be isolated from patient's serum without associated light chains. In several instances where the gene encoding the shortened heavy chain gene has been characterised, the truncation originated from deletions and/or insertions within the rearranged variable region genes (V) that in addition harbor somatic point mutations. One possibility is that several types of oncogene translocations happen as a by-product of somatic hypermutation [1]. It has been established the γ-HCD immunoglobulins are the products of aberrant biosynthesis, for example, deletions, splice site correction, and amino-terminal proteolysis [2]. Structural analysis of the defective gamma heavy chain in 23 patients showed some common features. In most cases, the variable region sequence was short and interrupted by large deletions, usually including the C_H1 domain. Normal sequence began at the hinge region or at the C_H2 domain [3].

Genetic subtypes of multiple myeloma (MM) have been identified which have different biological features and heterogeneity in clinical outcomes [4]. New gene sequencing techniques have yielded new insights into the pathogenesis and evolution of the disease and potential individualised treatment by novel targeted approaches [5].

We report two cases of γ-HCD: one case in a patient with lymphadenopathy and a second case in a patient with a history of Waldenstrom's macroglobulinemia (WM). Further, we review previous case series on γ-HCD. These two cases were diagnosed using the techniques of capillary zone electrophoresis, immunofixation, and "HevyLite" measurement.

Use of newer commercially available techniques simplified the diagnosis of γ-HCD. In one patient, there was no evidence of previous chemotherapy. The second patient developed γ-HCD during treatment for WM.

2. Case Report

2.1. Case 1. An 88-year-old woman presented with a change in the bowel habit. A colonoscopy showed some diverticular disease. The CT scan showed splenomegaly and some lymphadenopathy particularly in the region of the splenic hilum. The liver, kidney, pancreas, and adrenals were normal. She had a past history of osteopenia, type II diabetes, and fragility fracture. She was taking vitamin B12, vitamin D, and bisphosphonates. There was no history of sweating, weight loss, bruising, or recent infections. Her biochemistry and hematology at diagnosis and 3 months after diagnosis are summarised in Tables 1 and 2.

Gel protein electrophoresis and immunofixation (Figure 1(a)) and capillary zone electrophoresis and immunotyping (Figures 2(a) and 2(b)) (Sebia, UK) identified 2 γ-heavy chains. Both methods were negative for kappa and lambda light chains. Differing sensitivities of heavy and light chain reagents can cause false-negative results for light chain immunofixation, and the results were confirmed by a second gel electrophoresis (Helena, UK) method. Urine immunofixation identified a γ-heavy chain (Figure 3(a)).

Total IgG (determined by immunoturbidimetry on the Binding Site SPA-plus analyser) was elevated at 38.7 g/L (RR 7–16), with decreased levels of IgA and IgM (Table 1). IgG1 subclass levels were elevated, and other subclass levels were lower than the reference range (Table 3). Serum-free light chain ratios (determined by the Binding Site method, UK) were within the reference range (Table 4). HevyLite (Binding Site, UK) measurements are specific for individual heavy chains with either kappa or lambda light chains and can provide more specific information than individual immunoglobulin quantitation. Observed increased heavy chain pair ratios (e.g., IgMkappa/IgMlambda) can be indicative of clonal expansion. IgGkappa/IgGlambda ratios were within the reference range confirming the absence of clonal expansion of IgGkappa/IgGlambda intact immunoglobulins (Table 5).

In a previous study, HevyLite reagents which did not recognise intact IgG immunoglobulin ratios ((IgGkappa + IgGlambda)/total IgG) were used as indirect measures of heavy chain fragmentation [6]. The ratio of 0.04 in this patient was less than the average value of 0.18 found in the previous study [6].

Bone marrow biopsy showed subtle infiltrates by low-grade B-NHL, associated with groups of clonal plasma cells, which expressed neither kappa nor lambda chain but stained with IgG heavy chain (Figures 4(a)–4(g)). Lymphatic infiltrate was surrounded by a rim of CD138+ plasma cells. Though there was equal expression of kappa and lambda light chains, the sum of kappa- and lambda-positive cells appeared to be much less than the number of CD138+ cells which indicated that most plasma cells do not express light chains.

The patient is currently monitored on a 3-monthly basis.

2.2. Case 2. Patient 2 is an 81-year-old lady under treatment for WM (IgMkappa paraprotein). Details of her treatment are given in Figure 5. Capillary zone electrophoresis prior to the development of γ-HCD is shown in Figure 6(a). Gamma heavy chain developed during treatment and an unusually diffuse γ-heavy chain band was identified by gel electrophoresis (Figure 1(b)) and capillary zone electrophoresis (Figures 6(b) and 6(c)) (Sebia, UK) and confirmed by a second gel electrophoresis method (Helena, UK). Urine immunofixation identified the γ-heavy chain and kappa light chain (Figure 3(b)).

Her biochemistry and hematology prior to the development of γ-HCD and during follow-up are given in Tables 1 and 2. HevyLite measurements confirmed an IgMkappa paraprotein, and ratios of IgGkappa/IgGlambda were within the reference range, confirming increased IgG measurements were due to the IgG heavy chain (Table 5). The ratio of ((IgGkappa + IgGlambda)/total IgG) was 0.096.

The serum-free light chain ratio was elevated secondary to the presence of IgMkappa paraprotein (Table 4). Her total IgG levels were increased at 35.1 g/L, at diagnosis of γ-HCD, with suppressed IgA and an IgMkappa paraprotein of 10.7 g/L (Tables 1 and 2). IgG1 subtype was elevated, and other IgG subtypes were either decreased or at the lower reference range (Table 3). She is currently under observation for ibrutinib treatment.

Her bone marrow results are shown in Figures 7(a) and 7(b) and in the Supplementary Material (available here). Lymphoma cells were CD5−, CD20+, and partially CD79a +, CD10+, CD23+, CD56+, and CD138+. A second CD56+ plasma cell clone most likely to be the γ-heavy chain producer was identified. Bone marrow histology identified lymphoplasmacytic lymphoma/WM, which appeared as IgM/kappa plus another population of scattered plasma cells, occasionally expressing IgG and/or lambda.

3. Discussion

Heavy chain diseases are rare B-cell lymphoproliferative disorders that are characterised by the production of immunoglobulin heavy chains without associated light chains. γ-HCD has a variety of clinical presentations. The Mayo Clinic reported a series of 23 patients of whom 70% had an underlying lymphoplasma cell proliferative disorder, 13% an autoimmune disorder, and 4% no underlying disease. Pathological diagnosis of underlying disease reported in the 23 patients was lymphoplasma cell proliferative disorder, lymphoma, chronic lymphocytic leukemia, plasmacytoma, and plasma cell proliferative disorder. The disease was associated with lymphadenopathy (34%), hepatomegaly (4%), splenomegaly (30%), or bone marrow involvement (30%). The median survival of the 23 patients was 7.4 years (range 1 month to more than 21 years) [7]. In a further series of 13 patients, 8 patients showed a lymphoplasmacytic neoplasm that was difficult to classify. In the remaining 5 patients, biopsy identified well-defined neoplasms: splenic diffuse red pulp and small B-cell lymphoma, splenic marginal zone lymphoma, MALT lymphoma, lymphoplasmacytic lymphoma/WM, and chronic NK cell lymphocytosis. In the 13 cases, the study reported the

Table 1: Hematology and biochemistry results.

Date	Hb, g/L (RR 115–164)	WBC, 10^9/L (4–11)	Platelet, 10^9/L (150–400)	Neutrophils, 10^9/L (2–7.5)	Creatinine, μmol/L (RR 44–80)	Calcium, mmol/L (RR 2.2–2.6)
Case 1						
At diagnosis	115	2.5	100	1.6	46	2.41
3 months following diagnosis	116	2.8	101	2.1	61	2.33
Case 2						
Postcladribine at time 0 days	120	5.0	239	3.1	71	
At 10-year follow-up and treatment	89	3.4	133	2.0	65	2.41

Case 2: records date back to time = 0 after chemotherapy.

Table 2: Monoclonal protein studies.

Date	Total protein, g/L (RR 60–80)	Albumin, g/L (RR 35–50)	Monoclonal band 1, g/L	Monoclonal band 2, g/L	IgG, g/L (RR 7–16)	IgA, g/L (RR 0.7–4.0)	IgM (RR 0.4–2.3)
Case 1							
At diagnosis	60	33	2.8 (type: γ-heavy chain in the alpha region)	18.5 (γ-heavy chain in the beta region)	38.7	0.19	0.26
3 months following diagnosis	63	33	3.21	21.17	39.7	0.15	0.24
Case 2							
At time 0	78	39	11.0 (IgMK)		11.6	0.8	
At 10-year follow-up, after several treatments	76	40	10.7 (IgMK)	17.8 (γ-heavy chain)	35.1	0.06	

Case 2: records on the patient date back to time = 0 after chemotherapy.

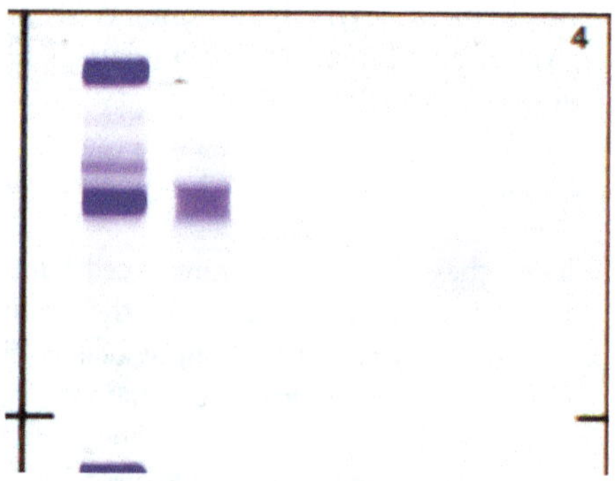

(a)

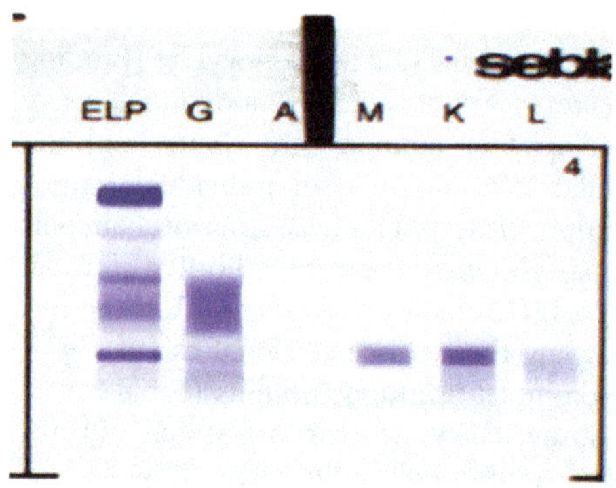

(b)

Figure 1: Serum electrophoresis and immunofixation. (a) Case 1: immunofixation shows staining in the gamma region, without a corresponding stain in the light chain region. Two bands are detected in the gamma region, a major and a second minor band. (b) Case 2: immunofixation shows a broad stain in the alpha-beta region, without a corresponding region in the light chain. Immunofixation further identifies an IgMkappa paraprotein. ELP = protein electrophoresis; G: immunofixation with anti-gamma chain; identifying gamma heavy chain; A: anti-alpha chain immunofixation; M: anti-mu chain immunofixation; K: anti-kappa chain immunofixation; L: anti-lambda chain immunofixation.

involvement of the lymph nodes (n = 7), spleen (n = 2), bone marrow (n = 8), and other extranodal tissues (n = 3). Patients showed a female predominance (85%) with frequent occurrence of autoimmune disease (69%) [8]. Iijima et al. [9] report a case γ-HCD and T-cell large granular lymphocytic leukemia. γ-HCD can exist in the absence of clinical symptoms similar to other forms of monoclonal gammopathy of undefined significance (MGUS) [10].

In our patients, two methods, capillary zone electrophoresis and gel electrophoresis, identified a gamma heavy chain with no corresponding light chain. Results from this report and previous reports [11] suggest that capillary zone

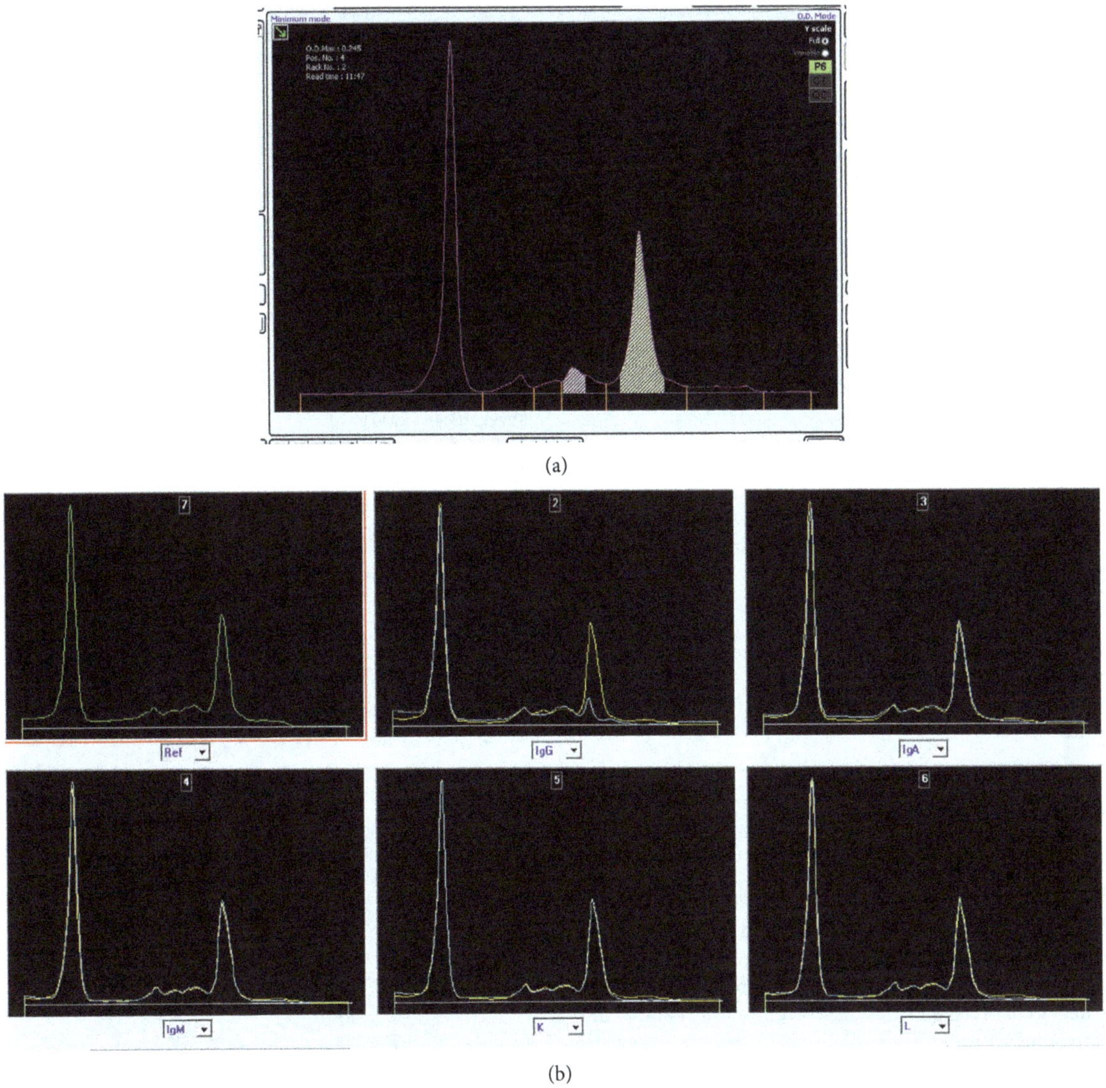

Figure 2: Capillary zone electrophoresis and immunotyping of Case 1. (a) Capillary zone electrophoresis showing a peak in the beta1 region and a minor peak in the alpha region. (b) Immunotyping showing a subtraction by the anti-IgG antibody, without a corresponding region in the light chain region, identifying a gamma chain peak. Ref: protein electrophoresis. IgG: immunosubtraction with anti-IgG antibody; IgA: immunosubtraction with anti-IgA antibody; IgM: immunosubtraction with anti-IgM antibody; K: immunosubtraction with anti-kappa antibody; L: immunosubtraction with anti-lambda antibody.

electrophoresis and immunotyping are able to detect and characterise γ-HCD in serum. γ-Heavy chain was identified in the urine of both patients, suggesting that the lower-molecular weight of the truncated heavy chain allowed renal clearance. In a modification of the immunofixation method, Gulli et al. [12] preincubated patient sera with anti-kappa and anti-lambda to precipitate intact immunoglobulins, except for free heavy chain, prior to immunofixation.

The intact IgGkappa/IgGlambda (HevyLite) measurement confirmed the presence of gamma heavy chain in the absence of associated kappa or lambda light chains. In a previous study, HevyLite assays showed that in 10/15 patients, substantial portions of IgG were not quantitated by antibodies to intact IgGkappa and IgGlambda immunoglobulins [6].

Serum IgG subtypes showed an increase in IgG1 subclass in both patients. In a previous report, serum IgG measured by nephelometry on the Beckman Coulter Immage analyser was below the reference range in a patient with γ-HCD [11]. Total IgG and IgG1 subclasses measured using the binding site reagent were increased in our patients. This has been previously illustrated by other groups [13]. The discrepant values observed between case reports can be the result of differences in analytical techniques, loss of antigenic domains due to truncation of the heavy chains, or analytical variation due to different detection antibody specificities.

There have been several advances in the diagnosis of multiple myeloma. New techniques may further enhance the diagnosis of γ-HCD. Capillary electrophoresis with immunotyping is able to characterise free heavy chains in serum, demonstrating the absence of intact IgG immunoglobulins by the HevyLite assay and the absence of serum-free light chains by serum-free light analysis are further valuable tools for

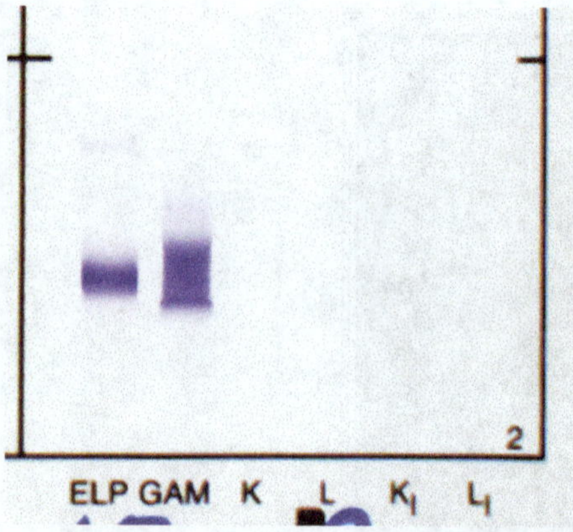

(a)

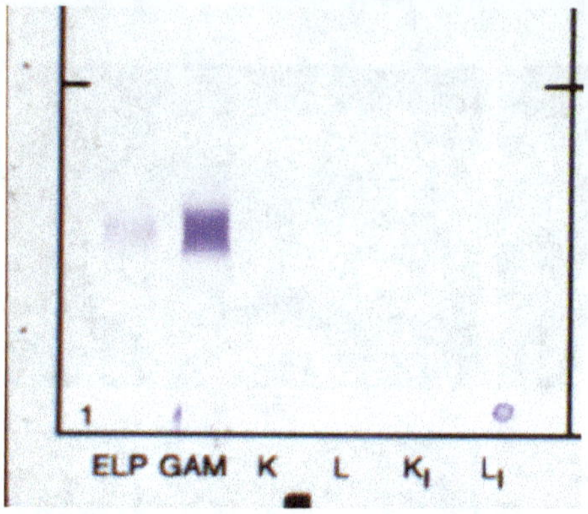

(b)

FIGURE 3: Urine electrophoresis and immunofixation. (a) Case 1: urine electrophoresis revealing a broad band and a minor band in the heavy chain region, without a corresponding band in the light chain region. (b) Case 2: urine electrophoresis revealing a broad band in the heavy chain region without a corresponding band in the light chain region. A further kappa light chain band is observed, corresponding to the IgMkappa band identified in the serum. ELP: reference track showing sample proteins; GAM: trivalent antiserum against gamma, alpha, and mu heavy chains; K and L: antisera against bound kappa and lambda light chains; K_I and L_I: antisera against free kappa and free lambda light chains.

TABLE 3: IgG subclasses.

	Case 1	Case 2
IgG1 (RR 3.8–9.29 g/L)	18.62	27.16
IgG2 (RR 2.42–7.0 g/L)	0.26	2.92
IgG3 (RR 0.22–1.76 g/L)	0.41	0.17
IgG4 (0.04–0.86 g/L)	<0.03	0.12

diagnosis. Serum/urine electrophoresis and immunofixation are analytical tools in the workup of γ-HCD patients.

Alpha (α), γ, and mu (μ) heavy chain diseases have been described. α-HCD, the most common of heavy chain diseases, appears to be a condition affecting primarily the secretory IgA system and mainly the digestive tract. α-HCD may present as a continuous sequence of events from an apparently reversible hyperplastic process to an overt neoplastic proliferation [14]. μ-HCD is the least common of the heavy chain diseases. Patients present with lymphoplasma cell proliferative disorder,

TABLE 4: Serum-free light chains.

Light chain type	Case 1	Case 2 (at time 0)
Kappa (3.3–19.4 mg/L)	18.47	33.94
Lambda 16.60 mg/L (5.7–26.3 mg/L)	16.8	18.77
Kappa/lambda ratio (0.26–1.65)	1.113	1.808

TABLE 5: HevyLite protein studies.

Heavy chain type	Case 1	Case 2
IgGkappa (3.84–12.07 g/L)	0.99	1.92
IgGlambda (1.91–6.74 g/L)	0.54	1.45
IgG K/L ratio (1.12–3.21)	1.83	1.32
IgA K (0.57–2.08 g/L)	0.23	<0.02
IgAL (0.44–2.04 g/L)	0.12	0.03
IgA K/L ratio (0.78–1.94)	1.92	Not available
IgMK = 0.27 g/L (0.19–1.63 g/L)	0.27	11.92
IgML = 0.04 g/L (0.12–1.01 g/L)	0.04	0.14
IgM K/L (1.18–2.74)	6.75	85.1

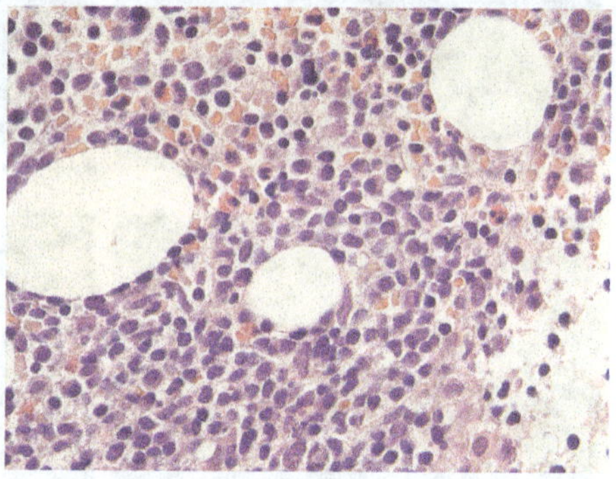

(a)

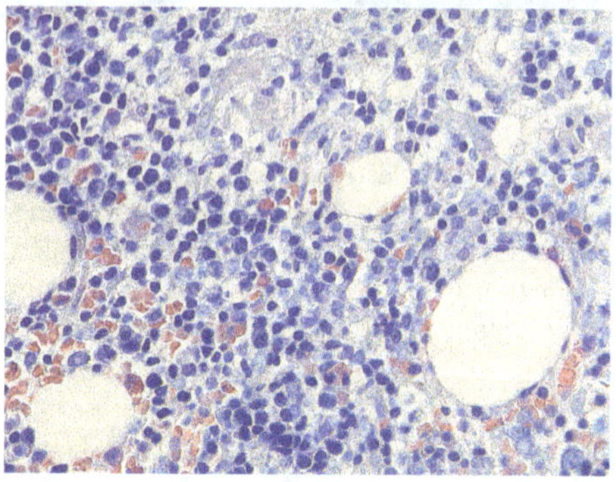

(b)

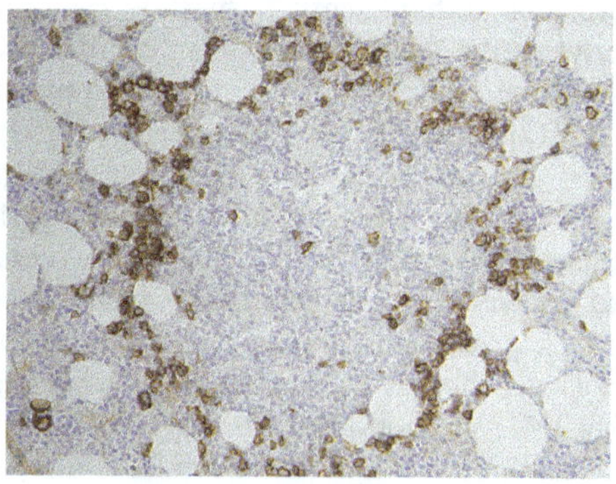

(c)

FIGURE 4: Continued.

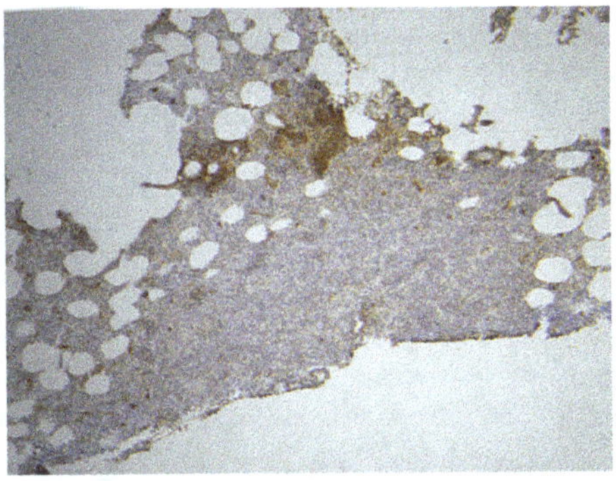

(d)

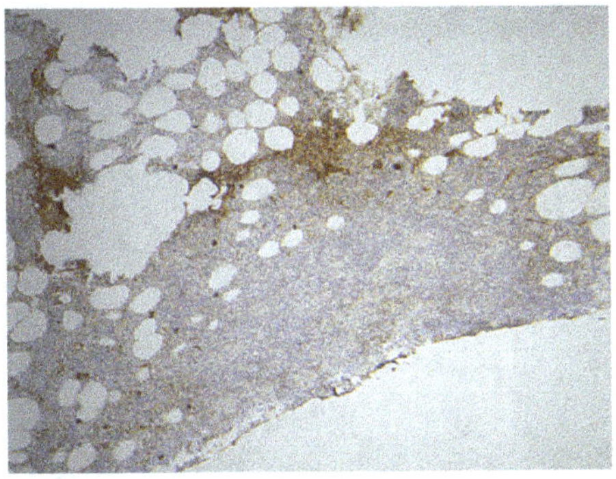

(e)

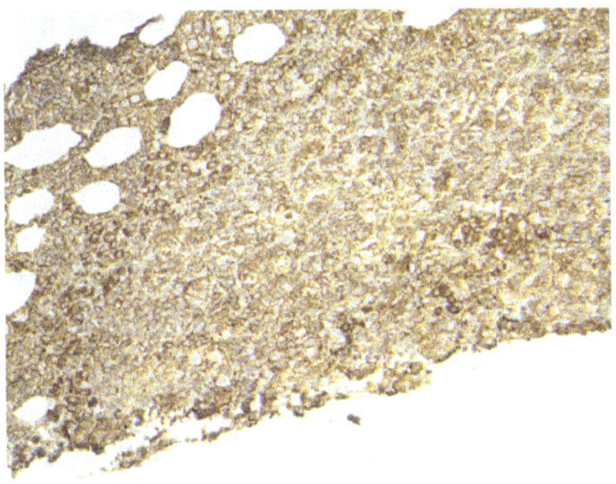

(f)

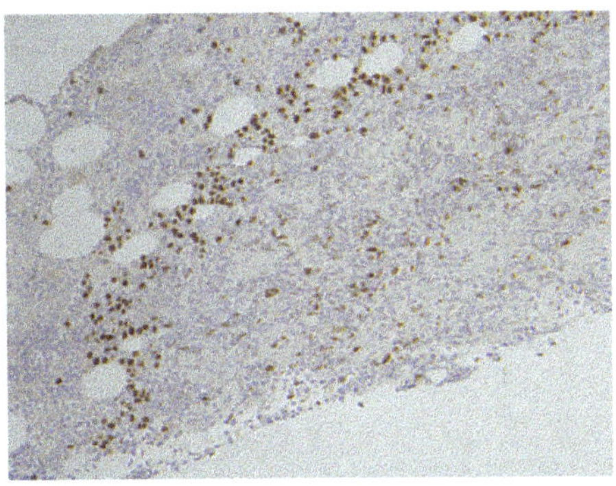

(g)

FIGURE 4: Bone marrow stain of Case 1. (a) Giemsa stain. (b) Small lymphocytes and scattered unusually small plasma cells. (c) CD138: plasma cells forming a characteristic corona around a lymphoid nodule. (d) Lambda stain—hardly any positive cells around the lymphoid nodule. (e) Kappa stain—hardly any positive cells around the lymphoid nodule. (f) IgG stain—a rim of strongly staining plasma cells. (g) Same area stained with MUM1 marker. Stains show there are IgG(+), kappa(−) and lambda (−) cells.

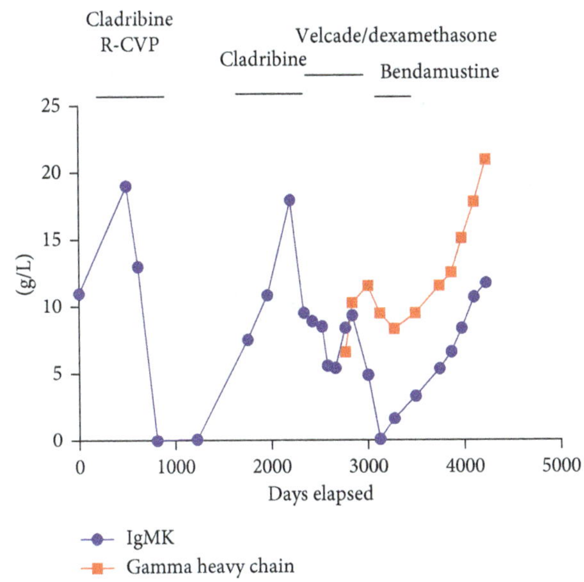

FIGURE 5: Paraprotein levels of Case 2 during treatment. Hospital records for the patient date back to time = 0 after chemotherapy. R-CVP = rituximab with cyclophosphamide, vincristine, and prednisolone.

and index of suspicion is high in patients with vacuolated plasma cells in the bone marrow [3].

The mechanism for the pathogenesis of γ-HCD is unclear. Bone marrow histology of the first patient with isolated γ-HCD suggested the presence of a clonal plasma cell which selectively secreted γ-heavy chain in the absence of kappa or lambda light chain. Genomic events that underlie the progression of MGUS to MM have been difficult to dissect. Both bone marrow microenvironment and genomic instability play a role in MM pathogenesis. Bone marrow biopsy in the second patient, with WM and γ-HCD, identified two possible malignant clones. It is worth noting that this patient's treatment included R-CVP, cladribine, and velcade. It is plausible that the treatment might have increased the transformation of the γ-HCD clone by increasing the instability of the MM cells. Clonal evolution in MM before and after therapy can follow several patterns. Branching clonal evolution involves one or more subclones that emerge at a later time point. Current therapeutic approaches have shortcomings, and understanding of MM tumorogenesis and progression may have implications for genomically guided precision treatment [15].

4. Conclusions

In summary, we report two cases of γ-HCD. The findings also provide information for practical guidance for the laboratory evaluation of γ-HCD. In the first case, γ-HCD developed as the presenting lymphoid malignancy. Bone marrow biopsy revealed an IgG heavy chain secreting clone. The second case was a composite lymphoid neoplasm of WM and γ-HCD. γ-HCD developed during treatment for WM. Bone marrow biopsy revealed the presence of two neoplastic lymphoid cell lines. The review of the literature

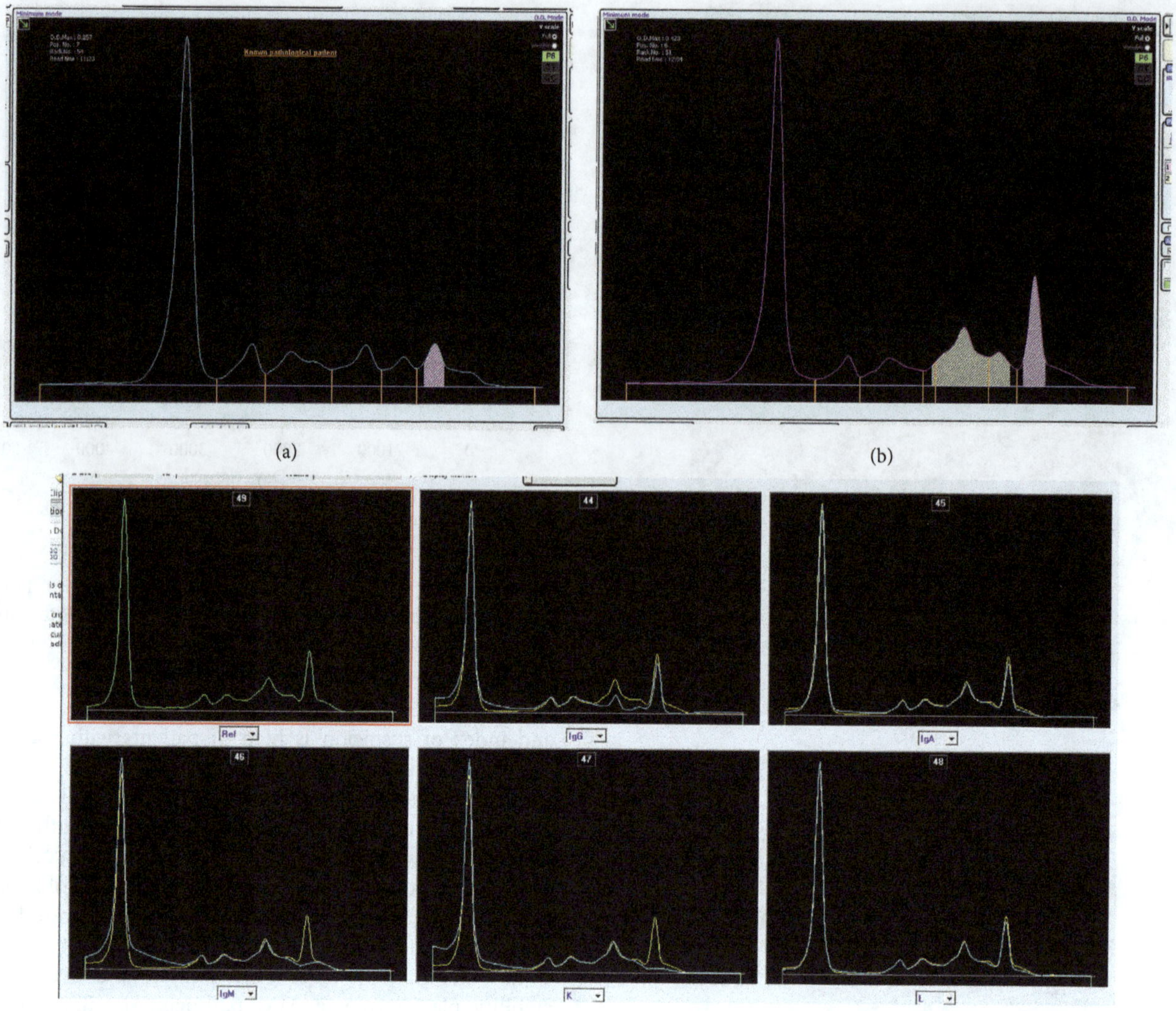

(a) (b) (c)

Figure 6: Capillary zone electrophoresis and immunotyping of Case 2. (a) Capillary zone electrophoresis prior to the appearance of the gamma heavy chain. A peak identified as the IgMkappa protein is detected in the gamma region. (b) Capillary zone electrophoresis identifies a broad peak in the beta region, identified as gamma heavy chain by immunotyping. (c) Immunotyping identifies a gamma heavy chain without a corresponding light chain and an IgMkappa paraprotein.

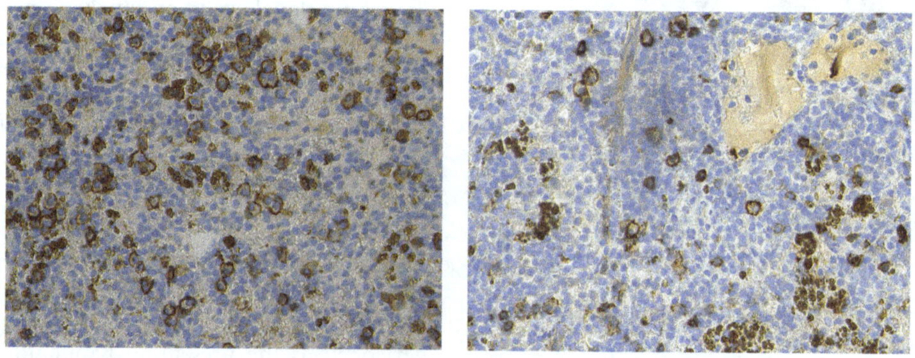

(a) (b)

Figure 7: Bone marrow stain of Case 2. (a) CD138 highlights plasma cells—here admixed with lymphocytes (which are CD138 negative). Note also granular golden-brown haemosiderin deposits. (b) CD56—some plasma cells are positive; this is an interesting finding, as plasma cells of lymphoplasmacytic lymphoma usually do not express this marker. It indirectly suggests that the "other clone" may be more of plasma cell myeloma-like (myeloma-like MGUS). Haemosiderin which is naturally yellow/brown is present as well.

suggests further studies are indicated to develop an understanding of the clonal evolution of γ-HCD.

Conflicts of Interest

The authors declare that they have no conflicts of interest.

References

[1] T. Goossens, U. Klein, and R. Küppers, "Frequent occurrence of deletions and duplications during somatic hypermutation: implications for oncogene translocations and heavy chain disease," *Proceedings of the National Academy of Sciences*, vol. 95, no. 5, pp. 2463–2468, 1998.

[2] A. Alexander, I. Anicito, and J. Buxbaum, "Gamma heavy chain disease in man. Genomic sequence reveals two noncontiguous deletions in a single gene," *Journal of Clinical Investigation*, vol. 82, no. 4, pp. 1244–1252, 1988.

[3] D. L. Wahner-Roedler and R. A. Kyle, "Heavy chain diseases," *Best Practice and Research Clinical Haematology*, vol. 18, no. 4, pp. 729–746, 2005.

[4] J. R. Sawyer, "The prognostic significance of cytogenetics and molecular profiling in multiple myeloma," *Cancer Genetics*, vol. 204, no. 1, pp. 3–12, 2011.

[5] C. Jiménez, M. Jara-Acevedo, L. A. Corchete et al., "A next-generation sequencing strategy for evaluating the most common genetic abnormalities in multiple myeloma," *Journal of Molecular Diagnostics*, vol. 19, no. 1, pp. 99–106, 2017.

[6] E. Kaleta, R. Kyle, R. Clark, and J. Katzmann, "Analysis of patients with γ-heavy chain disease by the heavy/light chain and free light chain assays," *Clinical Chemistry and Laboratory Medicine*, vol. 52, no. 5, pp. 665–669, 2014.

[7] D. L. Wahner-Roedler, T. E. Witzig, L. L. Loehrer, and R. A. Kyle, "Gamma-heavy chain disease: review of 23 cases," *Medicine*, vol. 82, no. 4, pp. 236–250, 2003.

[8] S. Bieliauskas, R. R. Tubbs, C. M. Bacon et al., "Gamma heavy-chain disease: defining the spectrum of associated lymphoproliferative disorders through analysis of 13 cases," *American Journal of Surgical Pathology*, vol. 36, no. 4, pp. 534–543, 2012.

[9] M. Iijima, N. Sekiguchi, A. Nagat et al., "Gamma heavy chain disease with T-cell large granular lymphocytic leukemia: a case report and review of the literature," *Internal Medicine*, vol. 55, no. 4, pp. 399–403, 2016.

[10] J. Van Keer, B. Meijers, M. Delforge, G. Verhoef, and K. Poesen, "Two cases of heavy chain MGUS," *Case Reports in Oncological Medicine*, vol. 2016, Article ID 8749153, 4 pages, 2016.

[11] P. Luraschi, "Heavy chain disease can be detected by capillary zone electrophoresis," *Clinical Chemistry*, vol. 51, no. 1, pp. 247–249, 2005.

[12] F. Gulli, C. Napodano, K. Pocino, A. Cuccaro, S. Hohaus, and U. Basile, "Heavy chain disease: our experience," *Clinical Chemistry and Laboratory Medicine*, vol. 56, no. 1, pp. e10–e12, 2017.

[13] W. Johannis, J. Blommer, A. R. Klatt, J. H. Renno, and K. Wielckens, "Gamma heavy chain disease in a patient with rheumatoid arthritis—a laboratory evaluation," *Biochemia Medica*, vol. 22, pp. 373–379, 2012.

[14] M. Seligmann, "Alpha-chain disease," *Journal of Clinical Pathology*, vol. 1–6, no. 1, pp. 72–76, 1975.

[15] N. J. Bahlis, "Darwinian evolution and tiding clones in multiple myeloma," *Blood*, vol. 120, no. 5, pp. 927-928, 2012.

Bradycardia during Induction Therapy with All-*trans* Retinoic Acid in Patients with Acute Promyelocytic Leukemia

Pin-Zi Chen, Yee-Jen Wu, Chien-Chih Wu, and Yu-Wen Wang

Department of Pharmacy, National Taiwan University Hospital, College of Medicine, National Taiwan University, 7 Chung Shan S. Rd., Taipei, Taiwan

Correspondence should be addressed to Yu-Wen Wang; enjoymyway@gmail.com

Academic Editor: Akimichi Ohsaka

A 41-year-old man with newly diagnosed acute promyelocytic leukemia (APL) received induction chemotherapy, containing all-*trans* retinoic acid (ATRA), idarubicin, and arsenic trioxide. On the 11th day of therapy, he experienced complete atrioventricular (AV) block; therefore, ATRA and arsenic trioxide were immediately postponed. His heart rate partially recovered, and ATRA was rechallenged with a half dose. However, complete AV block as well as differentiation syndrome recurred on the next day. ATRA was immediately discontinued, and a temporary pacemaker was inserted. Two days after discontinuing ATRA, AV block gradually improved, and ATRA was uneventfully rechallenged again. The Naranjo adverse drug reaction probability scale was 7 for ATRA, suggesting it was the probable cause of arrhythmia. A literature search identified 6 other cases of bradycardia during ATRA therapy, and all of them occurred during APL induction therapy, with onset ranging from 4 days to 25 days. Therefore, monitoring vital signs and performing electrocardiogram are highly recommended during the first month of induction therapy with ATRA. ATRA should be discontinued if complete AV block occurs. Rechallenging with ATRA can be considered in fully recovered and clinically stable patients.

1. Introduction

Acute promyelocytic leukemia (APL) is a subtype of acute myeloid leukemia (AML) with distinct morphology, clinical presentation, and cytogenetics. It is characterized by accumulation of abnormal promyelocytes in the bone marrow, potentially fatal coagulopathy, and translocation between chromosomes 15 and 17 [*t*(15;17)] [1, 2].

t(15;17) leads to the promyelocytic leukemia and retinoic receptor-α fusion gene (PML-RARα), which blocks the differentiation of myeloid cells at the promyelocytic stage. All-*trans* retinoic acid (ATRA or tretinoin) induces a configuration change of PML-RARα or its degradation. As a result of this treatment, abnormal promyelocytes can differentiate into mature myeloid cells, and coagulopathy is significantly reduced [1]. When ATRA combines with anthracycline-based chemotherapy, the complete remission rate is 90%–95%. Therefore, this approach is the standard induction therapy for newly diagnosed APL [1–3].

Arsenic trioxide (ATO) also promotes differentiation of APL cells by targeting the PML moiety and can be used as a synergistic therapy with ATRA [1, 4]. However, rapid differentiation of promyelocytes induced by ATRA or ATO may lead to leukocytosis and differentiation syndrome (DS), especially in patients with an initial white blood cell (WBC) count greater than 10,000/mm^3. DS is characterized by fever, dyspnea, respiratory distress, pulmonary infiltrates, and pleural or pericardial effusions. This condition is potentially life-threatening; therefore, when DS is suspected, it is crucial to immediately initiate high-dose steroid treatment and temporarily discontinue ATRA and/or ATO in severe DS [2, 5, 6]. Concurrent use of anthracycline-based chemotherapy can decrease the incidence of DS [1, 5, 6].

Other common adverse effects of ATRA include headache, dry skin, xerostomia, bone pain, and nausea [7]. Cardiovascular toxicities, such as arrhythmia, have rarely been reported and are often overlooked by clinical practitioners [8]. Here we report the clinical course of a patient with APL suffering from complete atrioventricular (AV) block during induction therapy with an ATRA-based regimen. Moreover, a literature review was conducted to summarize the clinical characteristics of ATRA-associated arrhythmia.

2. Case Report

A 41-year-old man without any underlying diseases such as cardiovascular disease was hospitalized for spontaneous gum bleeding, epistaxis, and lower limb ecchymosis. Laboratory data on the admission date showed leukocytosis (WBC, 15,820/mm^3; promyelocyte, 66%, with Auer rod), anemia (Hb, 9.5 g/dL), thrombocytopenia (PLT, 22,000/mm^3), and abnormal coagulation profile (fibrinogen, 29 mg/dL; fibrin degradation product (FDP), 68.5 mcg/mL; d-dimer, 19.81 mcg/mL; prothrombin time (PT), 20.5 sec; international normalized ratio (INR), 1.92; partial thromboplastin time (PTT), 29 sec). Other laboratory data were as follows: C-reactive protein (CRP), 8.97 mg/dL; total bilirubin (T-bil), 0.73 mg/dL; aspartate aminotransferase (AST), 60 U/L; alanine transferase (ALT), 100 U/L; and serum creatinine (Scr), 0.9 mg/dL. His baseline electrocardiogram (ECG) was normal (Figure 1(a)). Bone marrow aspiration and biopsy disclosed APL with PML-RARα. ATRA at a dose of 45 mg/m^2/day (40 mg twice daily) was administered. On the third day of therapy, oxygen saturation abruptly dropped to 90% without oxygen supplementation. Chest X-ray (CXR), ECG, and echocardiography did not show any abnormalities. In order to prevent DS, intravenous methylprednisolone was administered at a daily dose of 80 mg–120 mg according to the clinical signs and symptoms. Idarubicin (12 mg/m^2/dose) was administered starting on the fourth day for four doses. WBC progressively elevated to 46,830/mm^3; therefore, 1000 mg hydroxyurea twice daily was also added starting on the seventh day.

On the 11th day of therapy, WBC and promyelocyte decreased to 6,310/mm^3 and 14%, respectively. ATO infusion at a dose of 0.15 mg/kg was initiated; however, dizziness and chest pain occurred during infusion. ECG showed complete AV block with a heart rate (HR) of 40–50 beats/min (bpm) (Figure 1(b)). The electrolytes and liver function tests were all within normal limits (Na, 138 mmol/L; K, 4.6 mmol/L; Ca, 2.29 mmol/L; Mg, 0.95 mmol/L; T-bil, 0.77 mg/dL; AST, 15 U/L; ALT, 14 U/L). Thus, ATO and ATRA were immediately discontinued, and aminophylline was administered.

After interruption of ATRA for three doses, complete AV block persisted, but his HR partially recovered to 60 bpm. ATRA was rechallenged with 40 mg once daily on the 13th day of therapy under relatively stable vital signs. On the following morning, his HR decreased to 30 bpm and he required a nonrebreathing mask to maintain oxygen saturation. CXR showed bilateral pulmonary edema, and echocardiogram revealed a large amount of pericardial effusion with signs of cardiac tamponade. In addition, ECG showed complete AV block with QRS widening, and acute renal failure also occurred (Scr, 1.4 mg/dL; blood urea nitrogen (BUN), 45.2 mg/dL; Na, 133 mmol/L; K, 5.2 mmol/L; Ca, 2.22 mmol/L; Mg, 0.93 mmol/L; P, 4.9 mg/dL; T-bil, 1.22 mg/dL; ALT, 17 U/L). Therefore, ARTA was immediately postponed, and a temporary pacemaker was inserted. Steroid treatment was switched to dexamethasone (8 mg twice daily) because of suspected DS. Pericardiocentesis and thoracentesis were performed. Two days after stopping ATRA, ECG showed sinus bradycardia with a first-degree AV block and diffuse ST elevation. The Naranjo adverse drug reaction probability scale [9] indicated a score of 7 for ATRA, suggesting it was the probable cause of arrhythmia in this episode.

The PML-RARα mutant was still detected using polymerase chain reaction (PCR) of blood sampled on the 19th day of therapy. Consequently, ATRA was resumed the following day with 10 mg twice daily. His HR decreased from 70–90 bpm to 60–70 bpm with stable vital signs. ECG demonstrated sinus rhythm with first-degree AV block. The dose of ATRA was gradually titrated up to 30 mg twice daily on the 24th day. Sinus tachycardia with occasional premature ventricular complexes was noted. The pacemaker was removed on the 27th day. During follow-up, ECG showed normal sinus rhythm (Figure 1(c)), and echocardiogram revealed minimal pericardial effusion.

Complete molecular remission was documented by bone marrow aspiration done on the 38th day of therapy using flow cytometry and PCR for PML-RARα. Thereafter, the patient received three cycles of consolidation with ATRA-based chemotherapy. No further bradycardia episode was reported. The patient has been free of leukemia for 1.5 years after the diagnosis.

3. Discussion

The major etiologies of AV block include ischemic heart disease, cardiomyopathy, hyperkalemia, hypothyroidism or hyperthyroidism, and medications. This 41-year-old man did not have any underlying disease, and his baseline CXR, ECG, and echocardiography did not show any abnormalities. The serum potassium level was normal during the first-episode of complete AV block, and it was only mildly elevated and was corrected soon during the second episode of complete AV block. Although idarubicin and ATO have also been reported to cause arrhythmia in the literature, the second arrhythmia episode in this patient recurred only after ATRA rechallenge. Accordingly, ATRA was the most likely culprit drug for this adverse event.

The most common adverse effects of ATRA are headache, dry skin, xerostomia, bone pain, and nausea [7]. Arrhythmia is rarely reported. Therefore, we reported a case of this rare adverse reaction of ATRA and reviewed the literature for other cases. We searched literature reports on PubMed by using the following keywords: ("tretinoin" or "all-*trans* retinoic acid" or "ATRA") and ("bradycardia" or "tachycardia" or "arrhythmia"). Six other cases of bradycardia during ATRA induction therapy were found and summarized, along with the case reported here, in Table 1 [10–15].

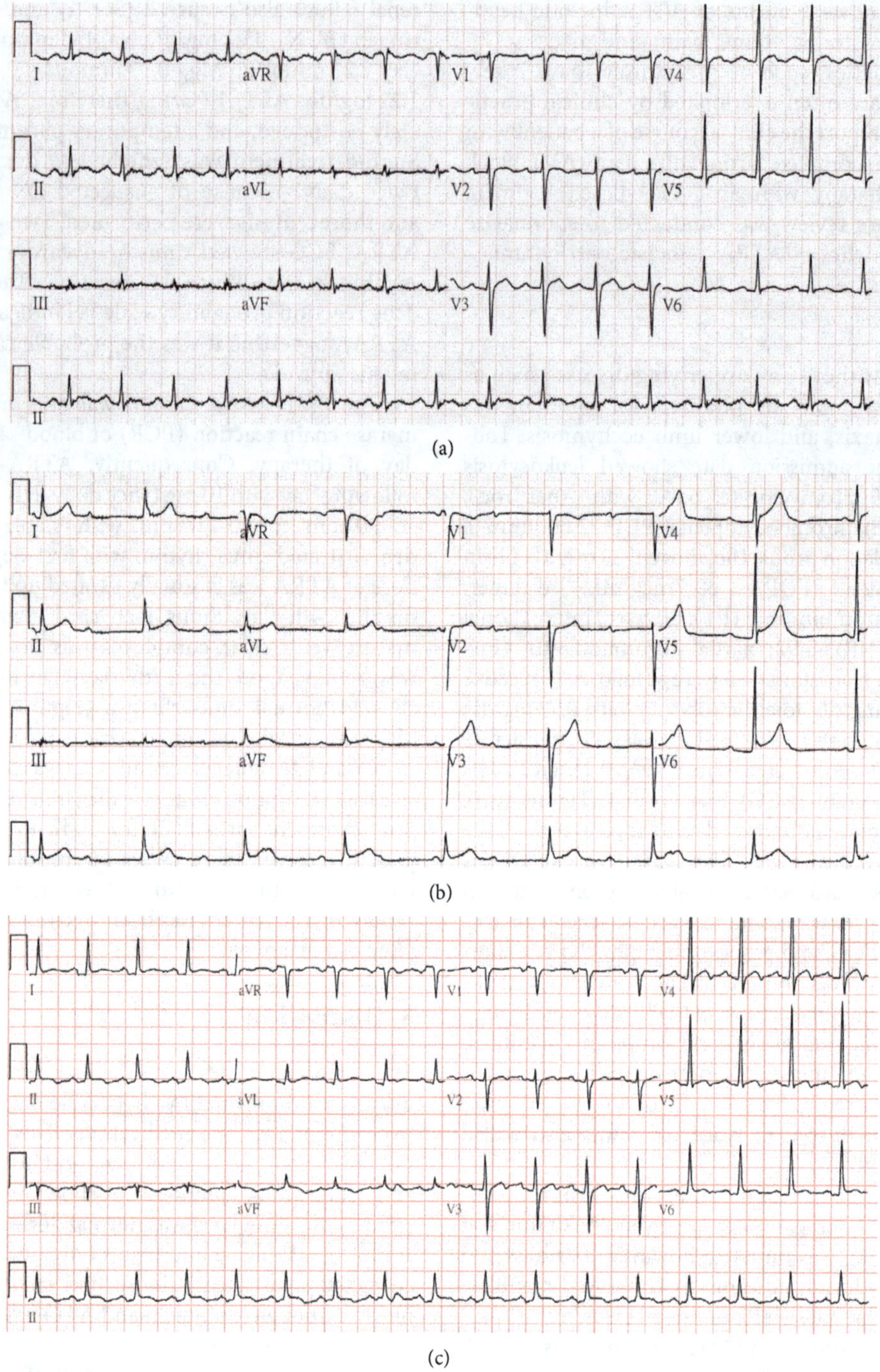

FIGURE 1: Serial electrocardiogram changes. (a) Normal sinus rhythm before the induction therapy (PR interval 206 ms, QTc 429 ms). (b) The 11th day of therapy, showing complete AV block (PR interval > 400 ms, QTc 395 ms). (c) Restoration of normal sinus rhythm after pacemaker removal (PR interval 192 ms, QTc 353 ms).

Median onset of bradycardia among the seven patients was 9 days (4–25 days). ECG abnormalities consisted of AV block, sinus bradycardia, and junctional bradycardia [10–15]. Arrhythmia resolved in two patients without interruption of ATRA [12, 14]. Sinus rhythm was restored in another four cases within 3–15 days after discontinuing ATRA [11, 13, 15]. Three of them required temporary pacemaker support [11, 15], and ATRA was rechallenged in two of them [15]. Interestingly, all of the incidents reported in the seven cases occurred during the induction therapy. Among the four cases with available information, three of them also experienced DS [12, 13].

The underlying mechanism of ATRA-related bradycardia has not been comprehensively studied. In 1995, Kang and Leaf demonstrated that ATRA significantly lowered the beating rate of cardiomyocytes and reduced the incidence and severity of ventricular tachyarrhythmia induced by isoproterenol in rats [16]. The inhibition of excitability may

TABLE 1: Case reports of all-*trans* retinoic acid-associated bradycardia.

	Age	Sex	Initial WBC (mm^3)	Indication of ATRA	ATRA dose (mg/m^2)	Concurrent chemotherapy	Onset (days)	ECG change	Pacemaker	Response after discontinuation of ATRA	Response after rechallenge	DS
Maruhashi et al. [10]	3	M	NA	Induction	45	NA	4	Sinus bradycardia	NA	Still arrhythmia	Arrhythmia augmented	NA
Yamauchi et al. [11]	46	M	NA	Induction	45	Enocitabine Mitoxantrone	25	CAVB	TPM	NSR after 15 days	NA	NA
Dhar and Barman [12]	16	F	2,000	Induction	45	NA	9	2nd degree AVB	No	ATRA was continued and steroid was given→NSR		Yes
McGregor et al. [13]	28	F	9,800	Induction	45→22.5	Idarubicin	5	Junctional bradycardia	No	NSR after 3 days	No more bradycardia	Yes
Karakatsanis et al. [14]	64	M	NA	Induction	NA	Idarubicin	8	Sinus bradycardia	No	ATRA was continued and bradycardia resolved spontaneously		NA
Shih and Wu [15]	57	M	1,600	Induction	45	NA	15	CAVB	TPM	Sinus rhythm after 4 days (under TPM)	75% dose→still AVB	No
This case	41	M	15,820	Induction	45	Idarubicin ATO	11	CAVB	TPM	HR partially recovered after interruption for 3 doses	50% dose→ CAVB with DS→hold ATRA, insert TPM→1st degree AVB→25% dose→bradycardia→75% dose→NSR	Yes

ATO: arsenic trioxide; ATRA: all-*trans* retinoic acid; AVB: atrioventricular block; CAVB: complete atrioventricular block; DS: differentiation syndrome; ECG: electrocardiogram; F: female; HR: heart rate; M: male; NA: not available; NSR: normal sinus rhythm; TPM: temporary pacemaker; WBC: white blood cell.

be mediated by the effect of ATRA on membrane ion channels, and this may result in conduction disturbance of the AV node [16]. Further studies are needed to elucidate the effect of ATRA on the AV node.

Another possible explanation of ATRA-related arrhythmia was leukemic cell infiltration in the myocardium. Second-degree AV block and pericardial effusion in a case with AML was reported by Hatake et al. On autopsy, focal leukemic cell infiltration in the His bundle was noted [17]. Therefore, eradication of leukemic cell could ameliorate the cardiac symptoms as reported in another case described by Civelek et al., wherein complete AV block spontaneously subsided after chemotherapy [18]. In reviewing the cases of ATRA-related arrhythmia, sinus bradycardia reported by Karakatsanis et al. also spontaneously subsided after chemotherapy without any specific intervention [14]. Moreover, all of the seven cardiac events occurred during induction chemotherapy course but not consolidation ones. These observations could possibly provide some evidence that the cardiac toxicity was partially caused by infiltration of leukemic cells in the myocardium.

As described above, APL patients receiving ATRA-based induction therapy may experience DS, which is characterized by fever, dyspnea, respiratory distress, pulmonary infiltrates, and pleural or pericardial effusions [5, 6]. The proposed pathophysiology involves tissue infiltration of APL cells. Besides infiltration of leukemic cells, ATRA also stimulates the production of chemokines and further increases lung infiltration of differentiating APL cells. Changes in cytokine production also occur in the liver, spleen, and heart [5]. According to these mechanisms, DS may also interfere with AV node conduction and result in bradyarrhythmia. In reviewing the incidents of ATRA-related bradycardia, three of four cases with available information also experienced DS [12, 13]. In Dhar's report, second-degree AV block simultaneously occurred with DS, and after steroid use, these manifestations resolved at the same time [12]. In our case, the AV block was more severe when DS occurred. Without the presentation of the DS, only mild bradycardia occurred under ATRA use. Therefore, DS may further deteriorate ATRA-related AV node conducting dysfunction. This clinical presentation strengthens the theory that DS may result in cardiac arrhythmia, which needs further study to elucidate the observation.

In conclusion, this case and literature review indicated that ATRA may cause conduction dysfunction-related arrhythmia, and it should be used more cautiously for APL patients during induction chemotherapy, especially those suffering from DS. The onset of bradycardia was usually within 1 month after initiation of ATRA. Therefore, closely monitoring vital signs and performing ECG are highly recommended during the first month of ATRA-based induction therapy. ATRA should be promptly discontinued if complete AV block occurs. In severe cases, temporary pacemaker insertion is indicated. After discontinuing ATRA, bradycardia may resolve gradually within 3–15 days. Since ATRA is the cornerstone in APL treatment, rechallenge can be considered in fully recovered and clinically stable patients.

Conflicts of Interest

All the authors declared no potential conflicts of interest with respect to the research, authorship, and/or publication of this article.

References

[1] Z. Y. Wang and Z. Chen, "Acute promyelocytic leukemia: from highly fatal to highly curable," *Blood*, vol. 111, no. 5, pp. 2505–2515, 2008.

[2] Network NCC, *Acute Myeloid Leukemia Version 1*, 2016, https://www.nccn.org/professionals/physician_gls/PDF/aml.pdf.

[3] M. A. Sanz and F. Lo-Coco, "Modern approaches to treating acute promyelocytic leukemia," *Journal of Clinical Oncology*, vol. 29, no. 5, pp. 495–503, 2011.

[4] H. J. Iland, K. Bradstock, S. G. Supple et al., "All-trans-retinoic acid, idarubicin, and IV arsenic trioxide as initial therapy in acute promyelocytic leukemia (APML4)," *Blood*, vol. 120, no. 8, pp. 1570–1580, 2012.

[5] J. E. Rogers and D. Yang, "Differentiation syndrome in patients with acute promyelocytic leukemia," *Journal of Oncology Pharmacy Practice*, vol. 18, no. 1, pp. 109–114, 2012.

[6] M. A. Sanz and P. Montesinos, "How we prevent and treat differentiation syndrome in patients with acute promyelocytic leukemia," *Blood*, vol. 123, no. 18, pp. 2777–2782, 2014.

[7] J. DiPiro, R. L. Talbert, G. Yee, B. Wells, and L. M. Posey, "Acute leukemias," in *Pharmacotherapy: A Pathophysiologic Approach*, B. B. Poon and A. H. Seung, Eds., McGraw-Hill Medical, New York, NY, USA, 9th edition, 2014.

[8] V. B. Pai and M. C. Nahata, "Cardiotoxicity of chemotherapeutic agents: incidence, treatment and prevention," *Drug Safety*, vol. 22, no. 4, pp. 263–302, 2000.

[9] C. A. Naranjo, U. Busto, E. M. Sellers et al., "A method for estimating the probability of adverse drug reactions," *Clinical Pharmacology and Therapeutics*, vol. 30, no. 2, pp. 239–245, 1981.

[10] K. Maruhashi, H. Wada, M. Taniguchi, and S. Koizumi, "Sinus bradyarrhythmia during administration of all-trans retinoic acid in a patient with acute promyelocytic leukemia," *Rinsho Ketsueki*, vol. 37, pp. 443–447, 1996.

[11] T. Yamauchi, H. Arai, M. Taga, N. Amaya, J. D. Lee, and T. Ueda, "Adams-stokes attack due to complete atrioventricular block in a patient with acute promyelocytic leukemia during remission induction therapy using all-trans retinoic acid," *Rinsho Ketsueki*, vol. 46, pp. 206–210, 2005.

[12] A. K. Dhar and P. K. Barman, "Retinoic acid syndrome–cardiac complication," *Journal of the Association of Physicians of India*, vol. 60, pp. 63–65, 2012.

[13] A. McGregor, E. Hurst, S. Lord, and G. Jones, "Bradycardia following retinoic acid differentiation syndrome in a patient with acute promyelocytic leukaemia," *BMJ Case Reports*, vol. 2012, p. bcr0220125848, 2012.

[14] S. Karakatsanis, M. Vardaka, P. Giannoulia, J. Apostolidis, and S. Delimpasi, "Bradycardia during induction therapy with all-trans retinoic acid (ATRA)," *Journal of BUON*, vol. 19, p. 315, 2014.

[15] C. H. Shih and H. B. Wu, "All-trans retinoic acid-induced, life-threatening complete atrioventricular block," *Journal of the Chinese Medical Association*, vol. 78, no. 5, pp. 316–319, 2015.

[16] J. X. Kang and A. Leaf, "Protective effects of All-trans-retinoic acid against cardiac arrhythmias induced by isoproterenol, lysophosphatidylcholine or ischemia and reperfusion,"

Journal of Cardiovascular Pharmacology, vol. 26, no. 6, pp. 943–948, 1995.

[17] K. Hatake, K. Saito, T. Saga, N. Akashi, and K Doishita, "A case of acute myelogenous leukemia with advanced atrioventricular block and pericardial effusion caused by leukemic cell infiltration," *Japanese Journal of Medicine*, vol. 21, no. 2, pp. 115–119, 1982.

[18] A. C. Civelek, J. A. Brinker, E. E. Camargo, J. M. Links, and H. N. Wagner, "Rest thallium-201 myocardial perfusion imaging in a patient with leukaemic infiltration of the heart," *European Journal of Nuclear Medicine*, vol. 19, no. 4, pp. 306–308, 1992.

Morphological Transformation of Myeloma Cells into Multilobated Plasma Cell Nuclei within 7 Days in a Case of Secondary Plasma Cell Leukemia that Finally Transformed as Anaplastic Myeloma

Akihito Fujimi,[1] Yasuhiro Nagamachi,[1] Naofumi Yamauchi,[1] and Yuji Kanisawa[2]

[1]*Department of Hematology, Sapporo Kiyota Hospital, Sapporo, Japan*
[2]*Department of Hematology and Oncology, Oji General Hospital, Tomakomai, Japan*

Correspondence should be addressed to Akihito Fujimi; akihito.fujimi@gmail.com

Academic Editor: Marie-Christine Kyrtsonis

A 48-year-old man was diagnosed with multiple myeloma (IgG-k) and was treated with high-dose dexamethasone as an induction therapy followed by thalidomide-based regimens. Approximately 22 months after the initial diagnosis, the patient developed secondary plasma cell leukemia (PCL) with a white blood cell (WBC) count of 20.2×10^9/L including 79.5% plasma cells. A G-banding chromosomal analysis in the bone marrow showed an t(11;14) abnormality of up to 5%, which was not detected at initial diagnosis. We immediately started bortezomib and dexamethasone therapy, but in just 7 days, the WBC count elevated to 48.5×10^9/L, and approximately 95% of them were medium-sized atypical lymphoid cells with multilobated nuclei. Although we subsequently initiated alternative regimens, the patient's condition deteriorated, and he died 4 months after developing PCL. Approximately 2 months before his death, the diameter of myeloma cells in the bone marrow enlarged by approximately twofold, and pleomorphic nuclei were present, indicating an anaplastic myeloma transformation. Concurrently, a 100% increase of the t(11;14) clone frequency was observed in the G-banding-analyzed bone marrow cells. Morphological transformation of myeloma cells into multilobated plasma cell nuclei can be considered as the starting point of the sequential process leading to anaplastic myeloma.

1. Introduction

Anaplastic myeloma is an extremely rare, but distinct, subtype of myeloma with poorly differentiated, pleomorphic, and significantly enlarged plasma cells [1–3]. The prognosis of anaplastic myeloma is extremely poor, with a mean survival of less than 3.5 months [2]. Another morphological variation of multiple myeloma described as multiple myeloma with cleaved, convoluted, or multilobated plasma cell nuclei has also been reported previously [4–13], having been frequently associated with plasma cell leukemia (PCL) [4–8] and with poor prognosis as well [6–10]. To date, the correlation between anaplastic myeloma and other morphological types of multiple myeloma has not been reported. Here, we present a case of secondary PCL, which morphologically transformed into multilobated plasma cell nuclei just 7 days after bortezomib and dexamethasone administration, and finally, transformed into anaplastic myeloma that simultaneously occurred with an expanded t(11;14) chromosomal abnormality.

2. Case Presentation

A 48-year-old man was diagnosed with multiple myeloma (IgG-k, Durie-Salmon IIIB, ISS III) in February 2008 and was treated with one course of high-dose dexamethasone as an induction therapy followed by TD (thalidomide and dexamethasone) therapy for the succeeding 4 months. G-banding chromosomal analysis at the initial diagnosis showed normal diploid cells. High-dose chemotherapy with

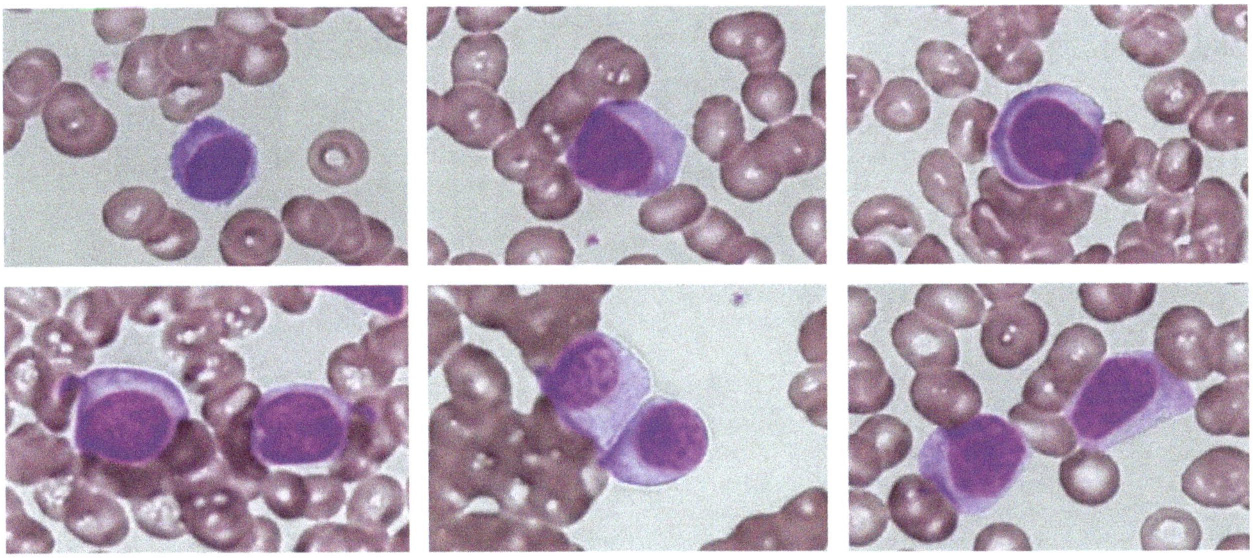

Figure 1: Morphological changes in myeloma cells immediately after the development of plasma cell leukemia. The WBC count was 20.2×10^9/L, and 79.5% of them were composed of typical myeloma cells (1,000x, May–Grünwald-Giemsa staining).

autologous peripheral blood stem cell transplantation was not performed as stem cell mobilization failed despite the use of high-dose cyclophosphamide and granulocyte colony-stimulating factor. As a result, thalidomide 50 mg was continued for 8 months and then switched to MPT (melphalan, prednisolone, and thalidomide) therapy after disease progression. In December 2009, after seven courses of MPT therapy, the patient developed secondary PCL (Figure 1). The following laboratory results were obtained: white blood cell (WBC) count, 20.2×10^9/L (plasma cells, 79.5%); hemoglobin level, 11.4 g/dL; platelet count, 2.9×10^4/L; and IgG, 3,770 mg/dL in the peripheral blood. Chromosomal analysis by G-banding showed t(11;14) abnormality of up to 5% in the bone marrow: 45, -X, -Y, add(1)(q32), -11, der(14)? t(11;14)(q13;q32), +2mar [1]/ 46, XY [19]. Extramedullary plasmacytoma was not observed on whole body computed tomography. About 2 weeks earlier, no evidence of PCL was noted in the peripheral blood: WBC count, 3.2×10^9/L (plasma cells, 0.0%); hemoglobin level, 12.3 g/dL; and platelet count, 9.6×10^4/L. BD (bortezomib 1.3 mg/m^2, days 1, 4, 8, 11 and dexamethasone 20 mg, days 1, 2, 4, 5, 8, 9, 11, 12 of 21) therapy was immediately initiated; however, only 7 days after, laboratory data revealed an increased WBC count (48.5×10^9/L) with approximately 95% of them being medium-sized atypical lymphoid cells with multilobated nuclei (Figure 2). During this period, no decrease in WBC count and no evidence of tumor lysis syndrome were observed. To elucidate the cell origin, a flow cytometry of the peripheral blood was performed, which showed the same phenotypes as the previously identified myeloma cells from the bone marrow. Namely, these cells expressed CD38, CD138, CD45, MPC-1, and cytoplasmic Igκ and did not express CD3, CD4, CD8, CD10, CD19, CD20, CD49e, CD56, and cytoplasmic Igλ. Although several regimens were given, such as 3 courses of VAD (vincristine, Adriamycin, and dexamethasone) and 4 subsequent courses of MMCP (ranimustine, melphalan, cyclophosphamide, and prednisolone), the patient's condition continuously deteriorated further, and he eventually died 4 months after developing PCL. Approximately 2 months before he died, the diameter of myeloma cells in the bone marrow increased twofold, and pleomorphic nuclei and vacuoles in the cytoplasm developed (Figure 3), indicating a transformation into anaplastic myeloma. Furthermore, a 100% increase of the t(11;14) clone frequency was observed in the bone marrow cells. The result of chromosomal analysis by G-banding was as follows: 45, -Y, del(X)(q?), ins(1;?)(q21;?), t(11;14)(q13;q32) [16]/ 45, sl, add(3)(q27), del(6)(q?) [2]/ 46, sl, +1, -ins(1;?), der(5)t(1;5)(q12;q35), +12 [1]/ 45, sl, +1, -ins(1;?), der(21)t(1;21)(q12;q22)[1]. Concurrently, the myeloma cells in the peripheral blood remained to be medium-sized atypical lymphoid cells with multilobated nuclei. Extramedullary plasmacytoma was not observed throughout the clinical course.

3. Discussion

Anaplastic myeloma can be diagnosed during the initial visit or may develop as the disease progresses [1–3], a characteristic similar to other low-grade lymphoid malignancies [14, 15]. Meanwhile, previous studies of myeloma cells with cleaved, convoluted, or multilobated nuclei reported that these cells have been present at the initial diagnosis in all cases [4–13]. In the present case, the development of secondary PCL, morphological transformation of myeloma cells into multilobated nuclei, and anaplastic transformation subsequently emerged in a short period of time, which resulted in the patient's death only 2 months after the anaplastic transformation. Therefore, the morphological transformation of myeloma cells into multilobated nuclei could be considered as the starting point of the sequential process leading to anaplastic transformation.

Interestingly, the morphological transformation of myeloma cells emerged in just 7 days in the current case.

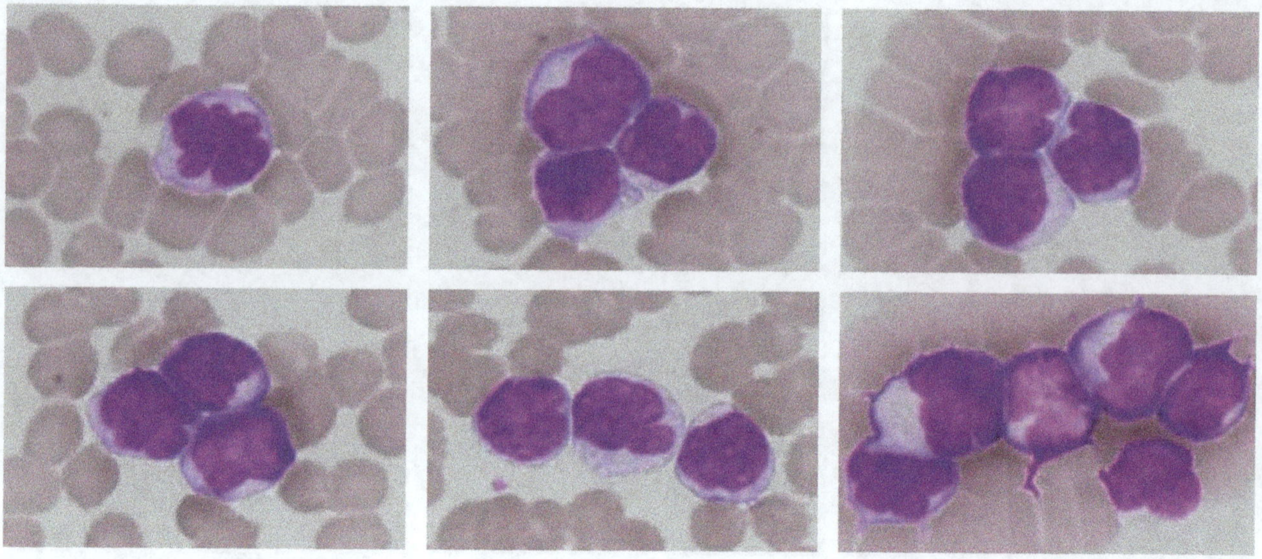

FIGURE 2: Morphological changes in myeloma cells seven days after initiating bortezomib and dexamethasone. The WBC count was elevated to 48.5×10^9/L, and 95% of them were composed of medium-sized atypical lymphoid cells with multilobated nuclei (1,000x, May–Grünwald-Giemsa staining).

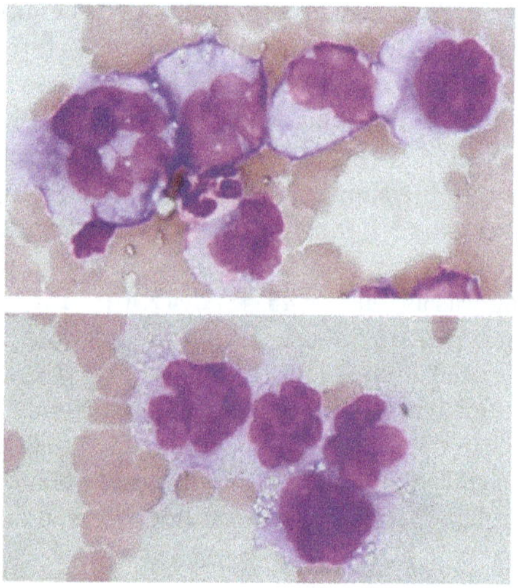

FIGURE 3: Morphological changes in myeloma cells two months after the development of secondary plasma cell leukemia. The diameter of the myeloma cells in the bone marrow significantly enlarged by approximately twofold, and pleomorphic nuclei and vacuoles in the cytoplasm were observed, indicating a transformation into anaplastic myeloma (1,000x, May–Grünwald-Giemsa staining).

Although the possibility that a small clone with multilobated nuclei expanded rapidly in a short period cannot be ruled out, we speculate that each myeloma cell simultaneously underwent a morphological transformation because the myeloma cell count increased only by 2.8-fold within 7 days versus the development of morphological transformation of myeloma cells in almost all the myeloma cells. About 2 weeks before the development of secondary PCL, no myeloma cells were evident in the peripheral blood, that is, the secondary PCL developed rapidly within 2 weeks. Thus, we suspect that these myeloma cells might have originated from a same clone in the bone marrow, and each of the cells might have aggressive characteristics resistant to BD therapy, with a predisposition for morphological transformation. Although the transformation happened just after the initiation of BD therapy, it might have occurred owing to the disease progression, and a possibility of the transformation being induced by BD therapy is low.

As the prognosis of anaplastic myeloma is poor, novel therapies, such as proteasome inhibitor or immunomodulatory drugs, are anticipated. Agrawal et al. reported a case of anaplastic myeloma with end-organ dysfunction effectively treated with bortezomib-based chemotherapy [16], whereas Ammannagari et al. reported two cases of anaplastic myeloma, of which one was resistant to bortezomib-based chemotherapy, and the other was resistant to bortezomib and lenalidomide combined chemotherapy [17]. In this case, bortezomib-based chemotherapy was ineffective for secondary PCL, and morphological transformation also occurred just after the treatment. At that time, lenalidomide was yet to be approved in Japan.

The treatment resistance and aggressive behavior of anaplastic myeloma can be associated with the high frequency of unfavorable cytogenetic abnormalities. Bahmanyar et al. reported that the prevalence of 1q21 amplification, 17p deletions, and t(4;14) in anaplastic myeloma was significantly higher than that in nonanaplastic myeloma [18]. They also reported that t(11;14) chromosomal abnormality was found in 18% cases of anaplastic myeloma, although it was not statistically significant compared with that of the nonanaplastic myeloma cases (13%) [18]. Some t(11;14)-associated anaplastic myeloma cases have also been reported. Maslovsky et al. reported a fulminant anaplastic myeloma case with complex karyotype, including t(11;14) [19], and Ammannagari et al. also reported an anaplastic myeloma case with t(11;14) refractory to bortezomib and lenalidomide combined chemotherapy [17]. In the present case, t(11;14) chromosomal abnormality that was not detected during initial diagnosis emerged concurrently with the occurrence of secondary PCL and progressed rapidly along with the anaplastic transformation. In the era of novel therapies, t(11;14) chromosomal abnormality is not considered as an unfavorable karyotype of multiple myeloma [20]; however, it was detected in a substantial proportion of primary or secondary PCL cases, which is an aggressive subset of multiple myeloma [21]. Thus, t(11;14) chromosomal abnormality is suspected to be associated with the morphological transformation of myeloma cells into anaplastic type.

This is the first reported case of myeloma cells being morphologically transformed into multilobated nuclei during the clinical course and simultaneously followed by anaplastic myeloma transformation. Further investigation regarding the morphological transformation of myeloma cells and the possible correlation with t(11;14) chromosomal abnormality is required.

Conflicts of Interest

The authors declare that there are no conflicts of interest regarding the publication of this article.

References

[1] K. Foucar, M. Raber, E. Foucar, B. Barlogie, C. M. Sandler, and R. Alexanian, "Anaplastic myeloma with massive extramedullary involvement. Report of two cases," *Cancer*, vol. 51, no. 1, pp. 166–174, 1983.

[2] S. L. Allen and M. Coleman, "Aggressive phase multiple myeloma: a terminal anaplastic transformation resembling high-grade lymphoma," *Cancer Investigation*, vol. 8, no. 3-4, pp. 417–424, 1990.

[3] S. Sethi and I. Miller, "Plasma cell myeloma with anaplastic transformation," *Blood*, vol. 128, no. 16, p. 2106, 2016.

[4] G. Beltran and W. J. Stuckey, "Nuclear lobulation and cytoplasmic fibrils in leukemic plasma cells," *American Journal of Clinical Pathology*, vol. 58, no. 2, pp. 159–164, 1972.

[5] J. Saumya, M. Feroze, N. K. Supriya, and K. A. Aisabi, "Plasma cell leukemia with pleomorphic plasma cells-a case report," *Indian Journal of Pathology and Microbiology*, vol. 49, no. 3, pp. 438-439, 2006.

[6] L. R. Zukerberg, J. A. Ferry, M. Conlon, and N. L. Harris, "Plasma cell myeloma with cleaved, multilobated, and monocytoid nuclei," *American Journal of Clinical Pathology*, vol. 93, no. 5, pp. 657–661, 1990.

[7] M. J. Grange, B. Fantin, C. Carbon, and J. Hakim, "A case of multiple myeloma with multilobulated and convoluted plasma cell nuclei," *Nouvelle Revue Française D'Hématologie*, vol. 34, no. 5, pp. 385–387, 1992.

[8] J. Richter, A. Swedin, T. Olofsson, B. Johansson, M. Akerman, and I. Winqvist, "Aggressive course of primary plasma cell leukemia with unusual morphological and cytogenetic features," *Annals of Hematology*, vol. 71, no. 6, pp. 307–310, 1995.

[9] D. H. Buss, G. D. Reynolds, and M. R. Cooper, "Multiple myeloma associated with multilobated plasma cell nuclei," *Virchows Archiv. B, Cell Pathology Including Molecular Pathology*, vol. 55, no. 5, pp. 287–292, 1988.

[10] A. Islam, S. Noyes, and E. S. Henderson, "A case of aggressive multiple myeloma with convoluted and multilobated plasma cell nuclei and no visible nucleoli," *British Journal of Haematology*, vol. 76, no. 2, pp. 306-307, 1990.

[11] M. Djaldetti and U. H. Lewinski, "Nuclear hypersegmentation in the myeloma cells of a patient with multiple myeloma," *Scandinavian Journal of Haematology*, vol. 31, no. 2, pp. 144–148, 1983.

[12] A. B. Olujohungbe, W. D. Brace, C. J. Laversuch, F. E. Cotter, and C. D. Reid, "Sternal-clavicular plasmacytomas with atypical morphology," *British Journal of Haematology*, vol. 78, no. 2, pp. 290-291, 1991.

[13] M. Nara, K. Suzuki, Y. Inoue, H. Enomoto, T. Saito, and S. Fujioka, "A case of multiple myeloma with nuclear hypersegmentation after MP/VAD/VCAP-IFN therapies with a good prognosis," *Acta Haematologica*, vol. 90, no. 2, pp. 102-103, 1993.

[14] T. A. Eyre and A. Schuh, "An update for Richter syndrome—new directions and developments," *British Journal of Haematology*, vol. 178, no. 4, pp. 508–520, 2017.

[15] C. Casulo, W. R. Burack, and J. W. Friedberg, "Transformed follicular non-Hodgkin lymphoma," *Blood*, vol. 125, no. 1, pp. 40–47, 2015.

[16] M. Agrawal, J. Kanakry, C. A. Arnold et al., "Sustained remission and reversal of end-organ dysfunction in a patient with anaplastic myeloma," *Annals of Hematology*, vol. 93, no. 7, pp. 1245-1246, 2014.

[17] N. Ammannagari, K. Celotto, V. Neppalli, K. Lee, and S. A. Holstein, "Anaplastic multiple myeloma: an aggressive variant with a poor response to novel therapies," *Clinical Lymphoma Myeloma and Leukemia*, vol. 16, no. 9, pp. e129–e131, 2016.

[18] M. Bahmanyar, X. Qi, and H. Chang, "Genomic aberrations in anaplastic multiple myeloma: high frequency of 1q21 (CKS1B) amplifications," *Leukemia Research*, vol. 37, no. 12, pp. 1726–1728, 2013.

[19] I. Maslovsky, G. Lugassy, R. Blumental, A. Ducach, O. Yehuda, and D. Abeliovich, "Multiple chromosomal abnormalities in fulminant anaplastic myeloma," *Clinical and Laboratory Haematology*, vol. 21, no. 3, pp. 207–210, 1999.

[20] A. Palumbo, H. Avet-Loiseau, S. Oliva et al., "Revised international staging system for multiple myeloma: a report from International Myeloma Working Group," *Journal of Clinical Oncology*, vol. 33, no. 26, pp. 2863–2869, 2015.

[21] F. lbarracin and R. Fonseca, "Plasma cell leukemia," *Blood Reviews*, vol. 25, no. 3, pp. 107–112, 2011.

17

$\gamma\delta$ T-Cell Acute Lymphoblastic Leukemia/ Lymphoma: Discussion of Two Pediatric Cases and its Distinction from Other Mature $\gamma\delta$ T-Cell Malignancies

Eric X. Wei,[1] Vasiliki Leventaki,[2] John K. Choi,[2] Susana C. Raimondi,[2] Elizabeth M. Azzato,[2] Sheila A. Shurtleff,[2] Menchu G. Ong,[1] Diana M. Veillon,[1] James D. Cotelingam,[1] and Rodney E. Shackelford[1]

[1]*Department of Pathology and Translational Pathobiology, LSU Health Shreveport, Shreveport, LA, USA*
[2]*Department of Pathology, St. Jude Children's Research Hospital, Memphis, TN, USA*

Correspondence should be addressed to Eric X. Wei; ericxwei@yahoo.com

Academic Editor: Marie-Christine Kyrtsonis

Gamma delta ($\gamma\delta$) T-cell antigen receptor (TCR) expression and its related T-cell differentiation are not commonly reported in T-cell acute lymphoblastic leukemia/lymphoma (T-ALL). Here we report two pediatric T-ALL cases and present their clinical features, histology, immunophenotypes, cytogenetics, and molecular diagnostic findings. The first patient is a two-year-old girl with leukocytosis, circulating lymphoblasts, and a cryptic insertion of a short-arm segment at 10p12 into the long-arm segment of 11q23 resulting in an MLL and AF10 fusion transcript, which may be the first reported in $\gamma\delta$ T-ALL. She responded to the chemotherapy protocol poorly and had persistent diseases. Following an allogeneic bone marrow transplant, she went into remission. The second patient is an eleven-year-old boy with a normal white cell count, circulating blasts, and a normal karyotype, but without any immature cellular markers by flow cytometric analysis. He responded to the chemotherapy well and achieved a complete remission. These cases demonstrate the diverse phenotypic, cytogenetic, and molecular aspects of $\gamma\delta$ T-ALL. Early T-precursor- (ETP-) ALL and their differential diagnosis from other mature $\gamma\delta$ T-cell leukemia/lymphomas are also discussed.

1. Introduction

Gamma delta ($\gamma\delta$) T-cell neoplasms are characterized by the expression of the $\gamma\delta$ T-cell antigen receptors (TCRs), are rare, and include a variety of clinicopathologic entities. T-cell acute lymphoblastic leukemia (T-ALL) with expression of alpha beta ($\alpha\beta$) or $\gamma\delta$ TCR has been previously described in about 35% T-ALL cases, while $\gamma\delta$ T-ALL cases represented 9–12% of T-ALL including children and adults [1]. Mature T-cell neoplasms with TCR $\gamma\delta$ expression include hepatosplenic T-cell lymphoma, skin and mucosal $\gamma\delta$ T-cell lymphoma, and $\gamma\delta$ T-cell large granular lymphocytic (T-LGL) leukemia [2, 3]. The 2016 revision of the WHO classification of lymphoid neoplasms emphasizes the primary cutaneous $\gamma\delta$ T-cell lymphoma [4]. $\gamma\delta$ T-cell lymphomas, other than hepatosplenic T-cell lymphoma and primary cutaneous $\gamma\delta$ T-cell lymphoma, are often classified within subcategories of T-cell lymphomas. $\gamma\delta$ T-ALL is uncommon with only 2% of all acute lymphoblastic leukemia (ALL) cases showing expression of the $\gamma\delta$ TCR [1]. $\gamma\delta$ TCR expression and T-cell differentiation are not frequently reported in T-ALL [1, 5]. We report clinicopathological features of two pediatric cases of $\gamma\delta$ T-ALL and discuss the differential diagnosis of other types of $\gamma\delta$ T-cell leukemia/lymphoma.

2. Case Presentation

The first case is a 2-year-old Caucasian girl, previously in good health, who suddenly presented at the LSU hospital with fever, shortness of breath, rhinorrhea, cyanosis, and hepatosplenomegaly by chest X-ray. She had anemia

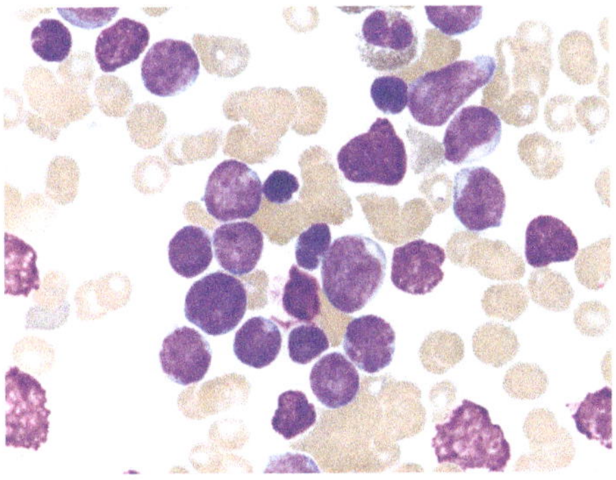

FIGURE 1: Bone marrow aspirate smear from patient #1, Wright-Giemsa, 1000x.

and thrombocytopenia, with a white cell count (WBC) at 118.8 thousand/μL and 73% lymphoid cells. Flow cytometry of peripheral blood showed a $\gamma\delta$ T-cell proliferation. Molecular studies revealed clonal TCR γ- and β-chain gene rearrangements by PCR. The patient was started on intravenous fluids and antibiotics. She did not undergo a liver or spleen biopsy. Her white cell count decreased to 56.8 thousand/μL the next day and she was transferred to St. Jude Children's Research Hospital (SJCRH). Bone marrow evaluation showed 90% lymphoblasts, exhibiting slightly open chromatin and irregular nuclear contours (Figure 1). Flow cytometry of bone marrow showed T lymphoblasts expressing surface CD3 (variable) and cytoplasmic CD3, CD5, CD7 (bright), CD34, CD45 (dim), and TCR $\gamma\delta$. The blasts were negative for CD1a, CD2, CD4, CD8, CD10, CD56, HLA-DR, TCR $\alpha\beta$, TdT, and MPO (Figure 2). Cytogenetic studies of the bone marrow showed that 90% of the metaphases had an abnormal karyotype: 47, XX, t(4;10)(q28;p12), cryp ins(11;10)(q23;p12p12), +17 (Figure 3(a)). FISH assays using the BCR-ABL1 and TLX3 probes were normal. FISH was also performed using the break-apart AF10 (10p12) probe (research use only) on sequential G-banded to FISH metaphases, and it was found that the probe was rearranged where the telomeric 3′ AF10 moved to the 4q confirming t(4;10). Of interest, the centromeric 5′ AF10 signal is inserted into the 11q23 region (Figure 3(b)). By FISH, MLL was not rearranged (Figure 3(c)). The reason MLL was not rearranged or separated because the insertion was very tiny and did not separate enough the 5′ from the 3′ signal. Overall, FISH results indicate a cryptic insertion; that is, a segment of 10p12 had been donated to the recipient 11q23. Molecular studies by real-time RT-PCR assay confirmed an *MLL/MLLT10 (MLL/AF10)* fusion transcript (Figure 4). The patient received treatment per Total XVI (TOTXVI) protocol.

At day 15 following induction, flow cytometry revealed residual disease with 35% blasts in bone marrow. Following reintensification I therapy, the patient had significantly decreased blast percentages but remained persistently positive for minimal residual disease (MRD), with the last MRD before bone marrow transplant (BMT) at 0.018% by flow cytometry. She eventually underwent allogeneic BMT. She had been on day +126 after transplant, remained MRD negative, and had been followed up at the LSU hospital.

The second case is an 11-year-old African American boy with an asthma history who complained of cough, chest tightness, and one-week back pain. His chest X-ray did not show a mediastinal mass. CBC showed a normal white cell count, mild thrombocytopenia, and increased circulating blasts, which appeared to be lymphoblasts morphologically. Flow cytometry revealed approximately 32% circulating $\gamma\delta$ T-cell lymphoblasts. After maintenance on intravenous fluid and allopurinol therapy, he was transferred to SJCRH for chemotherapy. His bone marrow showed 89% blasts that were small to medium in size with a high nuclear to cytoplasmic ratio, fine chromatin, round to slightly irregular nuclei, and scant cytoplasm (Figure 5). Flow cytometric analysis of the bone marrow confirmed the presence of T lymphoblasts that were positive for surface CD3 (variable), cytoplasmic CD3, CD5 (dim), CD7, CD45 (dim), CD79a, and TCR $\gamma\delta$. They were negative for CD1a, CD2, CD4, CD8, CD10, CD34, TdT, MPO, and TCR $\alpha\beta$ (Figure 6). Cytogenetic studies performed on the bone marrow showed normal a male karyotype without numerical or structural abnormalities. The patient received treatment per Total XVI (TOTXVI) protocol and achieved MRD negativity after induction on day 42. Following remission subsequent to chemotherapy, the patient had been followed up at the LSU hospital.

3. Discussion

The differential diagnosis of these two pediatric cases includes skin and mucosal $\gamma\delta$ T-cell lymphoma in leukemic phase, hepatosplenic T-cell lymphoma, $\gamma\delta$ T-cell large granular lymphocytic (T-LGL) leukemia, and $\gamma\delta$ T-ALL [2, 4, 6]. Peripheral $\gamma\delta$ T-cell lymphoma is a subtype of peripheral T-cell lymphoma, occurring mainly in skin and mucosal regions, often harboring cytotoxic activity. In the skin, $\gamma\delta$ T-cell lymphoma can be divided into mycosis fungoides-like and primary cutaneous $\gamma\delta$ T-cell lymphoma, presenting with Sézary syndrome in blood involvement [2, 4, 7]. Mucosal $\gamma\delta$ T-cell lymphoma may occur in the nasopharynx, lung, gastrointestinal tracts, and other organs, with intestinal $\gamma\delta$ T-cell lymphoma being type II enteropathy associated [2, 6, 8, 9].

Hepatosplenic T-cell lymphoma is a type of $\gamma\delta$ T-cell lymphoma with extranodal and systemic involvement [2,

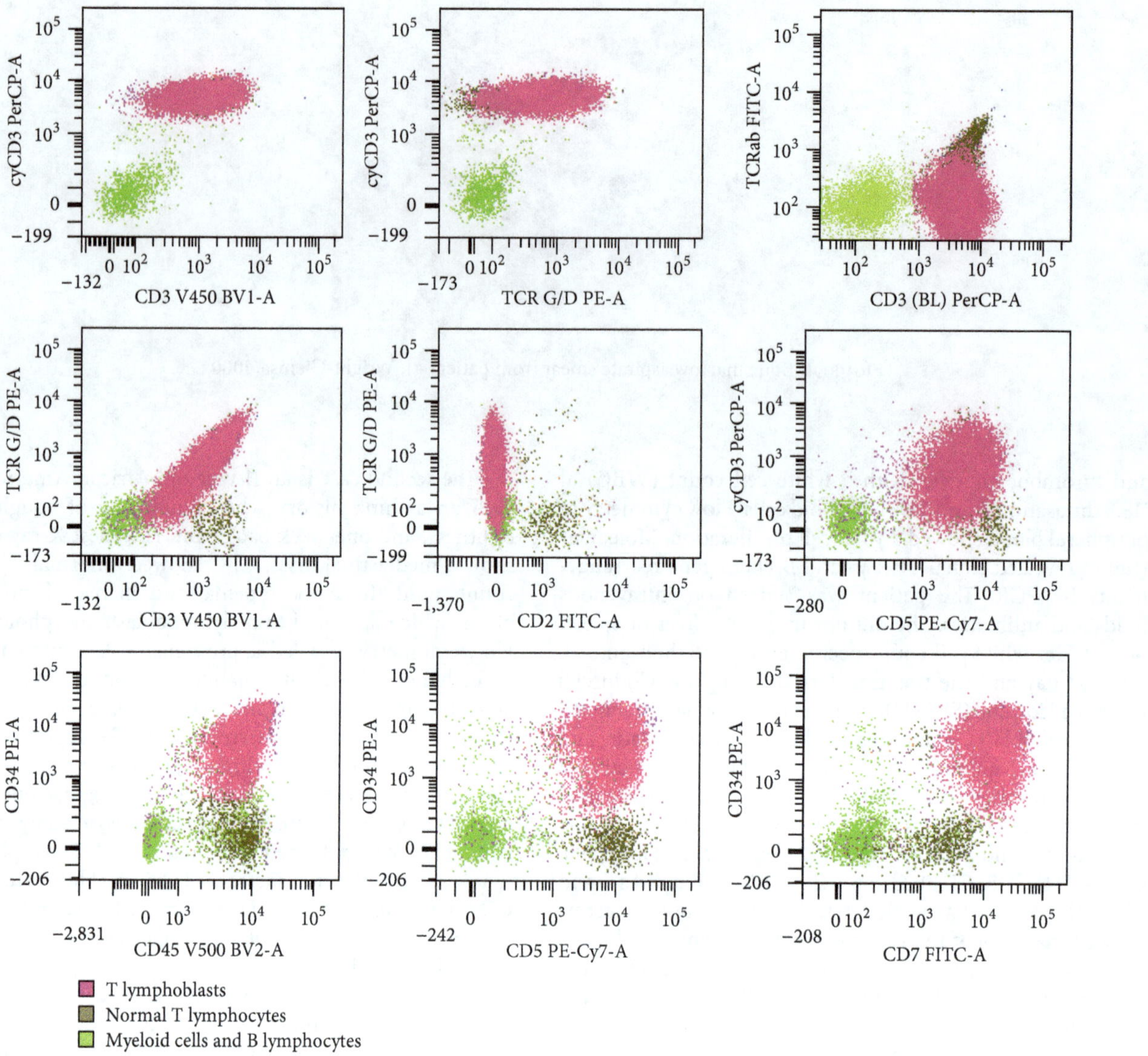

FIGURE 2: Representative flow cytometric histograms of bone marrow aspirate from patient #1.

3, 6, 10, 11]. It tends to occur in younger patients with hepatosplenomegaly, systemic symptoms, and cytopenia. The neoplastic cells involve the cords and sinuses of spleen, liver, and bone marrow [12]. The tumor cells are intermediate in size, with condensed chromatin, indistinct nucleoli, and absence of azurophilic granules [11, 12]. Phenotypically, the lymphoma cells are usually positive for CD2, CD3, CD7, CD56, and TCR $\gamma\delta$ and negative for CD4, CD5, CD8, and TCR $\alpha\beta$. Although the first patient showed hepatosplenomegaly with a $\gamma\delta$ T-cell phenotype, she had marked leukocytosis at the beginning of her disease course, with lymphoblastic appearing neoplastic cells positive for CD5 and CD34 and negative for CD2. Thus, the diagnosis of hepatosplenic T-cell lymphoma is not supported.

In spite of the fact that the majority of T-LGL leukemia cases are of $\alpha\beta$ type, there are rare cases of $\gamma\delta$ T-LGL leukemia [2, 13]. In comparison to its $\alpha\beta$ counterpart, $\gamma\delta$ T-LGL leukemia patients are prone to having rheumatoid arthritis, lower absolute neutrophil counts, more severe thrombocytopenia, and a higher probability of CD4 and CD8 double negativity. However, both groups of T-LGL leukemia frequently have anemia, an indolent clinical course, and a similar overall survival [2, 13].

T-ALL comprises approximately 20% of all ALL cases [1, 2, 14]. Overall, $\gamma\delta$ T-ALL is similar to $\alpha\beta$ T-ALL in the majority of clinical and hematological aspects [4, 14]. T-ALL is more common in children and younger adults, with a male preponderance. The bone marrow is affected in almost all T-ALL cases, and mediastinal or thymic involvement is common. They tend to have a high leukocyte count, lymphadenopathy, and hepatosplenomegaly. Morphologically, the lymphoblasts are intermediate in size and have delicate chromatin, inconspicuous nucleoli, and scant cytoplasm. Immunophenotypically, they are often positive for CD1a, CD2, surface and/or cytoplasmic CD3, CD5, CD7, CD10, CD34, CD45, and TdT but are negative for B cell and myeloid

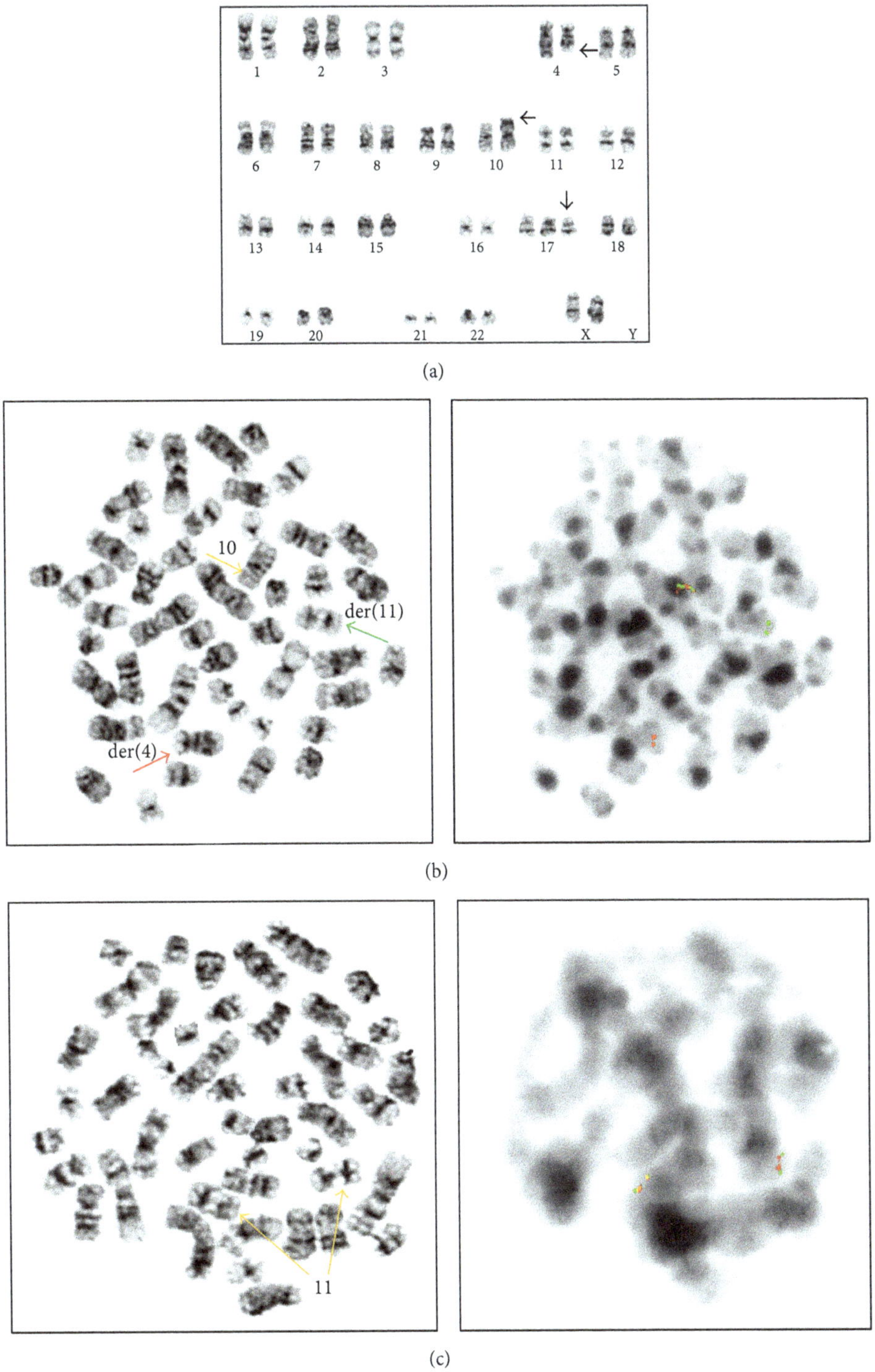

FIGURE 3: Cytogenetic and FISH results from patient #1. (a) Conventional karyotype with 47, XX, $t(4;10)(q28;p12)$, +17. (b) Break-apart AF-10 probe on sequential G-banded to FISH metaphases shows that telomeric $3'$ AF10 moves to the 4q28, and the centromeric $5'$ AF10 signal inserts into the 11q23 region. (c) The MLL FISH is not rearranged. In (a), the arrows to 4p28 and 10p12 are for indication of $t(4;10)(q28;p12)$; the arrow to chromosome 17 is for indication of +17.

markers. They may be CD4 and CD8 double negative, double positive, or only positive for CD4 or CD8. With cytoplasmic CD3 as the most specific T-cell marker expressed in all maturation stages, there are pro-T (CD7+), pre-T (CD2+ and/or CD5+ and/or CD8+), cortical T (CD1a+), and medullary T (surface CD3+, CD1a−) subtypes of T-ALL based on progressive stages of differentiation [14]. The expression levels of TCR $\alpha\beta$ or TCR $\gamma\delta$ in association with different differentiating stages are rarely reported [1]. T-ALL almost always shows clonal TCR gene rearrangements and

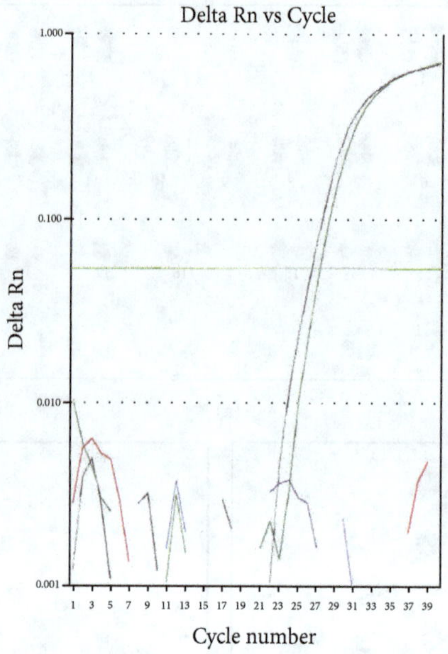

FIGURE 4: Real-time RT-PCR showing the *MLL/MLLT10* fusion transcripts from patient #1. Delta Rn = normalized fluorescence reporter signal minus baseline; cycle number = cycle of PCR; purple is the positive control; green is the patient; red is no-template control; blue is the negative control (HL60 cell line).

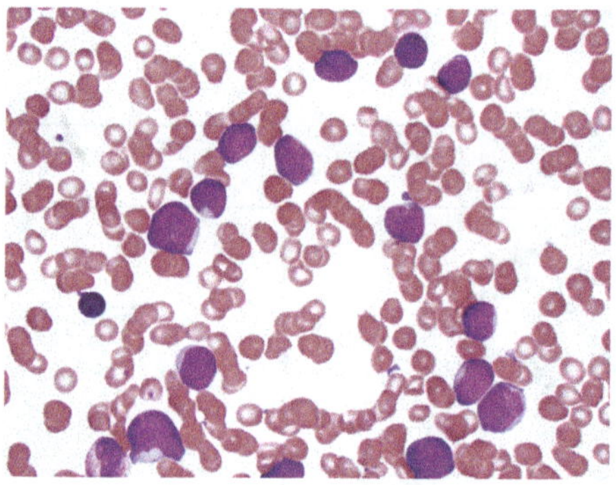

FIGURE 5: Bone marrow aspirate smear from patient #2, Wright-Giemsa, 1000x.

often carries an abnormal karyotype and an unfavorable prognosis. Early T-precursor- (ETP-) ALL, expressing stem cell or myeloid markers, has a much poorer clinical outcome compared to other T-ALL [14]. Numerous genes have been implicated for the pathogenesis and prognosis for T-ALL, including *NOTCH1, TAL1, and HOX1* [5, 14]. $\gamma\delta$ T-ALL is a rare variant of T lineage lymphoblastic leukemia/lymphoma. Compared to $\alpha\beta$ T-ALL, $\gamma\delta$ T-ALL tends to present with lower hemoglobin concentrations in children, more frequent splenomegaly and higher WBC in adults, and higher percentages of the CD45RA−/CD45RO+ phenotype in both children and adults [1]. Although $\gamma\delta$ T-ALL usually shows TCR gamma and TCR delta chain gene rearrangements, TCR beta chain and biclonal rearrangements involving both Vδ1 and Vδ2 segments have also been reported [5]. Both of these two pediatric $\gamma\delta$ T-ALL patients were likely in medullary (mature) T-ALL stage at presentation with variable surface CD3 expression. Neither of our patients has ETP-ALL due to the strong CD5 expression in the first patient and lack of immature or myeloid markers in the second patient. The cryptic insertion involving MLL and AF10 resulting in the expression of the fusion transcript has rarely been reported in T-ALL [15]. To our knowledge, such cryptic insertion with *MLL/MLLT10* fusion may be the first reported in $\gamma\delta$ T-ALL. Previous studies have shown a higher percentage of $\gamma\delta$ T-ALL, at 9~12%, in comparison with the very low proportion of $\gamma\delta$ T-cells in the normal thymus, which is at 1% [1]. The reason for this phenomenon is unclear. It is possible that $\gamma\delta$ T-cells have a higher chance of progression to malignancy compared to $\alpha\beta$ T-cells or a subset of $\gamma\delta$ T-ALL may originate from extrathymic tissues [1]. Even though normal $\gamma\delta$ T-cells are more commonly double negative for CD4 and CD8, a significant percentage of $\gamma\delta$ T-ALL may exhibit CD4, CD8, or both CD4 and CD8, which may be due to antigen evolution during malignant transformation [1]. $\gamma\delta$ T-ALL may represent a subcategory of acute lymphoblastic leukemia

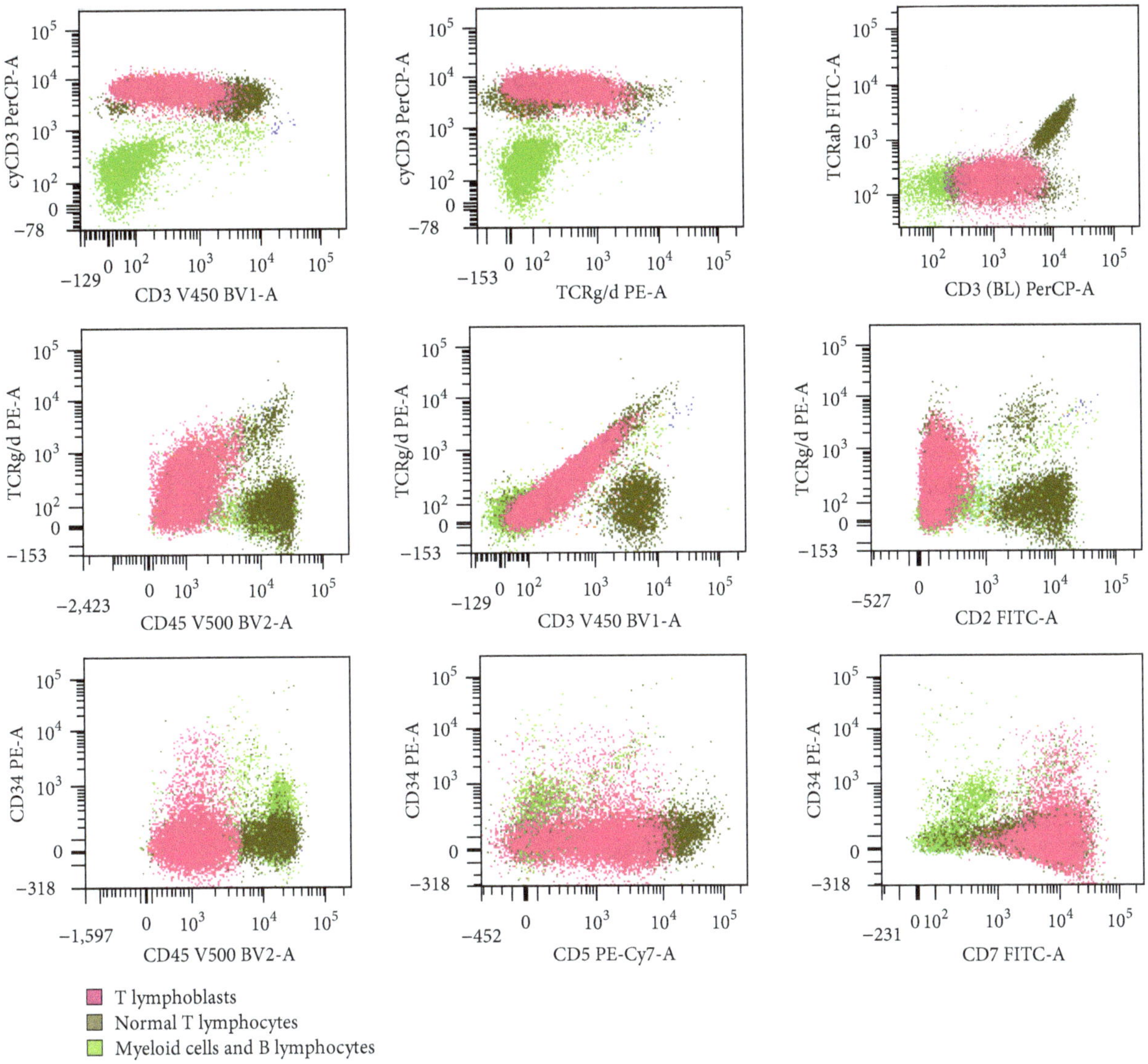

FIGURE 6: Representative flow cytometric histograms of bone marrow aspirate from patient #2.

with slightly distinctive clinical and laboratory features. More studies are needed to further investigate such subtypes of T-ALL, including their pathological diagnosis and clinical management.

Conflicts of Interest

The authors declare that there are no conflicts of interest regarding the publication of this paper.

References

[1] D. M. Matos, E. G. Rizzatti, M. Fernandes, V. Buccheri, and R. P. Falcao, "Gammadelta and alphabeta T-cell acute lymphoblastic leukemia: comparison of their clinical and immunophenotypic features," *Haematologica*, vol. 90, pp. 264–266, 2005.

[2] P. Gaulard, K. Belhadj, and F. Reyes, "γδ T-cell lymphomas," *Seminars in Hematology*, vol. 40, no. 3, pp. 233–243, 2003.

[3] C. Tripodo, E. Iannitto, A. M. Florena et al., "Gamma-delta T-cell lymphomas," *Nature Reviews Clinical Oncology*, vol. 6, no. 12, pp. 707–717, 2009.

[4] S. H. Swerdlow, E. Campo, S. A. Pileri et al., "The 2016 revision of the World Health Organization classification of lymphoid neoplasms," *Blood*, vol. 127, no. 20, pp. 2375–2390, 2016.

[5] H. Zheng, X. Wang, Y. Ma et al., "The TCR γδ repertoire and relative gene expression characteristics of T-ALL cases with biclonal malignant vδ1 and Vδ2 T cells," *DNA and Cell Biology*, vol. 33, no. 1, pp. 49–56, 2014.

[6] F. Vega, L. J. Medeiros, and P. Gaulard, "Hepatosplenic and other γδ T-cell lymphomas," *American Journal of Clinical Pathology*, vol. 127, no. 6, pp. 869–880, 2007.

[7] E. D. Merrill, R. Agbay, R. N. Miranda et al., "Primary cutaneous T-cell lymphomas showing gamma-delta (γδ) phenotype and predominantly epidermotropic pattern are clinicopathologically distinct from classic primary cutaneous γδ T-cell lymphomas," *American Journal of Surgical Pathology*, vol. 41, no. 2, pp. 204–215, 2017.

[8] A. L. Wilson, S. H. Swerdlow, G. K. Przybylski et al., "Intestinal $\gamma\delta$ T-cell lymphomas are most frequently of type II enteropathy-associated T-cell type," *Human Pathology*, vol. 44, no. 6, pp. 1131–1145, 2013.

[9] T. Tanaka, H. Yamamoto, A. A. Elsayed et al., "Clinicopathologic spectrum of gastrointestinal T-cell lymphoma reappraisal based on T-cell receptor immunophenotypes," *American Journal of Surgical Pathology*, vol. 40, no. 6, pp. 777–785, 2016.

[10] A. J. M. Ferreri, S. Govi, and S. A. Pileri, "Hepatosplenic gamma-delta T-cell lymphoma," *Critical Reviews in Oncology/Hematology*, vol. 83, no. 2, pp. 283–292, 2012.

[11] M. Yabe, L. J. Medeiros, G. Tang et al., "Prognostic factors of hepatosplenic T-cell lymphoma clinicopathologic study of 28 cases," *American Journal of Surgical Pathology*, vol. 40, no. 5, pp. 676–688, 2016.

[12] M. Yabe, L. J. Medeiros, S. A. Wang et al., "Distinguishing between hepatosplenic T-cell lymphoma and $\gamma\delta$ T-cell large granular lymphocytic leukemia," *American Journal of Surgical Pathology*, vol. 41, no. 1, pp. 82–93, 2017.

[13] M. Yabe, L. J. Medeiros, S. A. Wang et al., "Clinicopathologic, immunophenotypic, cytogenetic, and molecular features of T-cell large granular lymphocytic leukemia: an analysis of 14 patients suggests biologic differences with T-cell large granular lymphocytic leukemia," *American Journal of Clinical Pathology*, vol. 144, no. 4, pp. 607–619, 2015.

[14] M. J. You, L. J. Medeiros, and E. D. Hsi, "T-lymphoblastic leukemia/lymphoma," *American Journal of Clinical Pathology*, vol. 144, no. 3, pp. 411–422, 2015.

[15] K. Matlawska-Wasowska, H. Kang, M. Devidas et al., "MLL rearrangements impact outcome in HOXA-deregulated T-lineage acute lymphoblastic leukemia: A Children's Oncology Group Study," *Leukemia*, vol. 30, no. 9, pp. 1909–1912, 2016.

18

Chronic Myelomonocytic Leukemia following Multicentric Castleman Disease

Feng Li, Xiaomei Zhang, Yanting Guo, Yuandong Zhu, Yicun Wu, and Yun Ling

Department of Hematology, The First People's Hospital of Changzhou, The Third Affiliated Hospital of Soochow University, Changzhou, Jiangsu, China

Correspondence should be addressed to Yun Ling; a110426007@hotmail.com

Academic Editor: Sergio Storti

Multicentric Castleman disease (MCD) is a rare nonmalignant lymphoproliferative disorder presenting systemic symptoms such as fever, night sweats, fatigue, anemia, effusions, and multifocal lymphadenopathy. The etiology of MCD has not been clarified to date. The coexistence of MCD with chronic myelomonocytic leukemia (CMML) has been rarely reported. Although the pathogenesis remains unclear, this association probably reflects an incidental and fortuitous finding rather than the alteration of a common pluripotent stem cell precursor. Herein, we report on one case of MCD coexisting with CMML and elucidate the underlying mechanism of pathology in some aspects.

1. Introduction

MCD is a rare polyclonal B lymphoproliferative disorder that straddles the intersections of hematology, oncology, rheumatology, and virology. MCD manifests with a heterogeneous group of disorders with various etiologies that demonstrate episodic systemic inflammatory symptoms, reactive proliferation of morphologically benign lymphocytes, and multiple organ system impairment [1, 2].

Chronic myelomonocytic leukemia (CMML) is a clonal stem cell disorder with features that overlap those of myelodysplastic syndromes (MDSs) and myeloproliferative neoplasms (MPNs) with a variable but overall poor prognosis. It occurs almost exclusively in the elderly with a median age at diagnosis varying between 65 and 75 years. Similar to MDS, the pathogenesis of CMML appears to be multifactorial and linked to altered genetic, molecular, microenvironmental, and immunologic state in different individuals.

Patients with MCD have a significantly high risk of developing severe pancytopenia, multiorgan failure, and lymphoma compared with healthy controls [3]. On the contrary, it is quite a rare event for MCD to progress to CMML, which belongs to different pathogenic cell types. In the present case, we first describe a MCD patient, who progressed to CMML and was sensitive to decitabine therapy.

2. Case Report

The patient, a 44-year-old woman, was admitted to our center in December 2011 suffering from cough, asthma, and asthenia. Peripheral blood studies showed severe iron-deficiency anemia, elevations of C-reactive protein, and polyclonal hypergammaglobulinemia. Computed tomogram demonstrated diffuse (lung, axillary, and mediastinal) lymphadenopathy, interstitial pneumonitis, and splenomegaly (Figures 1(a) and 1(b)). Histology of left pulmonary nodule accessed by thoracic surgery revealed atretic follicles with plasmacytosis, prominent paracortical vascularity, and sinus histiocytosis with an overall appearance consistent with MCD (Figures 1(c) and 1(d)). Immunohistochemistry for IgG and CD138 was positive, and IgG4 was negative (Figures 1(e) and 1(f)). Based on clinical and pathological suspicion of Castleman disease, further testing revealed high interleukin-6 (IL-6) of 23.0 pg/mL and normal IgG4 of 1.28 g/L. The patient's serum tested negative for HIV, and no cytomegalovirus, Epstein–Barr virus, or human herpes

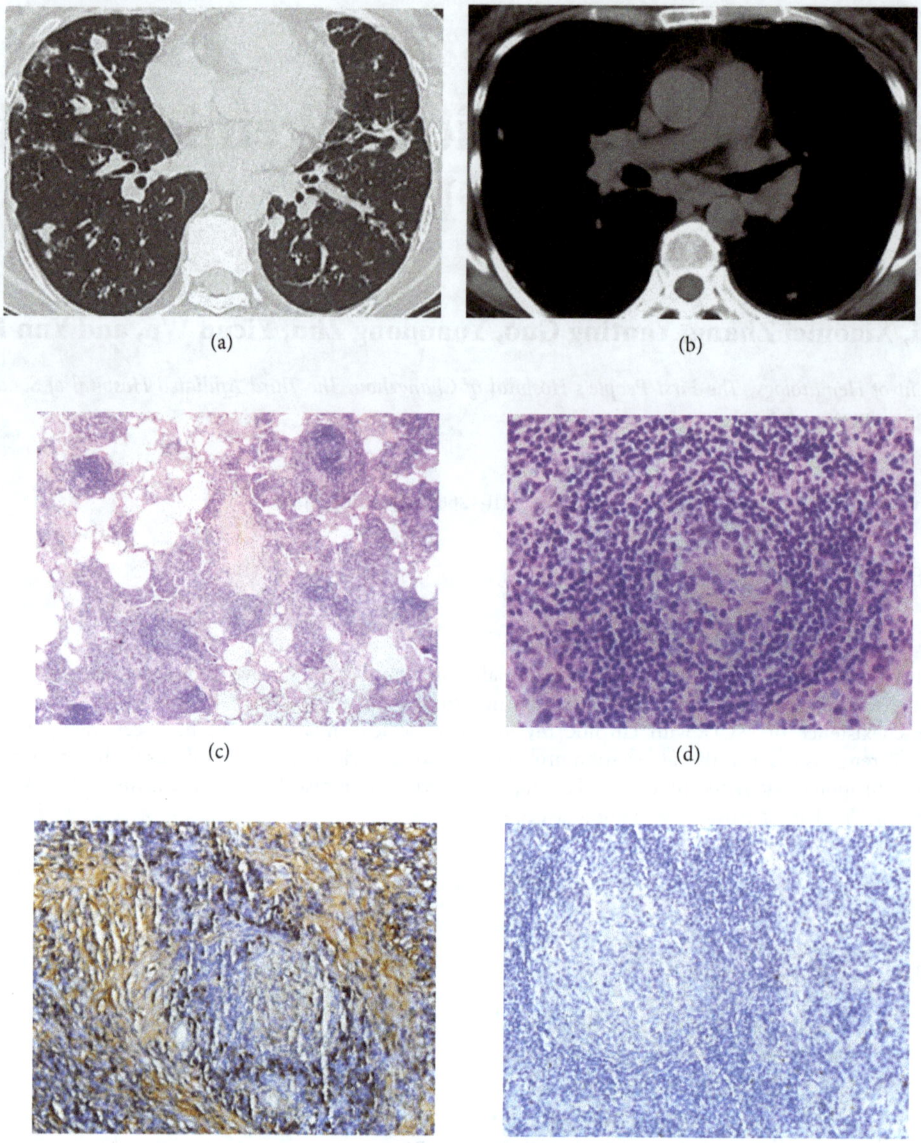

(a) (b) (c) (d) (e) (f)

Figure 1: (a) and (b) HRCT of the chest at diagnosis shows bilateral centrilobular nodules, thickening of the interlobular septa, and mediastinal lymphadenopathy. (c) and (d) Histological findings of the pulmonary nodule show infiltration of polyclonal plasma cells around the bronchovascular bundles and in the interfollicular areas of the nodes (H&E, 50x and 200x). (e) and (f) Sheets of mature plasma cells are present within the interfollicular region and are highlighted by positive immunostaining of IgG- and IgG4-negative plasma cells (immunohistochemistry, 200x).

virus-8 (HHV-8) replication was detected. She was diagnosed with HIV-negative and HHV-8-negative multicentric Castleman disease of plasma cell variant. She was started on monotherapy chemotherapy with low-dose cyclophosphamide, accompanied by oral steroids from March 2012.

Unfortunately, she was later readmitted to our hospital for severe abdominal pain and skin and mucous membrane bleeding in August 2015 with a history of type-II diabetes for two years. Just one month ago, she followed the doctors' advice of cessation of the cyclophosphamide for severe anemia (Hb, 4.4 g/dL). Continued monitoring of routine blood count showed normocytic normochromic anemia (Hb, 6.0–8.0 g/dL), severe thrombocytopenia (PLT, 10,000–20,000/μL), and mild leukocytosis (10,000–12,000/μL), while monocytes were at normal levels. Bone marrow (BM) study showed an increased number of megakaryocytes, and myeloid series hypercellularity and dysplastic change were evident. Abdominal CT showed severe splenomegaly and multifocal and wide-area infarction. Subsequently, she underwent laparoscopic splenectomy, and the pathological section demonstrated the structural breakdown and significant hypercellularity (Figures 2(a) and 2(b)). In next nine months, there was a stable increase of WBC (20,000–100,000/μL), especially peripheral blood monocytes (1,500–10,000/μL), which was

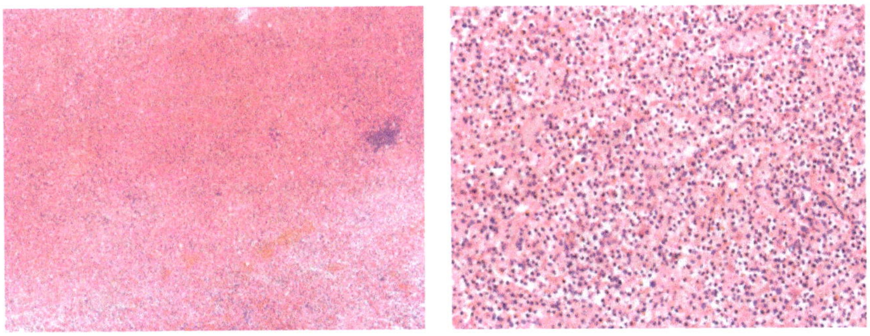

(a) (b)

Figure 2: (a) and (b) Pathological section demonstrated the structural breakdown and significant hypercellularity with hyperplastic granulopoiesis (H&E, 50x and 200x).

still accompanied by decreased platelet counts (15,000–60,000/μL) and anemia (Hb, 6.0–8.0 g/dL). At this period, BM examination was again performed and revealed a significant increase in monocytes (12%) and prominent dysplastic changes in myeloid lineages. High expression levels of CD13, CD33, CD14, CD64, and CD56 were detected in her bone marrow cells. The karyotype was normal, and BCR/ABL fusion gene was not detected by the fluorescent in situ hybridization. At the same time, molecular studies were negative for TET2, SRSF2, ASXL1, and SETBP1 mutations, which are reported in about 90% of patients with CMML. According to World Health Organization (WHO) classification, a diagnosis of CMML and MCD, which were simultaneously present, was made. Then, she received frontline treatment with decitabine (DAC, 20 mg/m^2 for 5 d in a 4-week cycle) for CMML. Surprisingly, after just one cycle, the WBC count had declined to 15,000/μL and the Hb increased to 9.0 g/dL and PLT to 220,000/μL (Figure 3). She also was recommended allogeneic hematopoietic stem cell transplant (HSCT) as the only potentially curative option.

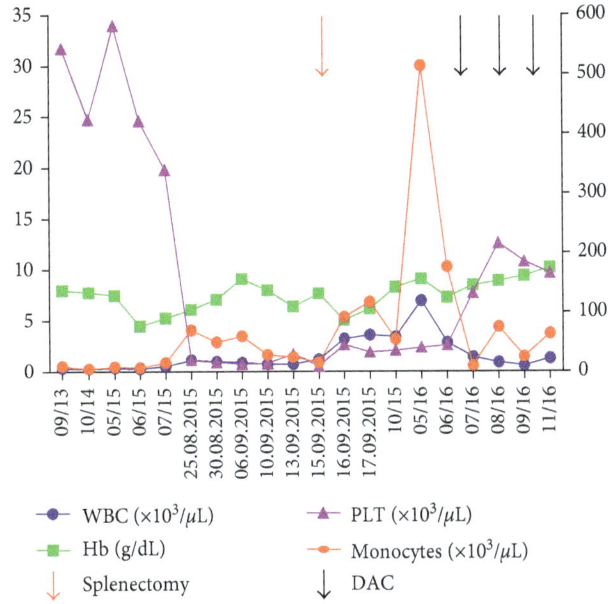

Figure 3: Blood counts of the patient during chronic treatment with prednisone and cyclophosphamide to MCD and conservative treatment with DAC. WBC and PLT used right-sided y-axis, while left-sided y-axis was used for Hb and monocytes.

3. Discussion

MCD is a rare nonmalignant lymphoproliferative disorder, and the population incidence has not been established. Little is known about the clinical abnormalities, disease associations, treatments, and outcomes. Systemic manifestations such as fever, night sweats, fatigue, anemia, and multifocal lymphadenopathy appear as a result of excessive IL-6 and other proinflammatory cytokines [2, 4]. Three treatment strategies have been used based on our understanding of MCD: anti-inflammatory and immunosuppressive therapies, cytotoxic elimination of cells responsible for hypercytokinemia, and blockade of IL-6 signaling with mAbs [5–7]. In addition, glucocorticoids have frequently been used in MCD. The response rate is usually high (60–70%), but symptoms typically recur with decreasing dose. Autologous stem cell transplantation has been successful in challenging cases [8]. Recently, one study found that multicentricity, histopathological type, and anemia are significant risk factors for shortened progression-free survival [9]. This case just only received monotherapy chemotherapy and prednisone and got long survival.

The current diagnostic criteria of CMML have recently been updated by the 2016 WHO classification. Persistent monocytosis defined both as an absolute count > 1,000/μL and as a proportion > 10% of WBC count is the cornerstone of diagnosis. CMML has a tendency to transform to acute myeloid leukemia (AML). Given the overlap with MDS and MPN, management and response evaluation for patients with CMML is often extrapolated from these diseases. However, internationally validated treatment algorithms for CMML are still lacking, and treatment remains loosely codified. The hypomethylating agents (HMA) azacitidine (AZA) and DAC seem active in CMML, though they have mostly been explored retrospectively, reporting overall response rates in the 40–70% range [10, 11]. For this case, the management of cytopenias is similar to that for MDS based on the MDS-like features and had a good response for DAC.

To our knowledge, there have been some studies founding that subjects with CMML have a high prevalence of chronic inflammatory or autoimmune disorders, especially systemic vasculitis, connective tissue diseases, and immune thrombocytopenia (ITP) [12–14]. This is in line with chronic inflammation acting as a trigger and driver of clonal evolution in CMML, implying an increased risk of CMML in patients with inflammatory and/or autoimmune diseases [15]. The reasons for this increased risk are unknown but may be due to immune deregulation with aberrant immune responses and impaired tumor immune surveillance.

MCD has an inherent tendency to progress to lymphoma, and the driving molecular aberrations involved in transformation remain obscure [16, 17]. Autoimmune manifestations and the discovery of autoreactive T cells and pathogenic autoantibodies in MCD patients would support it being an autoimmune disorder [1, 3]. However, it has been widely recognized that CMML is complicated with various types of autoimmune disorders. From these results, it was highly likely that Castleman disease is the underlying disease which triggers CMML for immune factors. Success in the setting of autoimmune dysfunction and thrombocytopenia has resulted in off-label use of the agents for patients with CMML, which verify our assumption in some ways. Alternatively, a study on therapy-related CMML concludes that chemotherapy and radiation are risk factors for the development of CMML. Therefore, we could not rule out in this case that chemotherapy is a risk factor for the development of CMML.

In summary, we report a rare case of MCD subsequently founding to have CMML, who responded with repeated long-lasting remissions to prednisone and decitabine therapy. Moreover, the findings in our study suggest a causal association between MCD and subsequent development of CMML for chronic inflammation/autoimmunity. The intrinsic immune pathogenesis of this unusual phenomenon remains to be further investigated.

Conflicts of Interest

The authors declare no conflicts of interest.

Authors' Contributions

Feng Li and Xiaomei Zhang contributed equally to this work.

References

[1] D. C. Fajgenbaum, F. van Rhee, and C. S. Nabel, "HHV-8-negative, idiopathic multicentric Castleman disease: novel insights into biology, pathogenesis, and therapy," *Blood*, vol. 123, no. 19, pp. 2924–2933, 2014.

[2] H. Kawabata, N. Kadowaki, M. Nishikori et al., "Clinical features and treatment of multicentric Castleman's disease : a retrospective study of 21 Japanese patients at a single institute," *Journal of Clinical and Experimental Hematopathology*, vol. 53, no. 1, pp. 69–77, 2013.

[3] F. van Rhee, K. Stone, S. Szmania, B. Barlogie, and Z. Singh, "Castleman disease in the 21st century: an update on diagnosis, assessment, and therapy," *Clinical Advances in Hematology and Oncology*, vol. 8, no. 7, pp. 486–498, 2010.

[4] D. M. P. Cronin and R. A. Warnke, "Castleman disease: an update on classification and the spectrum of associated lesions," *Advances in Anatomic Pathology*, vol. 16, no. 4, pp. 236–246, 2009.

[5] T. W. Muskardin, B. A. Peterson, and J. A. Molitor, "Castleman disease and associated autoimmune disease," *Current Opinion in Rheumatology*, vol. 24, no. 1, pp. 76–83, 2012.

[6] A. Gonzalez Garcia, M. A. Moreno Cobo, and J. L. Patier de la Pena, "Current diagnosis and treatment of Castleman's disease," *Revista Clinica Espanola*, vol. 216, no. 3, pp. 146–156, 2016.

[7] H. E. El-Osta and R. Kurzrock, "Castleman's disease: from basic mechanisms to molecular therapeutics," *Oncologist*, vol. 16, no. 4, pp. 497–511, 2011.

[8] Y. Tal, G. Haber, M. J. Cohen et al., "Autologous stem cell transplantation in a rare multicentric Castleman disease of the plasma cell variant," *International Journal of Hematology*, vol. 93, no. 5, pp. 677–680, 2011.

[9] L. Yu, M. Tu, J. Cortes et al., "Clinical and pathological characteristics of HIV- and HHV-8-negative Castleman disease," *Blood*, vol. 129, no. 12, pp. 1658–1668, 2017.

[10] L. Ades, M. A. Sekeres, A. Wolfromm et al., "Predictive factors of response and survival among chronic myelomonocytic leukemia patients treated with azacitidine," *Leukemia Research*, vol. 37, no. 6, pp. 609–613, 2013.

[11] A. Alfonso, G. Montalban-Bravo, K. Takahashi et al., "Natural history of chronic myelomonocytic leukemia treated with hypomethylating agents," *American Journal of Hematology*, vol. 92, no. 7, pp. 599–606, 2017.

[12] D. Peker, E. Padron, J. M. Bennett et al., "A close association of autoimmune-mediated processes and autoimmune disorders with chronic myelomonocytic leukemia: observation from a single institution," *Acta Haematologica*, vol. 133, no. 2, pp. 249–256, 2015.

[13] E. Grignano, A. Mekinian, T. Braun et al., "Autoimmune and inflammatory diseases associated with chronic myelomonocytic leukemia: a series of 26 cases and literature review," *Leukemia Research*, vol. 47, pp. 136–141, 2016.

[14] J. Hadjadj, M. Michel, M. P. Chauveheid et al., "Immune thrombocytopenia in chronic myelomonocytic leukemia," *European Journal of Haematology*, vol. 93, no. 6, pp. 521–526, 2014.

[15] M. V. Elbaek, A. L. Sorensen, and H. C. Hasselbalch, "Chronic inflammation and autoimmunity as risk factors for the development of chronic myelomonocytic leukemia?," *Leukemia and Lymphoma*, vol. 57, no. 8, pp. 1793–1799, 2016.

[16] S. Haque and R. van Kirk, "Three patients with both Hodgkin's lymphoma and Castleman's disease: clinicopathologic correlations and lack of association with HHV-8," *Indian Journal of Medical and Paediatric Oncology: Official Journal of Indian Society of Medical & Paediatric Oncology*, vol. 30, no. 2, pp. 76–79, 2009.

[17] U. Zanetto, F. P. Pagani, and C. Perez, "Interfollicular Hodgkin's lymphoma and Castleman's disease," *Histopathology*, vol. 48, no. 3, pp. 317–319, 2006.

19

Coexistent Breast Cancer and Essential Thrombocythemia: How we Addressed the Therapeutic Challenges

Karan Seegobin,[1] **Bharatsinh Gharia**,[2] **Satish Maharaj**,[1] **and Lara Zuberi**[2]

[1] *Department of Internal Medicine, University of Florida College of Medicine, Jacksonville, FL 32209, USA*
[2] *Department of Hematology and Oncology, University of Florida College of Medicine, Jacksonville, FL 32209, USA*

Correspondence should be addressed to Karan Seegobin; karanseegobin@hotmail.com

Academic Editor: Sergio Storti

Essential thrombocythemia (ET) occurring with breast cancer is uncommon; the therapeutic approach varies and poses a challenge. A 65-year-old female presented to us after being diagnosed with hormone positive, HER2-negative infiltrating ductal carcinoma. She had a platelet count of 600 thou/cu mm. Her JAK2 mutation was positive. Bone marrow biopsy showed increased megakaryocytes. She was diagnosed with ET in the setting of breast cancer. She underwent breast conservation surgery after which aspirin was resumed. Anticipating thrombocytopenia during chemotherapy and given the absence of data combining hydroxyurea with standard chemotherapy used for breast cancer, we felt it prudent to delay cytoreductive therapy for her ET until after completion of breast cancer treatment. Her average platelet count during chemotherapy was 480 thou/cu mm with the lowest being 377 thou/cu mm. Her platelet count remained at goal between 300 and 350 thou/cu mm after four months of hydroxyurea.

1. Background

Essential thrombocythemia (ET) is a myeloproliferative neoplasm (MPN) [1]. Patients with this condition have an increased risk to develop a second cancer including both haematological [2] and nonhaematological [2, 3] risks. However, breast cancer in the MPN population is not increased in comparison with the general population [4]. Physicians are faced with several therapeutic challenges when ET coexists with another tumour, in particular solid tumours. These should be managed on an individual basis. Physicians should take into consideration the risk of thrombosis, characteristics of the cancer, and the therapeutic approach for the tumour whether surgical, chemotherapy, or both.

2. Case

A 65-year-old female presented with a breast lump, diagnosed to be oestrogen and progesterone receptor positive, HER2 negative, and T1cN1bM0 moderately differentiated infiltrating ductal carcinoma. She had a platelet count of 600 thou/cu mm. There was no history of thrombotic or bleeding episodes.

Further testing showed that JAK2 mutation was positive and t(9;22) mutation was negative. Her bone marrow biopsy showed increased megakaryocytes. Her other lab workup was unremarkable including iron panel and liver function tests. She had no splenomegaly on ultrasound. She was diagnosed with ET in the setting of breast cancer.

Aspirin was commenced but held seven days prior to her breast conservation surgery, restarted postoperatively and continued thereafter. Postoperative thromboprophylaxis with low-molecular weight heparin (LMWH) was continued until the patient was fully ambulatory. Aspirin was restarted on day 7 after the surgery. Anticipating thrombocytopenia during chemotherapy, and given the absence of data combining hydroxyurea with standard chemotherapy used for breast cancer (in this case docetaxel and cyclophosphamide), we felt it prudent to delay cytoreductive therapy for her ET until after completion of breast cancer treatment. Her indication for cytoreductive therapy was >60 years. She was treated with adjuvant docetaxel and cyclophosphamide and continued on aspirin 81 mg for the entire duration of her chemotherapy. She tolerated the 6 cycles of chemotherapy well.

Following the completion of her chemotherapy, she was started on letrozole and radiotherapy with the aim to continue the letrozole for 5 years. Hydroxyurea (500 mg) was also started and titrated to a goal to 400–450 thou/cu mm platelets. Zoledronic acid was started for osteoporosis prevention.

Her average platelet count during chemotherapy was 480 thou/cu mm with the lowest being 377 thou/cu mm (Table 1). Her platelet count remained at goal between 300 and 350 thou/cu mm after four months of hydroxyurea (Table 2). Throughout her treatment, there were no bleeding or thrombotic complications. After one year on letrozole, hydroxyurea, and aspirin, the patient was doing well without complications with platelet counts at goal.

3. Discussion

ET is a myeloproliferative neoplasm and is unique among them because of its natural history, which is compatible with a normal lifespan [1]. It is diagnosed by having platelets more than 450 thou/cu mm in the absence of reactive cause, absence of iron deficiency, presence of JAK2 V617F assay, and haemoglobin less than 14 g/dL in women in the absence of splenomegaly [1, 5]. It is a diagnosis of exclusion, representing clonal or autonomous thrombocytosis not classifiable as any of the following diseases: polycythaemia vera, primary myelofibrosis, chronic myeloid leukaemia, or myelodysplastic syndrome [1]. By this criterion, our patient was diagnosed. Other mutations associated with ET are CALR and MPL which carry prognostic significance [6].

Patients with ET have an increased risk to develop a second cancer, with both haematological and non-haematological cancers being reported [2].

All patients are managed with aspirin provided there exists no contraindications [7]. It has been shown to reduce the risk of arterial and venous thrombosis in low-risk patients [8]. The indications for cytoreductive therapy include those with a history of thrombosis or age greater than 60 years [7]. The degree of thrombocytosis has not been shown to be a reliable indicator of thrombotic risk [7]. Patients with JAK 2 positivity has been shown to have a greater chance of arterial and venous thrombosis [7]. Hydroxyurea is the only cytoreductive agent proven to reduce thrombotic events in a randomized controlled trial and is the first-line cytoreductive agent [9].

The goal of cytoreductive therapy is to resolve symptoms and normalize the platelet count [7].

Although perioperative thrombotic and bleeding complications appear increased in ET patients, it is not clear whether this can be ameliorated by therapeutic intervention [10]. The management is difficult because there are no definite guidelines available in the literature discussing this issue [11].

Determining the method of cytoreduction is a challenge, as it is important to achieve a balance between such dangerous postoperative complications as vascular thrombosis and excessive haemorrhage [11]. In one report, hydroxyurea was the drug of choice to achieve effective cytoreduction in patients with symptoms of ET—who are intended to undergo cardiac surgery [11]. For patients receiving cytoreductive therapy who are undergoing elective surgery, the blood count is optimized preoperatively, and interruptions in therapy are kept to a minimum [7]. Postoperative thromboprophylaxis is recommended according to usual guidelines for the specific procedure [7]. For patients not receiving cytoreductive treatment, temporary therapy is considered on a case-by-case basis, after assessment of the patient's thrombotic risk profile, degree of thrombocytosis, and the nature of the surgery [7].

Other malignancies such as tongue cancer, gastric cancer, and colon cancer have been reported in the setting of ET [12–14]. ET is likely a coincidental finding in this breast cancer case.

Thrombocytopenia is a well-known side effect of chemotherapy [15, 16]. Considering this, we completed the course of chemotherapy prior to starting hydroxyurea for the patient's essential thrombocythemia. As expected, our patient's platelets counts had a downward trend during her course of chemotherapy.

One study conducted on low-risk ET patients showed that antiplatelet therapy reduces the incidence of venous thrombosis in JAK2-mutated patients and the rate of arterial thrombosis in those with cardiovascular risk factors [8]. Aspirin was continued during her chemotherapy treatment, and the patient was monitored closely for bleeding complications. Hydroxyurea was not started during chemotherapy as she did not have a history of thrombotic complications, and we expected her platelet count to drop during the chemotherapy treatment. She did not suffer from thrombotic or bleeding complications during her chemotherapy treatment. A decision to institute cytoreductive therapy should be based on an individual basis.

Survival of ET patients does not substantially differ from that of the general population [17]. On the contrary, the outlook for women with breast cancer varies by the stage of cancer [18]. In general, the survival rates are higher for women with earlier stage cancers [18]. The outlook for each woman is specific to her circumstances [18]. The 5-year relative survival rate for women with stage 0 or stage I breast cancer is close to 100% [18]. For women with stage II breast cancer, the 5-year relative survival rate is about 93% [18]. ET and breast cancer are two malignant disorders with favourable outcomes, and therefore, treatment for one should not preclude treatment for the other.

It is important to recall that letrozole and other aromatase inhibitors can increase the risk of venous thromboembolism (VTE) [19]. Furthermore, in our patient, ET increases her risk for VTE, thus the importance of hydroxyurea to keep platelets at goal cannot be overstated. We have not found any cases of adverse drug interactions between letrozole and hydroxyurea. Furthermore, our patient has been doing well without any adverse effects of such drug

Table 1: Complete blood count (CBC) before, during, and after chemotherapy.

CBC	Before chemotherapy	After 4 cycles of chemotherapy	After 5 cycles of chemotherapy	After 6 cycles of chemotherapy	Two months after completion of chemotherapy
White cell count ($\times 10^3/\mu L$)	6	3	3	6	7
Haemoglobin (g/dL)	13	12	12	13	12
Platelet (thou/cu mm)	631	592	497	377	457

Table 2: Complete blood count after hydroxyurea.

CBC	Two months after starting hydroxyurea	Four months after starting hydroxyurea
White cell count ($\times 10^3/\mu L$)	7	6
Haemoglobin (g/dL)	12	12
Platelet (thou/cu mm)	326	325

combinations. Solid tumours and chemotherapy both increase risk of blood clots [20, 21]. VTE is one of the causes of mortality reported in patients on chemotherapy, though this is less likely in an early stage cancer with low disease burden [21]. In our patient, the risk of VTE from her early stage breast cancer and chemotherapy would likely compound the risk from the underlying myeloproliferative neoplasm, so it is likely essential to counsel these patients on reducing risk by optimizing mobility. Additionally, antithrombotic prophylaxis should be considered during chemotherapy. While it is not routinely recommended in the outpatient setting, it should be considered for high risk patients [22]. The current guidelines indicate that low-molecular weight heparin is the first choice [22]. In our case, we continued postoperative VTE prophylaxis until the patient was fully ambulant; however, every case should be reviewed in a holistic way with consideration given to extending VTE prophylaxis if required. In patients undergoing major abdominal or pelvic surgery with high-risk features, VTE prophylaxis is recommended up to 4 weeks and in other cases, extended up to 6 months [22]. These patients should be periodically reassessed at each follow-up visit to review their risk for VTE [22].

4. Conclusion

(i) Physicians are faced with several therapeutic challenges when ET coexists with solid tumours.

(ii) These should be managed on an individual basis.

(iii) One should take into consideration the risk of thrombosis and the therapeutic approach for solid tumours in the management of these patients.

(iv) Extended VTE prophylaxis during chemotherapy may be needed in select cases.

(v) ET and breast cancer both have favourable outcomes, and therefore, treatment for one should not preclude treatment for the other.

Conflicts of Interest

The authors declare that they have no conflicts of interest.

Authors' Contributions

The idea for reporting this case was that of Lara Zuberi. Further intellectual content and editing was done by all authors. All authors read, edited, and approved the final contents. Karan Seegobin took responsibility for the integrity of the contents.

References

[1] J. L. Spivak and R. T. Silver, "The revised World Health Organization diagnostic criteria for polycythemia vera, essential thrombocytosis, and primary myelofibrosis: an alternativeproposal," *Blood*, vol. 112, no. 2, pp. 231–239, 2008.

[2] H. C. Hasselbalch, "Perspectives on the increased risk of second cancer in patients with essential thrombocythemia, polycythemia vera and myelofibrosis," *European Journal of Haematology*, vol. 94, no. 2, pp. 96–98, 2015.

[3] L. Masarova, M. Cherry, K. J. Newberry et al., "Secondary solid tumors and lymphoma in patients with essential thrombocythemia and polycythemia vera—single center experience," *Leukemia & Lymphoma*, vol. 57, no. 1, pp. 237–239, 2016.

[4] A. R. Landtblom, H. Bower, T. M. Andersson et al., "Second malignancies in patients with myeloproliferative neoplasms: a population-based cohort study of 9379 patients," *Leukemia*, 2018.

[5] D. A. Arber, A. Orazi, R. Hasserjian et al., "The 2016 revision to the World Health Organization classification of myeloid neoplasms and acute leukemia," *Blood*, vol. 127, no. 20, pp. 2391–2405, 2016.

[6] J. Asp, B. Andréasson, U. Hansson et al., "Mutation status of essential thrombocythemia and primary myelofibrosis defines clinical outcome," *Haematologica*, vol. 101, no. 4, pp. e129–e132, 2016.

[7] P. A. Beer, W. N. Erber, P. J. Campbell, and A. R. Green, "How I treat essential thrombocythemia," *Blood*, vol. 117, no. 5, pp. 1472–1482, 2011.

[8] E. Rumi and M. Cazzola, "How I treat essential thrombocythemia," *Blood*, vol. 128, no. 20, pp. 2403–2414, 2016.

[9] S. Cortelazzo, G. Finazzi, M. Ruggeri et al., "Hydroxyurea for patients with essential thrombocythemia and a high risk of thrombosis," *New England Journal of Medicine*, vol. 332, no. 17, pp. 1132–1137, 1995.

[10] M. Ruggeri, F. Rodeghiero, A. Tosetto et al., "Postsurgery outcomes in patients with polycythemia vera and essential thrombocythemia: a retrospective survey," *Blood*, vol. 111, no. 2, pp. 666–671, 2008.

[11] E. Ziadinov, H. Al-Sabti, M. Al-Toubi, and M. S. Siddiqi, "Pretreatment with hydroxyurea of the patient with essential thrombocythemia followed by coronary artery bypass surgery," *Oman Medical Journal*, vol. 29, no. 4, pp. 294-295, 2014.

[12] R. G. Mihăilă, S. Marchian, and R. Mihăilă, "A rare case of thrombocytosis with duble malignant etiology—pathogenetic interrelationships and consequences," *Scholars Journal of Medical Case Reports*, vol. 3, no. 8, pp. 684–686, 2015.

[13] H. Kondo, Y. Sakai, and T. Takaso, "Coexistence of essential thrombocythemia and gastric cancer," *Rinsho Ketsueki*, vol. 34, no. 2, pp. 224–228, 1993.

[14] E. Kondo, M. Ueda, T. Yamashita, Y. Nakajima, S. Rin, and M. Fujita, "Therapeutic experience with tongue cancer in a patient who had essential thrombocythemia: a case report," *Japanese Journal of Oral and Maxillofacial Surgery*, vol. 58, no. 3, pp. 123–127, 2012.

[15] J. Puente, E. Grande, A. Medina, P. Maroto, N. Lainez, and J. A. Arranz, "Docetaxel in prostate cancer: a familiar face as the new standard in a hormone-sensitive setting," *Therapeutic Advances in Medical Oncology*, vol. 9, no. 5, pp. 307–318, 2017.

[16] A. L Hepburn, S. Narat, and J. C. Mason, "The management of peripheral blood cytopenias in systemic lupus erythematosus," *Rheumatology*, vol. 49, no. 12, pp. 2243–2254, 2010.

[17] F. Cervantes, "Management of essential thrombocythemia," *Hematology*, vol. 2011, no. 1, pp. 215–221, 2011.

[18] American Cancer Society, *Breast Cancer Facts & Figures 2015-2016*, American Cancer Society, Inc., Atlanta, GA, USA, 2015.

[19] J.-M. A. Nabholtz, "Long-term safety of aromatase inhibitors in the treatment of breast cancer," *Therapeutics and Clinical Risk Management*, vol. 4, no. 1, pp. 189–204, 2008.

[20] S. Sallah, J. Y. Wan, and N. P. Nguyen, "Venous thrombosis in patients with solid tumors: determination of frequency and characteristics," *Thrombosis and Haemostasis*, vol. 87, no. 04, pp. 575–579, 2002.

[21] G. J. Caine, P. S. Stonelake, G. Y. H. Lip, and S. T. Kehoe, "The hypercoagulable state of malignancy: pathogenesis and current debate," *Neoplasia*, vol. 4, no. 6, pp. 465–473, 2002.

[22] G. H. Lyman, K. Bohlke, A. A. Khorana et al., "Venous thromboembolism prophylaxis and treatment in patients with cancer: American Society of Clinical Oncology clinical practice guideline update 2014," *Journal of Clinical Oncology*, vol. 33, no. 6, pp. 654–656, 2015.

20

EBV-Associated Lymphoproliferative Disorder and Hemophagocytic Lymphohistiocytosis in a Patient with Severe Celiac Disease

John Jacob Kinross-Wright,[1] Kalyan Chakravarthy Potu,[1] Brandy Pownell,[2] Randall Lamfers,[1] and Jonathan S. Bleeker[3]

[1]*Department of Internal Medicine, Sanford USD School of Medicine, Sioux Falls, SD, USA*
[2]*Department of Pathology, Sanford USD School of Medicine, Sioux Falls, SD, USA*
[3]*Division of Hematology and Oncology, Sanford USD School of Medicine, Sioux Falls, SD, USA*

Correspondence should be addressed to Jonathan S. Bleeker; jonathan.bleeker@sanfordhealth.org

Academic Editor: Simon Davidson

Background. Epstein-Barr virus- (EBV-) associated lymphoproliferative disease (LPD) is a rare condition, usually occurring in immunocompromised patients. We report a case of EBV-associated LPD in a patient with severe celiac disease, the first report to describe this syndrome in a patient with this diagnosis. *Case Summary.* A 69-year-old Caucasian woman with recent diagnosis of celiac sprue presented to our hospital with persistent diarrhea, abdominal pain, weight loss, and fatigue despite adherence to gluten-free diet for a number of weeks prior to presentation. She underwent evaluation for occult malignancy and was found to have diffuse intra-abdominal mesenteric lymphadenopathy on CT scan. Biopsy of mesenteric nodes revealed an EBV positive, CD20 positive mixed lymphoproliferative process with T-cell predominance, but without a monoclonal cell population felt to be consistent with EBV-associated LPD. Bone marrow biopsy revealed hemophagocytic lymphohistiocytosis, complicating her course. She was treated with steroids and rituximab but continued to decline, eventually developing MSSA bacteremia and succumbing to her disease. *Conclusion.* To our knowledge, this is the first report of the constellation of celiac sprue, EBV-associated LPD, and hemophagocytic lymphohistiocytosis. Providers caring for patients with severe, uncontrolled celiac disease and adenopathy should consider EBV-associated LPD.

1. Introduction

Epstein-Barr virus (EBV), also called human herpes virus 4 (HHV-4), is one of the eight known human herpes viruses [1]. It was discovered in 1964 by electron microscopy of African Burkitt lymphoma cells [2]. Antibodies to EBV have been demonstrated in all population groups worldwide; approximately 90 percent of adults worldwide are EBV-seropositive [3].

The majority of EBV infections are subclinical [3]. Infectious mononucleosis is the most common clinical manifestation of EBV infection [4]. Epstein-Barr virus (EBV) has been implicated in the pathogenesis of B-cell lymphomas, T-cell lymphomas, Hodgkin lymphoma, and nasopharyngeal carcinomas and has associated with the development of EBV-associated lymphoproliferative disorders (LPD) as well. EBV-associated LPD occur in a spectrum, ranging from polyclonal B-cell proliferation to clonal, malignant B-cell lymphoma and most commonly occur in immunocompromised patients, especially in posttransplant and HIV-positive patients. [3, 5, 6] EBV-associated LPD are increasingly being recognized in the elderly population as well, likely due to age-related immunosenescence [7]. However, the constellation of celiac sprue, EBV-associated LPD, and hemophagocytic lymphohistiocytosis is unique in the literature.

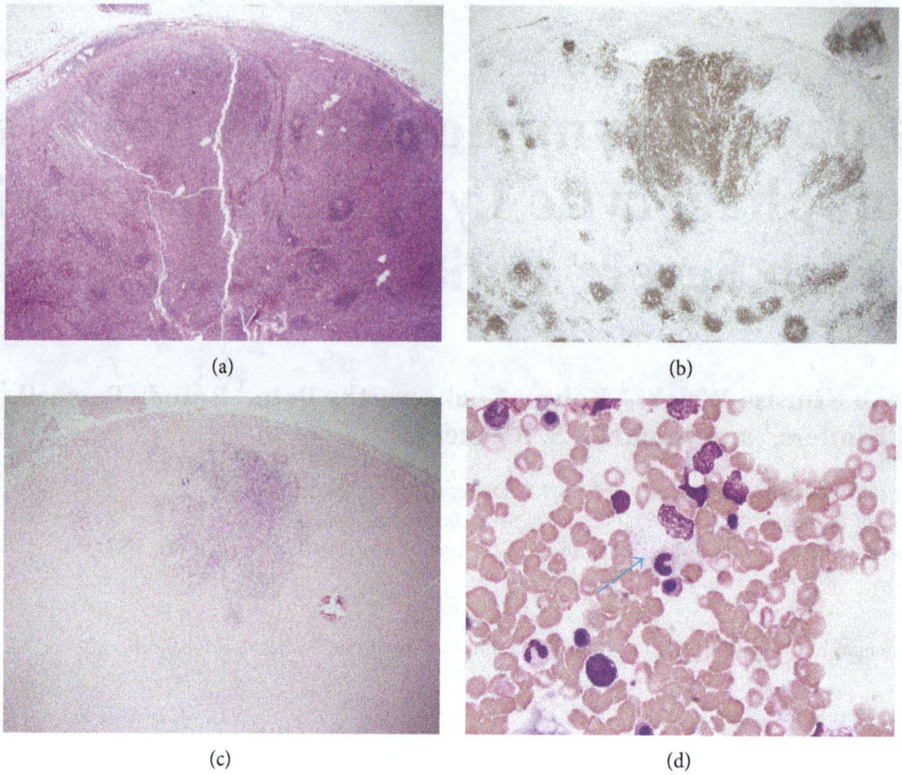

Figure 1: (a) Hematoxylin and eosin (H&E) stained mesenteric lymph node reveals effacement of nodal architecture by paracortical expansion of an atypical lymphoid population. Scattered small lymphoid follicles are noted (2x). (b) A CD20 immunohistochemical stain highlights sheets of monotonous, medium-sized cells, identifying the cells as B-lymphocytes (2x). (c) EBER, a nuclear stain for EBV-encoded RNA, is expressed by the B-lymphocyte population and scattered throughout the paracortical expansion, suggesting an EBV-related lymphoproliferative disorder (2x). (d) H&E staining of the bone marrow aspirate shows a hemophagocytic histiocyte (arrow), which contains a leukocyte and appears to be in the process of engulfing a red blood cell (100x).

2. Case Report

A 69-year-old Caucasian female with recently diagnosed celiac sprue presented with fever, nausea, abdominal pain, diarrhea, and weight loss despite adherence to a gluten-free diet. Past medical history included hypothyroidism, hypertension, and atrial fibrillation. She initially presented to an outside facility several months prior to presentation to our facility where she had a small bowel biopsy showing villous blunting consistent with celiac sprue as well as positive autoantibodies for gliadin and tissue transglutaminase. She was started on a gluten-free diet and discharged. Despite adhering to the gluten-free diet, she lost approximately 15 pounds over the month prior to presentation at our facility.

Given persistent symptoms, she was admitted to our institution, where initial blood work noted pancytopenia, elevated serum ferritin, elevated serum triglycerides, and low serum fibrinogen, raising clinical concern for hemophagocytic lymphohistiocytosis (HLH). Computed tomography (CT) of the chest, abdomen, and pelvis noted extensive lymphadenopathy throughout the abdomen with the largest nodes including a 2.9 cm mesenteric node in the left abdomen, a 2.4 cm node near the left iliac crest, and a 3.4 cm mass adjacent to the cecum.

A needle biopsy of an intra-abdominal lymph node demonstrated a lymphoproliferative process, with a predominance of CD4-positive T-lymphocytes. Following needle biopsy, an excisional biopsy was obtained revealing a polymorphic-type EBV-positive lymphoproliferation with extensive paracortical T-cell hyperplasia. The paracortical expansion was comprised of predominantly CD4-positive polymorphic T cells that stained positively for CD2, CD3, and CD5, with partial loss of CD7 (Figure 1(a)). A monotonous population of CD20-positive B cells was also identified that coexpress MUM-1 and was positive for EBER (Epstein-Barr virus encoded messenger RNA) (Figures 1(b) and 1(c)). T-cell receptor gene rearrangement studies by PCR were not performed; however, gene rearrangement studies for TCR-gamma/delta and TCR-betaF1 by immunohistochemistry were performed. TCR-betaF1 was positive in the polymorphic T-cell population within the paracortical expansion. TCR-gamma/delta stained a small subset of T cells. The final diagnosis was a CD20-positive, EBV-positive lymphoproliferative disorder, which did not meet criteria for frank lymphoma and was not monoclonal in nature.

Following the diagnosis of EBV-associated LPD, peripheral blood EBV DNA quantitation via PCR was markedly positive at 9367 copies/mL (<200 copies/mL); to our knowledge, the patient's EBV status was unknown until this point. Subsequent bone marrow biopsy was performed to further evaluate her pancytopenia. This revealed marked hemophagocytic changes consistent with HLH (Figure 1(d)). She was started on a course of rituximab and methylprednisolone for EBV-associated LPD with HLH. She subsequently developed methicillin-sensitive *Staphylococcus aureus (MSSA)* bacteremia, further worsening her clinical status. Following development of bacteremia, the patient and her family decided to pursue comfort care, and she succumbed while receiving comfort cares 25 days after initial presentation to our hospital.

3. Discussion

We describe a case of EBV-associated LPD, a rare disorder which typically occurs in immunocompromised patients and has been most commonly described in posttransplant and HIV-positive patients. To our knowledge, this is the first case report to describe EBV-associated LPD disorder associated with celiac disease.

Celiac disease has been associated with many different subtypes of lymphoma [8, 9], although lymphoma remains an uncommon complication in this population. Enteropathy-associated T-cell lymphoma (EATL) is a distinct lymphoma subtype highly associated with celiac disease, although B-cell lymphoma in association with celiac disease has also been described [10]. Patients with celiac-associated B cell lymphoma may have a better prognosis than those with EATL [11].

To our knowledge, EBV-associated LPD has not been described in a patient with celiac disease, although EBV has been implicated in some cases of EATL [10] and active EBV has been detected in small bowel biopsies in up to 70% of patients with refractory celiac disease [12]. In this case, the strength of the link between the diagnosis of celiac disease and the EBV-associated LPD is somewhat difficult to discern, as the patient also had multiple other factors potentially causing relative immunosuppression including malnutrition secondary to celiac disease as well as age-related immunosenescence, but this case should alert clinicians to the possibility of EBV-associated LPD when presented with a patient with celiac disease and associated adenopathy concerning for lymphoma.

In patients with early, nonclonal EBV-associated LPD on immunosuppression either following solid organ transplant or due to a chronic autoimmune condition, modulation of immunosuppression is the initial management recommendation. Modulation of immunosuppressive therapy induces tumor regression in 25%–50% of patients [13–15]. In patients with a polyclonal EBV-associated LPD, rituximab is often added to modulation of immunosuppression [16, 17], as rituximab is generally well tolerated and rapidly depletes mature B-lymphocytes, the major reservoir of EBV [18]. In patients with monoclonal EBV-associated LPD or disease refractory to rituximab and modulation of immunosuppression, rituximab is typically combined with chemotherapy directed at the particular lymphoma subtype described [17]. In this case, given her frail state at diagnosis and patient hesitance regarding more aggressive therapy, treatment with rituximab was combined with high dose steroids as opposed to multiagent chemotherapy. Unfortunately, the patient developed a significant infectious complication and succumbed to her disease prior to an opportunity to assess her response to the above therapy.

Another confounding feature of this case is the concurrent diagnosis of HLH. HLH has been well described in concert with both B-cell lymphomas [19] and EBV infection [20] as a trigger for HLH. Our patient met 5/8 of the diagnostic criteria for HLH (fever, pancytopenia, hypertriglyceridemia, elevated serum ferritin, and hemophagocytosis on histopathological examination of bone marrow) [21]. Serum soluble IL2 receptor level was not checked as our patient already met the diagnostic criteria for HLH. The treatment regimen of HLH is chemo-immunotherapy based with the most commonly used regimen being etoposide, cyclosporin A, and dexamethasone [22]. Rituximab is also commonly utilized in the treatment of EBV-associated HLH [21].

In conclusion, we represent a case of EBV-associated LPD occurring in a patient with refractory celiac disease complicated by hemophagocytic lymphohistiocytosis. This case demonstrates the difficulty in diagnosis and management of EBV-associated LPD and will hopefully lead to increased awareness of this possible diagnosis amongst clinicians treating patients with refractory celiac disease.

Consent

Consent could not be obtained from the patient as she is deceased. The authors were able to obtain consent to publish from the patient's husband who is next of kin. The authors have made every effort to ensure patient anonymity. There is no reason to believe that the patient would have objected to publication.

Conflicts of Interest

The authors declare that there are no conflicts of interest regarding the publication of this article.

Authors' Contributions

John Jacob Kinross-Wright, Randall Lamfers, and Jonathan S. Bleeker were involved in managing the patient. John Jacob Kinross-Wright and Kalyan Chakravarthy Potu conducted the literature search and wrote the first draft. Brandy Pownell made the pathological diagnosis. Randall Lamfers and Jonathan S. Bleeker edited the manuscript. All authors read and approved the final manuscript.

Acknowledgments

The authors would like to thank the nursing staff who participated in the care of this patient and the patient's family.

References

[1] E. Kieff and A. B. Rickinson, "Epstein–Barr virus and its replication," in *Fields Virology*, D. M. Knipe, P. M. Howley,

D. E. Griffin et al, Eds., vol. 2, pp. 2603–2654, Lippincott Williams & Wilkins, Philadelphia, PA, USA, 5th edition, 2007.

[2] M. A. Epstein, B. G. Achong, and Y. M. Barr, "Virus particles in cultured lymphoblasts from Burkitt's lymphoma," *The Lancet*, vol. 283, no. 7335, pp. 702-703, 1964.

[3] J. I. Cohen, "Epstein–Barr virus infection," *New England Journal of Medicine*, vol. 343, no. 7, pp. 481–492, 2000.

[4] G. Henle, W. Henle, and V. Diehl, "Relation of Burkitt's tumor- associated herpes-type virus to infectious mononucleosis," *Proceedings of the National Academy of Sciences*, vol. 59, no. 1, pp. 94–101, 1968.

[5] O. A. Odumade, K. A. Hogquist, and H. H. Balfour Jr., "Progress and problems in understanding and managing primary Epstein–Barr virus infections," *Clinical Microbiology Reviews*, vol. 24, no. 1, pp. 193–209, 2011.

[6] L. Quintanilla-Martinez, S. Kumar, F. Fend et al., "Fulminant EBV(+) T-cell lymphoproliferative disorder following acute/chronic EBV infection: a distinct clinicopathologic syndrome," *Blood*, vol. 96, no. 2, pp. 443–451, 2000.

[7] S. D. Dojcinov, G. Venkataramn, S. Pittalug et al., "Age-related EBV-associated lymphoproliferative disorders in the Western population: a spectrum of reactive lymphoid hyperplasia and lymphoma," *Blood*, vol. 117, no. 18, pp. 4726–4735, 2011.

[8] G. K. T. Holmes, P. Prior, M. R. Lane, D. Pope, and R. N. Allan, "Malignancy in coeliac disease: effect of a gluten free diet," *Gut*, vol. 30, no. 3, pp. 333–338, 1989.

[9] C. Cellier, E. Delabesse, C. Helmer et al., "Refractory sprue, coeliac disease, and enteropathy-associated T-cell lymphoma. French Coeliac Disease Study Group," *The Lancet*, vol. 356, no. 9225, pp. 203–208, 2000.

[10] K. E. Smedby, M. Akerman, H. Hildebrand, B. Glimelius, A. Ekbom, and J. Askling, "Malignant lymphomas in coeliac disease: evidence of increased risks for lymphoma types other than enteropathy-type T cell lymphoma," *Gut*, vol. 54, no. 1, pp. 54–59, 2005.

[11] T. R. Halfdanarson, A. Rubio-Tapia, K. M. Ristow, T. M. Habermann, J. A. Murray, and D. J. Inwards, "Patients with celiac disease and B-cell lymphoma have a better prognosis than those with T-cell lymphoma," *Clinical Gastroenterology and Hepatology*, vol. 8, no. 12, pp. 1042–1047, 2010.

[12] V. Perfetti, F. Baldanti, M. V. Lenti et al., "Detection of active Epstein–Barr virus infection in duodenal mucosa of patients with refractory celiac disease," *Clinics and Research in Gastroenterology and Hepatology*, vol. 14, no. 8, pp. 1216–1220, 2016.

[13] C. V. Paya, J. J. Fung, M. A. Nalesnik et al., "Epstein–Barr virus-induced post- transplant lymphoproliferative disorders. ASTS/ASTP EBV-PTLD Task Force and The Mayo Clinic Organized International Consensus Development Meeting," *Transplantation*, vol. 68, no. 10, pp. 1517–1525, 1999.

[14] S. Choquet, V. Leblond, R. Herbrecht et al., "Efficacy and safety of rituximab in B-cell post-transplantation lymphoproliferative disorders: results of a prospective multicenter phase 2 study," *Blood*, vol. 107, no. 8, pp. 3053–3057, 2006.

[15] R. Reshef, S. Vardhanabhuti, M. R. Luskin et al., "Reduction of immunosuppression as initial therapy for posttransplantation lymphoproliferative disorder," *American Journal of Transplantation*, vol. 11, no. 2, pp. 336–347, 2011.

[16] H. Heslop, "How I treat EBV lymphoproliferation," *Blood*, vol. 114, no. 19, pp. 4002–4008, 2009.

[17] D. Direckx, T. Tousseyn, and O. Gheyens, "How I treat posttransplant lymphoproliferative disorders," *Blood*, vol. 126, no. 20, pp. 2274–2283, 2015.

[18] I. Kuehnle, M. H. Huls, Z. Liu et al., "CD20 monoclonal antibody (rituximab) for therapy of Epstein–Barr virus lymphoma after hemopoietic stem-cell transplantation," *Blood*, vol. 95, no. 4, pp. 1502–1505, 2000.

[19] M. Miyahara, M. Sano, K. Shibata et al., "B-cell lymphoma-associated hemophagocytic syndrome: clinicopathological characteristics," *Annals of Hematology*, vol. 79, no. 7, pp. 378–388, 2000.

[20] A. Filipovich, K. McClain, and A. Grom, "Histiocytic disorders: recent insights into pathophysiology and practical guidelines," *Biology of Blood and Marrow Transplantation*, vol. 16, no. 1, pp. S82–S89, 2010.

[21] J. I. Henter, A. Horne, M. Arico et al., "HLH-2004 : diagnostic and therapeutic guidelines for hemophagocytic lymphohistiocytosis," *Pediatric Blood & Cancer*, vol. 48, no. 2, pp. 124–131, 2007.

[22] E. Brisse, P. Matthys, and C. H. Wouters, "Understanding the spectrum of haemophagocytic lymphohistiocytosis: update on diagnostic challenges and therapeutic options," *British Journal of Hematology*, vol. 174, no. 2, pp. 175–187, 2016.

21

Multiple Myeloma Masquerading as Ovarian Carcinosarcoma Metastases: A Case Report and Review of the Approach to Multiple Myeloma Screening and Diagnosis

Robert Stuver[1] **Alec Petersen,**[2] **Thomas A. Guerrero-Garcia,**[3] **Ursula Matulonis,**[3] **Paul Richardson,**[3] **and Prabhsimranjot Singh**[3]

[1]Beth Israel Deaconess Medical Center, Department of Internal Medicine, 330 Brookline Avenue, Boston, MA 02215, USA
[2]Brigham and Women's Hospital, Department of Internal Medicine, 45 Francis Street, Boston, MA 02115, USA
[3]Dana Farber Cancer Institute, 450 Brookline Avenue, Boston, MA 02215, USA

Correspondence should be addressed to Robert Stuver; rnstuver@bidmc.harvard.edu

Academic Editor: Akimichi Ohsaka

Multiple myeloma is the most common plasma cell dyscrasia and causes 2% of all cancer deaths in Western countries. Ovarian carcinosarcomas are very rare gynecological malignancies and account for only 1–2% of all ovarian tumors. In this case, we report a 67-year-old woman with known relapsed ovarian carcinosarcoma who presented with headache and neck pain. She was found to have new lytic lesions in the cranial and thoracic regions. While these lesions were assumed to be metastases, a diligent approach detected an M-spike on serum protein electrophoresis and a monoclonal gammopathy with immunoglobulin G lambda monoclonal immunoglobulin on immunofixation. A bone marrow biopsy confirmed the diagnosis of multiple myeloma. To our knowledge, this is the first ever reported case of concomitant multiple myeloma and ovarian carcinosarcoma. Our case highlights the utmost importance of a systematic approach to lytic lesions and emphasizes the need to consider secondary malignancies in the evaluation of possible metastases. We used the International Myeloma Working Group guidelines for screening and diagnosing multiple myeloma, and we provide a thorough review of this updated approach.

1. Introduction

Multiple myeloma is the most common plasma cell dyscrasia and causes 2% of all cancer deaths in Western countries. Ovarian carcinosarcomas are very rare gynecological malignancies and account for only 1–2% of all ovarian tumors.

2. Case Presentation

A 67-year-old female with a history of ovarian carcinosarcoma presented to the hospital with one week of headache and neck pain.

Her malignancy had been diagnosed one year prior to presentation after she had presented to her primary care physician with abdominal pain. Radiographic imaging at that time showed a large pelvic mass, and the patient subsequently underwent radical cytoreductive surgery which included total abdominal hysterectomy, bilateral salpingo-oophorectomy, and omentectomy. Pathology showed a focal left ovarian carcinosarcoma with metastases to the right ovary, omentum, and posterior cul-de-sac. The patient underwent six cycles of carboplatin and paclitaxel.

Eight months after completion of chemotherapy, the patient presented to her oncologist with new right pelvic pain. Pelvic imaging showed a new, deep right pelvic mass, and the patient underwent surgical resection which confirmed disease recurrence. The patient was set to begin localized radiation therapy and further chemotherapy when she developed headache and neck pain and presented to the hospital.

Upon current presentation, she noted an intractable bandlike headache and neck pain. Physical examination revealed normal vital signs, a normal mental status assessment, and a nonfocal neurological examination. She had restricted range of motion at the neck and midline point tenderness in the upper thoracic spine.

Laboratory testing demonstrated a normal complete blood count, normal renal function, and normal serum electrolyte levels. Magnetic resonance imaging (MRI) of the head and spine were obtained and showed a lytic mass centered in the left clivus and occipital condyle, as well as an expansile soft tissue lesion in the T4 spinous process (Figure 1). A positron emission tomography-computed tomography (PET-CT) was also obtained (Figure 2). In the setting of known ovarian recurrence, these findings were assumed to be metastases.

However, a 1.83 g/dL M-spike (reference range: 0.80–1.70 g/dL) was detected on serum protein electrophoresis, and a monoclonal gammopathy with immunoglobulin G (IgG) lambda monoclonal immunoglobulin was seen on immunofixation. Lambda free light chains were elevated at 49.1 mg/L (reference range: 5.7–26.3 mg/L), and kappa free light chains were borderline decreased at 5.3 mg/L (reference range: 3.3–19.4 mg/L). The free kappa to free lambda ratio was abnormal at 0.12 (reference range: 0.26–1.65). No M-spike was detected on urine protein electrophoresis. A biopsy of the T4 lesion showed a plasma cell neoplasm, and a bone marrow biopsy showed a clonal population of >10%, confirming the diagnosis of multiple myeloma (Figure 3).

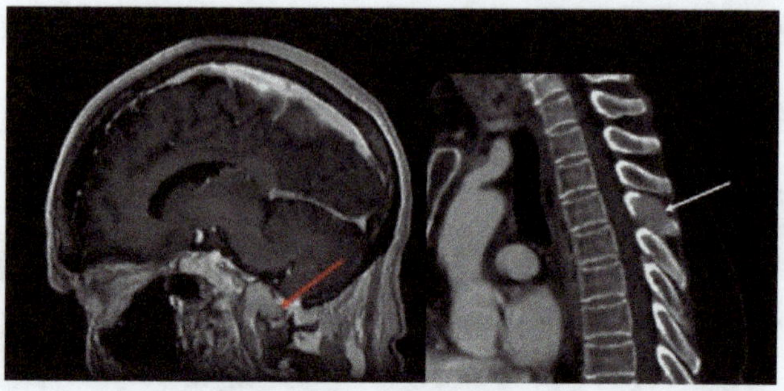

FIGURE 1: Magnetic resonance imaging (MRI) of the head and spine. MRI captured a 2.8 × 2.2 × 1.9-centimeter enhancing lytic mass centered in the left clivus and occipital condyle (red arrow). Additionally, an expansile soft tissue lesion was noted in the T4 spinous process (white arrow).

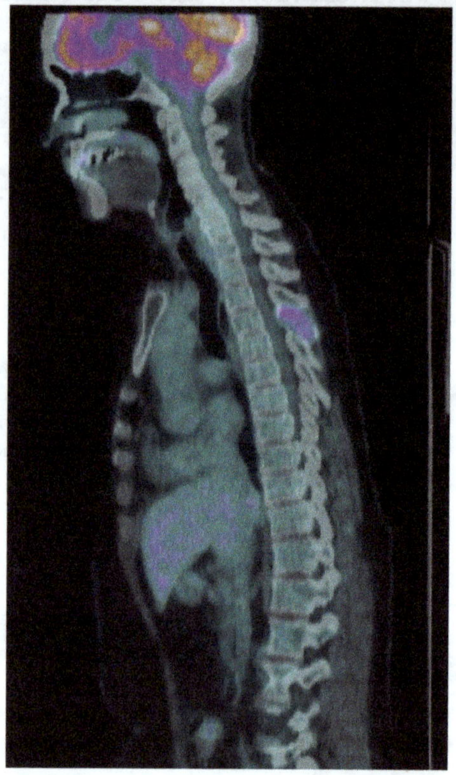

FIGURE 2: Positron emission tomography (PET). PET scan displayed a fluorodeoxyglucose (FDG)-avid lytic lesion in the left skull base where the previously noted mass on MRI was seen, as well as FDG uptake within the previously noted T4 lesion, seen here as the purple coloration within the T4 vertebral body.

3. Discussion

This case is a startling demonstration of the coexistence of a solid and liquid malignancy, and we are unaware of any other reports in the literature of a concomitant presentation of metastatic ovarian carcinosarcoma and multiple myeloma. At first, the clivus and T4 lesions were presumed to be metastases; however, due to the uncommon location of these lesions for ovarian metastases, an alternative workup was pursued, and this diligent approach allowed for the correct diagnosis. This case highlights the importance of not overlooking the possibility of secondary malignancies. Additionally, our case emphasizes the correct approach to the diagnosis of multiple myeloma and provides a platform to review this topic.

Much has changed within the last decade in regard to the recommended screening tests and formal diagnosis of multiple myeloma, and a succinct review is necessary. The preferred screening test for multiple myeloma has become the combination of serum protein electrophoresis (SPEP) and immunofixation (SIFE) with serum free light chain analysis (FLC), as recommended by the International Myeloma Working Group (IMWG) in their consensus guideline [1]. These tests should be strongly considered in any patient with lytic bone lesions of indeterminate origin. These assays rely upon excess free light chains produced by proliferating neoplastic plasma cells and the subsequent disturbance in normal free light chain ratios. Importantly, the combination of SPEP and SIFE with FLC has replaced the need for urine studies in the initial screening for plasma cell dyscrasias and is a marked change in the historical tradition of screening with protein electrophoresis and immunofixation of the serum and urine. The most important study to evaluate these screening tests and accentuate this paradigm shift was performed by Katzmann et al. [2]. This group used the Mayo Clinic plasma cell database to identify 428 patients with positive urine IFE who also had SPEP, SIFE, and FLC in their diagnostic workup. SPEP and SIFE alone would have missed the diagnosis in 28 patients (6.5%); serum FLC alone would have missed the diagnosis in 60 patients (14%); however, SIFE with FLC together identified 99.5% of

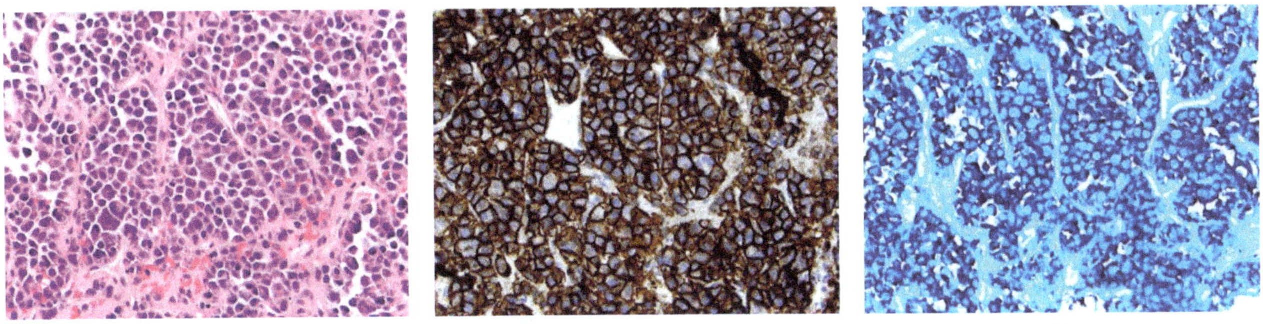

(a) (b) (c)

FIGURE 3: Bone marrow biopsy. (a) Staining with hematoxylin and eosin shows a population of abnormal plasma cells, many with binucleate and multinucleate forms. (b) Staining for CD138, a plasma marker, shows strong and diffuse positivity. (c) Fluorescence in situ hybridization (FISH) shows a monoclonal population with lambda light chain restriction, as essentially all cells are positive for lambda light chain and negative for kappa light chain.

patients with positive urine studies. Hill et al. performed a similar prospective study of 923 patients and found that no substantial pathology would have been missed by replacing urine studies with FLC as an initial screen [3]. These studies, along with several others on the matter [4–6], have led the IMWG to state that the serum FLC in combination with SPEP and SIFE yields a great enough sensitivity to negate the need for urine studies when screening for plasma cell dyscrasias [1]. Moreover, FLC has prognostic implications and has become standard in assessing treatment response, so its measurement at onset cannot be understated. This approach likely has cost benefits as well, as Katzmann et al. note that based on available Medicare reimbursement at that time, serum FLC is $31 less than urine studies ($38 as compared to $71). An important caveat to this approach is if light-chain amyloidosis is suspected, in which case urine studies should still be obtained.

Like screening, the formal diagnosis of multiple myeloma has undergone updates within the last decade that deserve attention [7]. These updates, published in 2014 by the IMWG, are largely based on improved serum and radiographic diagnostics, such as the serum FLC assay, that allow for a diagnosis of multiple myeloma before the inevitable appearance of end-organ disease. Under these criteria, a diagnosis still can be made using the historic definition of a clonal population of bone marrow plasma cells ≥10% or a biopsy-proven boney or extramedullary plasmacytoma plus evidence of end-organ damage, which remains the classic CRAB criteria—hypercalcemia, renal insufficiency, anemia, or bony lesions on skeletal radiography, CT, or PET-CT. However, diagnosis has been updated to include a clonal population of bone marrow plasma cells or a biopsy-proven boney or extramedullary plasmacytoma plus any one of the following three biomarkers of malignancy: (1) clonal bone marrow plasma cell (BMPC) percentage ≥60%, (2) involved to uninvolved serum FLC ratio ≥100%, or (3) >1 focal lesion > 5 mm on MRI.

Earlier diagnoses using the aforementioned biomarkers of malignancy have allowed for earlier application of disease-altering therapy, and therefore clinicians must be aware of these novel definitions. These biomarkers identify patients who would have previously been classified as having smouldering multiple myeloma but have a great enough probability of progression to multiple myeloma that they deserve treatment. The IMWG previously stated that if a biomarker is associated with roughly an 80% probability of progression to multiple myeloma within two years, positivity should be regarded as a diagnosis of multiple myeloma [7]. The inclusion of BMPC ≥60% as a biomarker is largely based on a review by Rajkumar et al. of 651 patients who had been given a diagnosis of smouldering multiple myeloma [8]. They found that 21 patients (3%) had a BMPC ≥60%, and 95% of these patients progressed to multiple myeloma within two years. A similar finding was reported by Kastritis et al. [9]. The inclusion of involved to uninvolved serum FLC ratio ≥100% as a biomarker is largely based on a retrospective study by Larsen et al. [10] of 586 patients with a diagnosis of smouldering multiple myeloma. They found that an involved to uninvolved serum FLC ratio ≥100% predicted a 72% risk of progression to multiple myeloma within two years. When the involved FLC was also ≥1000 milligrams per liter (mg/L), the risk increased to 82%. This led the IMWG to state that when involved to uninvolved serum FLC ratio is ≥100%, the involved FLC must also be ≥1000 mg/L to be considered a true biomarker of malignancy. Finally, the inclusion of >1 focal lesion on MRI as a biomarker is based on 2 studies that showed that more than 1 focal MRI lesion was a strong predictor of progression to multiple myeloma within 2 years [11, 12]. Taken together, these biomarkers of malignancy are landmark additions to the definition of multiple myeloma. In our patient, criteria were met by having a clonal bone marrow population of ≥10% and >1 focal MRI lesions; importantly, as our patient had no overt evidence of end-organ disease, a reliance on the CRAB criteria could have delayed diagnosis.

4. Discussion of Management

Management of this patient's dual malignancies presented a complex challenge. It was deemed that her metastatic ovarian carcinosarcoma demanded immediate therapy, and she therefore was initiated on carboplatin and pegylated liposomal doxorubicin. We knew that chemotherapy for her carcinosarcoma would also provide antimyeloma effects. She was also started on zoledronic acid every 4 weeks. The patient has since completed six cycles and has no radiographic evidence of recurrent ovarian malignancy on CT scanning. Her clivus lesion remains stable in size, her T4 lesion has decreased in size, and her IgG lambda has decreased greater than 50%, equating to a partial response. She will continue zoledronic acid with consideration for bortezomib-based therapy if disease burden worsens.

Conflicts of Interest

The authors declare that they have no conflicts of interest.

Acknowledgments

The authors thank William Wrobel for help with radiological images and Lisa Teot for help with pathological slides.

References

[1] A. Dispenzieri, R. Kyle, G. Merlini et al., "International myeloma working group guidelines for serum-free light chain analysis in multiple myeloma and related disorders," *Leukemia*, vol. 23, no. 2, pp. 215–224, 2009.

[2] J. A. Katzmann, A. Dispenzieri, R. A. Kyle et al., "Elimination of the need for urine studies in the screening algorithm for monoclonal gammopathies by using serum immunofixation and free light chain assays," *Mayo Clinic Proceedings*, vol. 81, no. 12, pp. 1575–1578, 2006.

[3] P. G. Hill, J. M. Forsyth, B. Rai, and S. Mayne, "Serum free light chains: an alternative to the urine Bence Jones proteins screening test for monoclonal gammopathies," *Clinical Chemistry*, vol. 52, no. 9, pp. 1743–1748, 2006.

[4] J. M. Abadie and D. D. Bankson, "Assessment of serum free light chain assays for plasma cell disorder screening in a veterans affairs population," *Annals of Clinical and Laboratory Science*, vol. 36, no. 2, pp. 157–162, 2006.

[5] N. A. Bakshi, R. Gulbranson, D. Garstka, A. R. Bradwell, and D. F. Keren, "Serum free light chain (FLC) measurement can aid capillary zone electrophoresis in detecting subtle FLC-producing M proteins," *American Journal of Clinical Pathology*, vol. 124, no. 2, pp. 214–218, 2005.

[6] G. Marien, E. Oris, A. R. Bradwell, N. Blanckaert, and X. Bossuyt, "Detection of monoclonal proteins in sera by capillary zone electrophoresis and free light chain measurements," *Clinical Chemistry*, vol. 48, no. 9, pp. 1600-1601, 2002.

[7] S. V. Rajkumar, M. A. Dimopoulos, A. Palumbo et al., "International myeloma working group updated criteria for the diagnosis of multiple myeloma," *The Lancet Oncology*, vol. 15, no. 12, pp. e538–e548, 2014.

[8] S. V. Rajkumar, D. Larson, and R. A. Kyle, "Diagnosis of smoldering multiple myeloma," *New England Journal of Medicine*, vol. 365, pp. 474-475, 2011.

[9] E. Kastritis, E. Terpos, L. Moulopoulos et al., "Extensive bone marrow infiltration and abnormal free light chain ratio identifies patients with asymptomatic myeloma at high risk for progression to symptomatic disease," *Leukemia*, vol. 27, no. 4, pp. 947–953, 2012.

[10] J. T. Larsen, S. K. Kumar, A. Dispenzieri, R. A. Kyle, J. A. Katzmann, and S. V. Rajkumari, "Serum free light chain ratio as a biomarker for high-risk smoldering multiple myeloma," *Leukemia*, vol. 27, no. 4, pp. 941–946, 2013.

[11] J. Hillengass, K. Fechtner, M. A. Weber et al., "Prognostic significance of focal lesions in whole-body magnetic resonance imaging in patients with asymptomatic multiple myeloma," *Journal of Clinical Oncology*, vol. 28, no. 9, pp. 1606–1610, 2010.

[12] E. Kastritis, L. A. Moulopoulos, E. Terpos, V. Koutoulidis, and M. A. Dimopoulos, "The prognostic importance of the presence of more than one focal lesion in spine MRI of patients with asymptomatic (smoldering) multiple myeloma," *Leukemia*, vol. 28, no. 12, pp. 2402-2403, 2014.

22

Sequential use of Second-Generation Tyrosine Kinase Inhibitor Treatment and Intensive Chemotherapy Induced Long-Term Complete Molecular Response in Imatinib-Resistant CML Patient Presenting as a Myeloid Blast Crisis

Masaaki Tsuji, Tatsuki Uchiyama, Chisaki Mizumoto, Tomoharu Takeoka, Kenjiro Tomo, and Tatsuharu Ohno

Department of Hematology and Immunology, Otsu Red Cross Hospital, 1-1-35 Nagara, Otsu-shi, Shiga, Japan

Correspondence should be addressed to Masaaki Tsuji; mtsuji@otsu.jrc.or.jp

Academic Editor: Kazunori Nakase

Myeloid blast crisis of chronic myeloid leukemia (CML-MBC) is rarely seen at presentation and has a poor prognosis. There is no standard therapy for CML-MBC. It is often difficult to distinguish CML-MBC from acute myeloid leukemia expressing the Philadelphia chromosome (Ph+ AML). We present a case in which CML-MBC was seen at the initial presentation in a 75-year-old male. He was treated with conventional AML-directed chemotherapy followed by imatinib mesylate monotherapy, which failed to induce response. However, he achieved long-term complete molecular response after combination therapy involving dasatinib, a second-generation tyrosine kinase inhibitor, and conventional chemotherapy.

1. Introduction

The prognosis of patients with myeloid blast crisis of chronic myeloid leukemia (CML-MBC) is extremely poor, with a median survival time of only a few months [1]. Imatinib monotherapy for CML-MBC produces comparable results to conventional chemotherapy, but the associated survival period remains short [2, 3]. A recent study showed that the use of imatinib has improved the outcomes of blast crisis of CML (CML-BC) to some extent, but the median survival time of patients with the condition is still short (6.5–10 months) [4]. The use of second-generation tyrosine kinase inhibitors (2nd TKIs) such as dasatinib and nilotinib to treat CML-MBC has also resulted in improved outcomes [5–9]. Furthermore, combination treatment with conventional chemotherapy and TKIs is currently being investigated and is expected to result in better outcomes [11–13].

When the proliferation of Philadelphia chromosome-positive (Ph+) blasts is detected at presentation, it can be difficult to distinguish between CML-MBC and Ph+ acute myeloid leukemia (AML). Although several studies have detected clinical, pathological, and cytogenetic differences between CML-MBC and Ph+ AML, it remains uncertain whether these differences represent true entity-defining characteristics or merely reflect a more rapid clinical presentation of the same disease [14, 15].

Here, we report a case in which a patient with conventional chemotherapy- and imatinib-resistant CML-MBC achieved a long-term complete molecular response (CMR) after sequential treatment with a 2nd TKI and conventional chemotherapy.

2. Case Report

A 75-year-old male was admitted to our hospital due to a month-long history of malaise. He had not previously suffered from hematological disorders. However, he had diabetes and was an active smoker. On physical examination, he exhibited mild splenomegaly but not lymphadenopathy. His initial white blood cell count was as follows: 113,500/μL

Table 1: Laboratory data on admission.

CBC		Chemistry		Bone marrow	
WBC	113,500/μl	LDH	2,162 U/l	NCC	1,30,000/μl
Blasts	83.0%	AST	74 U/l	Megakaryocytes	0.0/μl
Promyelocytes	1.0%	ALT	444 U/l	M/E	11.40
Myelocytes	2.0%	ALP	250 U/l	Blasts	83.8%
Metamyelocytes	2.0%	T-Bil	0.59 mg/dl	Promyelocytes	1.0%
Stabs	0.0%	T-Pro	6.0 g/dl	Myelocytes	1.0%
Segmented	2.0%	Na	139 mEq/l	Metamyelocytes	0.6%
Eosinophils	0.0%	K	4.3 mEq/l	Slabs	1.4%
Basophils	0.0%	Cl	107 mEq/l	Segmented	1.0%
Monocytes	32.0%	BUN	17.9 mg/dl	Eosinophils	0.0%
Lymphocytes	7.0%	Creatinine	1.18 mg/dl	Basophils	0.0%
Reticulocytes	5.5%	CRP	1.2 mg/dl	Monocytes	1.2%
RBC	$289 \times 10^4/\mu l$	—	—	Lymphocytes	2.0%
Hemoglobin	8.8 g/dl	—	—	G-banding	46,XY,*t*(9;22)(*q*34;*q*11.2)
PLT	$2.1 \times 10^4/\mu l$	—	—	Major bcr/abl mRNA	1.0×10^5 copies/μg RNA

CBC: complete blood cell count, WBC: white blood cells, RBC: red blood cells, PLT: platelets, LDH: lactate dehydrogenase, AST: alanine aminotransferase, ALT: aspartate aminotransferase, ALP: alkaline phosphatase, T-Bil: total bilirubin, T-Pro: total protein, BUN: blood urea nitrogen, CRP: C-reactive protein, NCC: nuclear cell count, and M/E: myeloid to erythroid ratio.

with 83% blasts, 1% promyelocytes, 2% myelocytes, 2% metamyelocytes, 0% stabs, 2% segmented neutrophils, 0% basophils, 0% eosinophils, 32% monocytes, and 7% lymphocytes. His hemoglobin level and platelet count were 8.8 g/dL and $2.1 \times 10^4/\mu L$, respectively. His serum lactate dehydrogenase level was 2,162 U/L. Bone marrow aspiration disclosed a hypercellular marrow with a blast cell frequency of 83.8% (Table 1). The blast cells were positive for myeloperoxidase (MPO). No dysplastic features were observed in the patient's erythroid or megakaryocyte cells. Flow cytometric analysis of the bone marrow blasts produced the following results: CD13+: 94.2%, CD33+: 25.0%, CD117+: 71.9%, MPO+: 4.6%, and human leukocyte antigen- (HLA-) DR+: 90.0%. A cytogenetic study of the same material revealed the following karyotype in 100% (20/20) of the cells: 46,XY,*t*(9;22)(*q*34;*q*11.2). Fluorescence in situ hybridization (FISH) using the bcr–abl probe produced positive results for both the interphase peripheral polymorphonuclear cells (74.4%) and mononuclear cells (94.1%). The patient's bone marrow cells contained 1.0×10^5 copies/μg RNA of the major BCR-ABL mRNA molecule, detected by real-time quantitative reverse transcription polymerase chain reaction (RQ-PCR) (Table 1). The results of the FISH analysis and splenomegaly were more suggestive of CML-MBC than de novo Ph+ AML. The patient initially received intensive chemotherapy with 50 mg/m^2 daunorubicin on days 1–3 and 100 mg/m^2 cytosine arabinoside (Ara-C) on days 1–7. He did not respond to induction chemotherapy. He subsequently received 600 mg/day imatinib alone. Three weeks after the initiation of imatinib therapy, the number of blast cells in the patient's peripheral blood was increased, indicating that the imatinib treatment had not resulted in hematological remission. At that time, imatinib and dasatinib were the only TKIs approved in Japan for use in CML-BC. Thus, dasatinib treatment (140 mg daily) was started. About 20 days later, the patient developed grade 3 pleural effusion as a side effect of dasatinib. After the discontinuation of dasatinib and diuretic treatment, he recovered. Dasatinib was restarted at a dose of 100 mg/day, and the patient achieved a complete hematological response (CHR) within 34 days. After 42 days, bone marrow aspiration was performed. Cytogenetic analysis of the bone marrow revealed the Ph chromosome in 80% (16/20) of the cells, and BCR-ABL was detectable at the molecular level (5.1×10^4 copies/μg RNA). The patient was treated with reinduction chemotherapy (12 mg/m^2 idarubicin on days 1–3 and 100 mg/m^2 Ara-C on days 1–5) after the cessation of dasatinib treatment. After the bone marrow had recovered, bone marrow aspiration confirmed that hematological, immunophenotypic, and cytogenetic remission had been achieved, and no BCR-ABL transcripts were detected by RQ-PCR-based analysis of the bone marrow aspirate. Furthermore, FISH analysis using the bcr–abl probe produced negative results for both the interphase peripheral polymorphonuclear cells and mononuclear cells. Consolidation chemotherapy was not administered because the patient developed a severe pulmonary infection. As no matched sibling donor was available, and the patient's comorbidities were correlated with a hematopoietic cell transplantation-specific comorbidity index of 3, he was not eligible for an allogeneic hematopoietic stem cell transplantation (allo-SCT). Therefore, dasatinib monotherapy was started at a dosage of 100 mg/day. About one month later, he developed bilateral pleural effusion as a side effect of the dasatinib therapy. After the discontinuation of the dasatinib and diuretic treatment, he recovered. Dasatinib treatment was reinitiated at a dose of 50 mg/day, but pleural effusion developed again. Moreover, grade 4 thrombocytopenia and grade 4 neutropenia also arose. Thus, dasatinib was replaced with nilotinib at a reduced dosage of 600 mg/day (Figure 1). At 3.5 years after the initiation of nilotinib treatment, no BCR-ABL transcripts were

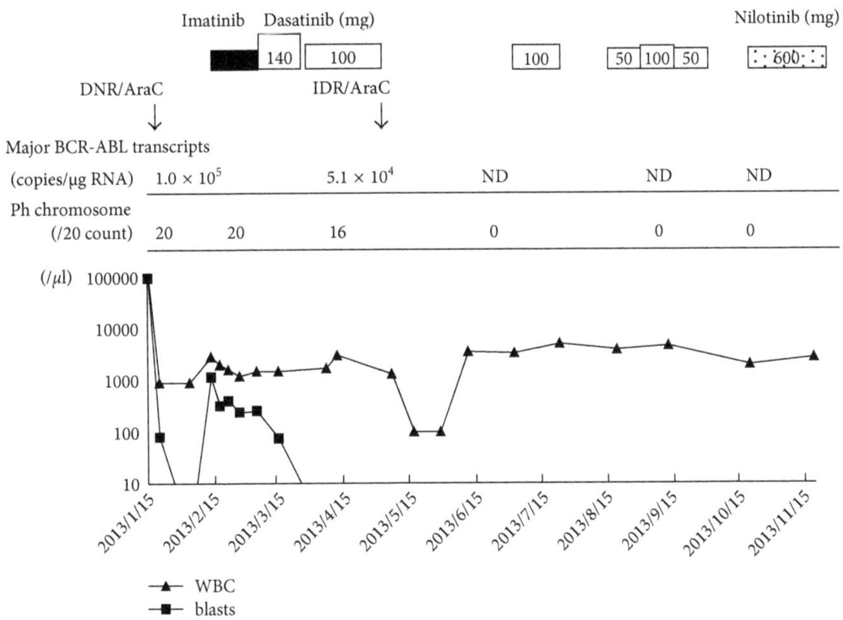

FIGURE 1: Clinical course. The kinetics of the hematological, cytogenetic, and molecular responses to tyrosine kinase inhibitors and conventional chemotherapy seen during the patient's clinical course are shown. Ara-C: cytosine arabinoside, DNR: daunorubicin, IDR: idarubicin, and ND: not detectable.

detected by RQ-PCR-based analysis of the patient's bone marrow aspirate. We also confirmed that there were no detectable BCR-ABL transcripts in the patient's peripheral blood (a molecular response of > MR4.5 according to the International Scale). He is still in CMR and is being treated with nilotinib at a daily dose of 600 mg.

3. Discussion

Myeloid blast crisis is the major remaining problem in the management of CML. In a multicenter study of imatinib monotherapy for CML-MBC, only 15.3% of the patients achieved CHR, and the median survival time was 6.9 months [2]. In another study with a 6-year follow-up period, 72 patients with CML-MBC were treated with imatinib alone at a dosage of 600 mg/day. CHR were achieved in 24% of cases, complete cytogenetic responses were achieved in 5% of cases, and the median survival time was 7 months [3]. Several studies have assessed the use of a combination of imatinib and conventional chemotherapy to treat CML-MBC. In a phase I/II trial involving 16 CML-MBC patients, 600 mg imatinib daily was combined with mitoxantrone and etoposide. The median overall survival time was 6.4 months [10]. Another study described the use of a combination of 600 mg imatinib and low-dose Ara-C and idarubicin in 19 CML-MBC patients. The median survival time was only 5 months [11]. Deau et al. reported the outcomes of 36 patients with CML-MBC that were treated with daunorubicin and Ara-C in combination with imatinib. The median overall survival time was 16 months, and the results were significantly improved by escalating the daily dose of daunorubicin [12]. These results suggest that the use of a more intensive induction regimen in combination with imatinib might improve the outcomes of CML-MBC.

The use of 2nd TKIs could overcome the refractoriness of CML-MBC to conventional chemotherapy, including imatinib therapy. Compared with imatinib therapy, several studies of CML-BC patients that were treated with dasatinib therapy showed hematological remission rates of 33% to 61%, major cytogenetic remission rates of 35% to 56%, and median survival times of 8 to 11 months [5–7]. In a CML-MBC cohort study, Saglio et al. found that the median overall survival time was 7.7–7.9 months [7]. Two studies of CML-BC patients that were treated with nilotinib therapy have been published [8, 9]. Giles et al. reported that CML-MBC patients exhibited a hematological remission rate of 60%, a major cytogenetic remission rate of 38%, and a median survival time of 10.1 months [9]. Thus, the combination of a 2nd TKI with conventional chemotherapy as a treatment for CML-MBC is of interest. A phase II study of Ph+ acute lymphoblastic leukemia and the lymphoid blast phase of CML involving patients that were treated with a combination of the hyper-CVAD (cyclophosphamide, vincristine, doxorubicin, and dexamethasone) regimen and dasatinib detected a complete cytogenetic remission rate of 84% and a complete molecular response rate of 42%. Although some grade 3 and 4 toxicities, including episodes of bleeding (34%), pleural effusion (15%), and pericardial effusion (6%), arose, the treatment regimen was well tolerated [16]. Milojkovic et al. reported that dasatinib can be safely combined with conventional chemotherapy, such as the FLAG-IDA (fludarabine, Ara-C, granulocyte colony-stimulating factor, and idarubicin) regimen, and this combination seems to induce deep remission in patients with CML-BC [13].

The incidence of Ph+ AML is reported to be 0.35–0.9% of all cases of AML. Whether Ph+ AML is distinct from CML-

MBC was disputed until recently. Various clinical characteristics have been suggested to be helpful for differentiating Ph+ AML from CML-MBC, including the absence of previous myeloproliferative disorders, the absence of evidence of chronic- or accelerated-phase CML, and a lack of clinical and laboratory features of CML, such as splenomegaly, basophilia, and a higher bone marrow myeloid/erythroid ratio. In addition, compared with CML-MBC, Ph+ AML is associated with very marked leukocytosis. In a FISH analysis of polymorphonuclear cells, the p210 BCR-ABL protein was found to be more common than the p190 BCR-ABL protein in Ph+ AML. The presence of additional cytogenetic aberrations, such as an extracopy of the Ph chromosome, trisomies 8 and 19, and isochromosome 17*q*, is more common in CML-MBC than in Ph+ AML. The coexistence of normal metaphases in addition to Ph+ metaphases at presentation is more characteristic of Ph+ AML than of CML-MBC. Moreover, the persistence of *t*(9;22) after induction therapy is more common in CML-MBC than in Ph+ AML [14]. A recent study showed that nucleophosmin 1 (NPM1) mutations are seen exclusively in Ph+ AML, whereas ABL1 mutations are exclusive to CML-MBC, suggesting that Ph+ AML is distinct from CML-MBC [15]. In our case, at the time that a dasatinib-induced CHR was achieved, cytogenetic analysis of the patient's bone marrow revealed the Ph chromosome in 80% (16/20) of the cells, and FISH analysis using the bcr–abl probe produced positive results for both the interphase peripheral polymorphonuclear cells and mononuclear cells. The patient's clinical course also supported a diagnosis of CML-MBC.

Our patient has been in CMR for more than three years. He has continued to take nilotinib after dasatinib, and intensive chemotherapy produced a CMR. Although an allo-SCT remains the only curative option for patients with CML-MBC, long-term remission may be expected by administering a combination of 2nd TKIs and intensive chemotherapy even without allo-SCT, given that the patient cannot tolerate the procedure or no suitable donor was available.

Conflicts of Interest

The authors declare that they have no conflicts of interest.

References

[1] H. M. Kantarjian, J. Shan, T. Smith et al., "Response to therapy is independently associated with survival prolongation in chronic myelogenous leukemia in the blastic phase," *Cancer*, vol. 92, no. 10, pp. 2501–2507, 2001.

[2] C. L. Sawyers, A. Hochhaus, E. Feldman et al., "Imatinib induces hematologic and cytogenetic responses in patients with chronic myelogenous leukemia in myeloid blast crisis: results of a phase II study," *Blood*, vol. 99, no. 10, pp. 3530–3539, 2001.

[3] R. Hahlann, S. Sausele, A. Voskanyan et al., "Management of CML-blast crisis," *Best Practice & Research in Clinical Hematology*, vol. 29, no. 3, pp. 295–307, 2016.

[4] F. Palandri, F. Castaqnetti, N. Testoni et al., "Chronic myeloid leukemia in blast crisis treated with imatinib 600 mg: outcome of the patients alive after a 6-year follow-up," *Haematologica*, vol. 93, no. 12, pp. 1792–1796, 2008.

[5] M. Talpaz, N. P. Shah, H. Kantarjian et al., "Dasatinib in imatinib-resistant Philadelphia chromosome-positive leukemias," *New England Journal of Medicine*, vol. 354, no. 24, pp. 2531–2541, 2006.

[6] J. Cortes, D. W. Kim, E. Raffoux et al., "Efficacy and safety of dasatinib in imatinib-resistant or -intolerant patients with chronic myeloid leukemia in blast phase," *Leukemia*, vol. 22, no. 12, pp. 2176–2183, 2008.

[7] G. Saglio, A. Hochhaus, Y. T. Goh et al., "Dasatinib in imatinib-resistant or imatinib-intolerant chronic myeloid leukemia in blast phase after 2 years of follow-up in a phase 3 study: efficacy and tolerability of 140 milligrams once daily and 70 milligrams twice daily," *Cancer*, vol. 116, no. 16, pp. 3852–3861, 2010.

[8] H. Kantarjian, F. Giles, L. Wunderle et al., "Nilotinib in imatinib-resistant CML and Philadelphia chromosome-positive ALL," *New England Journal of Medicine*, vol. 354, no. 24, pp. 2542–2551, 2006.

[9] F. J. Giles, H. M. Kantarjian, P. D. le Coutre et al., "Nilotinib is effective in imatinib-resistant or -intolerant patients with chronic myeloid leukemia in blastic phase," *Leukemia*, vol. 26, no. 5, pp. 959–962, 2012.

[10] S. Fruehauf, J. Topaly, E. C. Buss et al., "Imatinib combined with mitoxantrone/etoposide and cytarabine is an effective induction therapy for patients with chronic myeloid leukemia in myeloid blast crisis," *Cancer*, vol. 109, no. 8, pp. 1543–1549, 2007.

[11] A. Quintas-Cardama, H. Kantarjian, G. Garcia-Manero et al., "A pilot study of imatinib, low-dose cytarabine and idarubicin for patients with chronic myeloid leukemia in myeloid blast phase," *Leukemia & Lymphoma*, vol. 48, no. 2, pp. 283–289, 2007.

[12] B. Deau, F. E. Nicolini, J. Guilhot et al., "The addition of daunorubicin to imatinib mesylate in combination with cytarabine improves the response rate and the survival of patients with myeloid blast crisis chronic myelogenous leukemia (AFR01 study)," *Leukemia Research*, vol. 35, no. 6, pp. 777–782, 2011.

[13] D. Milojkovic, A. Ibrahim, A. Rcid, L. Forotri, J. Apperley, and D. Marin, "Efficacy of combining dasatinib and FLAG-IDA for patients with chronic myeloid leukemia in blastic transformation," *Hematologica*, vol. 97, no. 3, pp. 473-474, 2012.

[14] C. P. Soupir, J. A. Vergilio, P. Cin et al., "Philadelphia chromosome-positive acute myeloid leukemia. A rare aggressive leukemia with clinicopathologic features distinct from chronic myeloid leukemia in blast crisis," *American Journal of Clinical Pathology*, vol. 127, no. 4, pp. 642–650, 2007.

[15] S. Konoplev, C. C. Yin, S. M. Kornblau et al., "Molecular characterization of de novo Philadelphia chromosome-positive acute myeloid leukemia," *Leukemia and Lymphoma*, vol. 54, no. 1, pp. 138–144, 2013.

[16] O. Benjamini, T. L. Dumlao, H. Kantarjian et al., "Phase II trial of hyper CVAD and dasatinib in patients with relapsed Philadelphia chromosome positive acute lymphoblastic leukemia or blast phase chronic myeloid leukemia," *American Journal of Hematology*, vol. 89, no. 3, pp. 282–287, 2014.

23

Anti-CD20 Treatment of Autoimmune Hemolytic Anemia Refractory to Corticosteroids and Azathioprine

Alexandros Makis, Zoi Kanta, Dimitrios Kalogeropoulos, and Nikoloaos Chaliasos

Department of Pediatrics, University Hospital of Ioannina, Ioannina, Greece

Correspondence should be addressed to Alexandros Makis; amakis@cc.uoi.gr

Academic Editor: Tatsuharu Ohno

Autoimmune hemolytic anemia (AIHA) is a relatively uncommon hematological entity in children and sometimes is characterized by a severe course requiring more than one line course therapy. Treatment decisions depend on the severity and chronicity of the anemia and the characteristics of the autoantibodies. Immunosuppression with corticosteroids is the first-line treatment, especially in warm-reactive AIHA. Refractory cases are treated with immunosuppressive drugs, cytotoxic agents, androgens, or splenectomy, with various side effects and questionable efficacy. Another second-line option is rituximab, an anti-CD20 monoclonal antibody, which has been used as an off-label agent with encouraging results from small limited studies or case reports. Herein, we add our experience on the safety and clinical efficacy of rituximab by presenting the case of a boy with warm-type AIHA resistant to corticosteroids and azathioprine, successfully treated with rituximab. We also offer a review of the relevant literature.

1. Introduction

Autoimmune hemolytic anemia (AIHA) is rare in children, and it is characterized by the presence of autoantibodies (IgM and IgG) against erythrocyte membrane antigens, leading to their premature elimination by the macrophages of the reticuloendothelial system. AIHA is determined as primary or secondary depending on the presence of an underlying systemic illness, such as infections, autoimmune diseases, immunodeficiencies, malignancies, and drug exposure. Primary AIHA is subdivided in warm-reactive AIHA, paroxysmal cold hemoglobinuria, and cold agglutinin disease, according the type of antibody, its optimal binding temperature, and the fixation of the complement [1, 2].

Warm-type AIHA is the most common type accounting approximately for half of the pediatric cases. Warm-reactive autoantibodies, primarily IgG, attach on erythrocyte membrane antigens at 37°C, sometimes fix the complement, and lead to Fc receptor-mediated clearance by the macrophages in the spleen and other parts of the reticuloendothelial system [3]. Children present with anemia, jaundice, and mild splenomegaly. In most cases of warm-type AIHA, transfusions must be avoided due to the risk of further hemolysis, and the administration of corticosteroids, mainly prednisolone, is the best first-line option. However, if the anemia is severe (hemoglobin below 5 g/dL or is rapidly dropping), cardiovascular compromise might occur and erythrocyte transfusions are needed [4, 5].

In a significant proportion of children with warm-type AIHA (20%), the disease can have a chronic course with resistance or dependency to corticosteroids with subsequent side effects, requiring the use of second-line choices which have not been clearly established in children [4, 6]. More specifically, splenectomy and immunosuppressive drugs such as azathioprine, cyclophosphamide, cyclosporine, mycophenolate mofetil, or immunomodulating agents have been used as sole or combined options.

Rituximab, a chimeric monoclonal antibody targeting the CD20 antigen on B lymphocytes, has emerged as an off-label option in order to avoid splenectomy and the serious complications of corticosteroids and immunosuppressive drugs [7, 8]. In adults, a recent meta-analysis from several studies showed that the overall response rate and complete response rate were nearly 70% and 40%, respectively, for warm AIHA [9]. In children, the majority of the available publications are case reports or single-center uncontrolled studies [4, 7, 8, 10–14]. In a recent prospective national French study of 61 children, the 6-year relapse-free survival was 48% [15].

The purpose of this paper is to describe the case of a young boy with warm-reactive AIHA, refractory to corticosteroids, and azathioprine, who exhibited late response to rituximab and to present the relevant literature.

2. Case Report

A previously healthy 3.5-year-old male was referred to our department because of a five-day history of weakness and pallor. Two weeks before, a three-day history of diarrhea was mentioned. The past medical history is unremarkable, and no family history of hematological problems or autoimmune disorders was reported.

Physical examination revealed jaundice, pallor, and splenomegaly. The boy's heart rate was 125 beats/min, and a 2/6 systolic heart murmur was present. The initial laboratory investigation showed: hemoglobin 5.1 g/dL, absolute reticulocyte count $220 \times 10^3/\mu L$, mean corpuscular volume 75 fl, white blood cells $9.3 \times 10^9/L$, and platelets $255 \times 10^9/L$. The peripheral blood film showed polychromasia and spherocytes without schistocytes. Serum lactate dehydrogenase levels were 1540 U/L, total bilirubin 3.8 mg/dl, and indirect bilirubin 0.9 mg/dl. The renal and liver function tests showed calcium and phosphate were normal. Urine examination was negative for hemoglobin and myoglobin. The direct antiglobulin test (DAT) was strongly positive for IgG autoantibodies with no fixation of the complement. The results of antinuclear antibody and anti-deoxyribonucleic acid were negative. Serum C3 and C4 as well as IgG, IgM, and IgA levels were normal. Serology for cytomegalovirus, Epstein–Barr virus, *Mycoplasma pneumonia,* and human immunodeficiency virus were negative. Based on the symptoms, the clinical findings and the laboratory tests the warm type of AIHA was established.

Erythrocyte transfusion was firstly administered because of the severe anemia in order to avoid cardiovascular compromise. Intravenous methylprednisolone was also initiated at a dose of 3 mg/kg/day for the first 72 hours with excellent hematological response. When the boy was clinically stable, oral prednisolone at a dose of 2 mg/kg/day was then used for 4 weeks followed by a slow taper during the following 5 months. At that time, prednisolone was discontinued, and a relapse occurred after an upper respiratory infection as shown in Table 1.

For this reason, prednisolone was restarted at 2 mg/kg/day with a good hematological response. Due to the steroids side effects, the dose of prednisolone was slightly reduced two weeks later and a hematological deterioration occurred. After that, the dose was increased again to 2 mg/kg for 1-month period. The expected side effects, such as blood pressure above the 95th percentile, bilateral posterior subcapsular cataract, facial edema, and hairy back, were quite evident, and it was decided to slowly discontinue prednisolone and to administer azathioprine at a dose of 2 mg/kg/day.

Azathioprine was given for 4 months with a slight hematological deterioration despite the increase up to 3 mg/kg/day, as shown in Table 1, while the boy suffered from mumps, possibly due to the underlying immunosuppression. At this point, rituximab was initiated after informed written consent. The agent was given in 4 weekly doses at a dose of 375 mg/m^2, with no infusion-related side effects. Stable response was noticed 2 months after initiation of rituximab (Table 1). Immunoglobulin levels remained normal without the need for replacement therapy with intravenous immunoglobulin (IVIG). The DAT became negative 12 months later. The boy remains disease-free without relapses, 3 years after the first presentation.

3. Discussion

In our report, we describe the successful use of rituximab in a child with warm-type AIHA, priorly treated with corticosteroids and azathioprine. Rituximab was a valuable option that allowed corticosteroid and azathioprine discontinuation due to unresponsiveness and side effects.

Corticosteroids represent the most effective first-line treatment for warm AIHA and especially for the IgG-related type. Their action is associated with a decrease in hemolysis by blocking the mononuclear phagocytic Fc gamma receptor leading to a rapid response within 24 to 48 hours. They also have a late negative effect in the autoantibody production, but this demands several weeks [16, 17]. In cases with severe anemia, intravenous methylprednisolone is usually administered at a total dose of 1 to 2 mg/kg/day for the first 1 to 3 days. After the initial stabilization, a scheme of oral prednisone at a dose of 1 to 2 mg/kg/day is then preferred for two to four weeks, followed by a slow discontinuation over two to six months, with a good overall response rate of approximately 80 percent [1, 5, 18]. However, in some cases AIHA can be resistant and dependent to large doses of corticosteroids or to long-term therapy resulting in severe and adverse systemic effects, as was the case in our patient [17, 19].

In order to avoid the corticosteroid side effects, splenectomy or administration of immunomodulatory drugs can be used. However, these therapies are not consistently effective and present no negligible risk of infectious complications due to their profound immunosuppression.

Splenectomy is the surgical removal of the main site of erythrocyte destruction and autoantibody production. It is considered in children above the age of five, because in younger ages there is a significant risk of postsplenectomy sepsis caused by encapsulated bacterial organisms. Children with IgG-derived AIHA have a good response up to 65% [5, 20, 21]. Despite that, splenectomy as rarely an option, because several second-line drugs exist in order to avoid the long-term risks.

Several immunomodulatory agents are available for children with refractory disease, such cyclosporine, mycophenolate mofetil, azathioprine, rapamycin, danazol, cyclophosphamide,

Table 1: Hematological parameters and treatment during the course of the disease.

	Admission	4th day	4th week	3rd month	6th month	7th month	9th month	13th month	15th month	3rd year
Agent	Methylprednisolone (3 mg/kg/day)	Prednisolone (2 mg/kg/day)	Prednisolone (2 mg/kg/day)	Prednisolone (1 mg/kg/day)	—	Prednisolone (2 mg/kg/day)	Prednisolone (2 mg/kg/day)	—	—	—
	Transfusion						Azathioprine (2 mg/kg/day)	Azathioprine (3 mg/kg/day) Rituximab	—	—
Hb	5.1	9.2	11.5	12.3	12.8	7.3	11.6	9.8	12.9	13.2
Rets	220	120	92	79	75	186	95	115	83	62
DAT	+++ IgG	+++ IgG	+++ IgG	+++ IgG	+++ IgG	+++ IgG	+++ IgG	+++ IgG	+++ IgG	Negative
LDH	1540	720	523	310	285	1230	310	370	290	250
TBL	3.8	1.9	1.2	0.9	0.9	2.9	1.0	1.2	0.9	0.8

Hb (g/dl): hemoglobin; Rets (x $10^3/\mu L$): reticulocytes; DAT: direct antiglobulin test; LDH (U/L): lactate dehydrogenase; TBL (mg/dl): total bilirubin.

TABLE 2: Basic data from case reports and studies regarding the use of rituximab in children with primary or secondary autoimmune hemolytic anemia.

First author/year	Number of patients	Age	Primary/ secondary	Response	Time to response	Duration of response/ follow-up	IVIG	Complications
Quartier et al. [8]	6	7–35 mo	5/1	CR	4 min	15–22 min	Y	Pyelonephritis, febrile bronchitis
Zecca et al. [7]	1	18 mo	0/1	CR	2 w	5 min	Y	—
Motto et al. [31]	4	3.5–15 y	3/1	CR	NM	NM	Y	*Pneumocystis carinii* pneumonia, varicella pneumonia
McMahon et al. [32]	1	16 y	1/0	CR	4 w	19 mo	N	—
Hongeng et al. [33]	1	37 mo	0/1	CR	2 w	3 mo	Y	—
Kerridge et al. [34]	1	8 y	1/0	CR	3 w	14 mo	N	—
Zecca et al. [35]	15	0.3–13, 8 y	11/4	13 CR, 2 NR	5–72 d	7.3–27.6 mo	Y	Varicella infection
Gottardo et al. [36]	1	2 y	1/0	CR	1 w	19 mo	Y	—
Wakim et al. [37]	1	6 y	0/1	CR	1 min	16 mo	Y	—
Raj et al. [38]	1	14 y	0/1	CR	3 w	22 mo	N	—
van Daalen et al. [39]	4	3–16 y	4/0	3 CR, 1 NR	NM	NM	Y	—
Bonduel et al. [40]	1	13 mo	0/1	CR	4 w	5 mo	Y	—
Silvana et al. [41]	1	23 mo	0/1	CR	18 d	7 mo	Y	—
Kim et al. [42]	4	3–16 mo	0/4	CR	1–5 w	NM	Y	—
Schappi et al. [43]	1	16 mo	0/1	CR	10 w	18 mo	N	—
Rao et al. [10]	8	5–17 y	6/2	4 CR, 2 PR, 2 NR	NM	3–30 mo	Y	Mild infusion reactions
Beretta et al. [44]	1	8 mo	1/0	PR	2 relapses	7 mo	N	—
Simms-Waldrip et al. [45]	1	9 y	0/1	CR	3 w	4 mo	N	—
Svahn et al. [11]	4	1–9 mo	2/2	3 CR, 1 PR	1–8 min	21–80 mo	Y	—
Lucchini et al. [46]	1	3 y	1/0	CR	2 w	12 mo	N	—
Rao et al. [30]	3	1–9 y	0/3	NR	Relapses	-	Y	Neutropenia
Haller et al. [47]	1	4 mo	0/1	CR	3 w	12 mo	Y	—
Ansari et al. [12]	5	3–14 y	5/0	CR	NM	8–30 mo	N	Seizures during infusion, meningitis
van der Linde et al. [48]	1	2 y	1/0	PR	1 relapse, 11 min	6 y	N	—
Gupta et al. [13]	2	0.5/4 y	2/0	CR/PR	3 w	12 mo	N	—
Kuzmanovic and Jurisic [49]	1	5 mo	1/0	CR	3 w	12 mo	Y	—
Moriya et al. [50]	1	3 mo	1/0	CR	4 w	30 mo	N	—
O'Connell et al. [51]	1	4 y	0/1	PR	NM	NM	N	—
Makadia et al. [52]	1	4 mo	1/0	CR	4 w	6 mo	N	*Pneumocystis carinii* pneumonia
Faraci et al. [53]	7	2–6 mo	0/7	CR	1–3 m	3.5–140 mo	NM	—
Dev et al. [54]	1	9 y	1/0	CR	NM	12 mo	N	Respiratory tract infections
Sankaran et al. [4]	5	NM	NM	2 CR, 1 PR, 2 NR	NM	NM	NM	NM
Ducassou et al. [15]	61	3.3–14.9 y	46/15	40 CR, 6 PR, 15 NR	1–3 min	2.5–7.8 y	13 cases	3 allergic reactions, 1 neutropenia
Ajmi et al. [14]	1	10 y	1/0	CR	3 w	4 mo	N	—
Gonzalez-Vicent et al. [55]	40	NM	0/40	CR or PR	NM	NM	NM	—

vincristine, vinblastine, and eculizumab. Each of these agents is less effective than either corticosteroids or splenectomy. Cyclosporine, mycophenolate mofetil, azathioprine, and rapamycin act by targeting T-lymphocytes, cause immunosuppression, and have several hematological and renal side effects [22–24]. Clinical response may require several weeks, as happened in our case who also suffered from mumps due to the severe immunosuppression. In a recent study, rapamycin has been shown to be effective and safe in children with multiresistant AIHA [25]. Danazol is a synthetic androgen with multiple mechanisms of action which decreases autoantibody production and complement activation. Among their widely known implications, they affect hepatic transaminases and cause elevation of masculinizing hormones [26]. Cyclophosphamide, vincristine, and vinblastine are cytotoxic agents that diminish the autoantibody production. Limitation of their use in children is the myelosuppressive and mutagenic effects [27]. Eculizumab is a monoclonal antibody targeting C5 complement that has been recently shown to be effective in complement-mediated AIHA [28, 29].

Therefore, there is a great need for the introduction of new effective and safer pharmaceutical options. The anti-CD20 monoclonal antibody rituximab has been successfully used to treat children with refractory AIHA. The preferred scheme is four weekly intravenous infusions (375 mg/m^2/dose). During the last years, several reports have emerged, along with few single-center uncontrolled studies and one very recent prospective study [4, 7, 8, 10–15]. The basic characteristics of these case reports and studies are presented in Table 2. As it is apparent, rituximab is a valuable option in refractory primary AIHA as well as in secondary cases, such as after bone marrow transplantation, related to primary immunodeficiencies and Evan's syndrome. Although hematological responses are promising, secondary hypogammaglobulinemia and prolonged B lymphopenia will occur after rituximab therapy. Close monitoring of immunoglobulin levels is necessary. Therefore, in patients who present with severe or recurrent infections and concomitant low immunoglobulin levels, intravenous immunoglobulin (IVIG) may be useful as replacement therapy after rituximab use. In a few cases, IVIG supplementation was administrated for six months after rituximab treatment until the hypogammaglobulinemia resolved [30]. Generally, rituximab is considered a well-tolerated treatment as only a small number of children from the literature needed IVIG and prophylaxis for possible infectious complications [4, 15].

Very recently, a prospective national observational study was published by Ducassou et al. on the benefits of rituximab as a second-line treatment for AIHA in children [15]. For the first time in the literature, the investigators estimate the clinical value of rituximab by achieving a four-year median follow-up. The response was better in primary, isolated AIHA and in infants when used early in the course of treatment. Rituximab allowed steroid tapering in 60–70% of patients with 30% showing long-term response. Regarding safety, allergic reactions were rare and no case of progressive multifocal leucoencephalopathy was observed. The major safety problems were prolonged hypogammaglobulinaemia in few cases and severe neutropenia in one case. Therefore, it seems rational to propose rituximab as a second-line therapy, if response is not observed with first-line corticosteroids.

In conclusion, corticosteroids remain the cornerstone of the first-line therapeutic treatment for AIHA. Nevertheless, according to the existing literature data, the implementation of rituximab as a second-line therapy is relatively safe and can resolve difficult cases of AIHA resistant to corticosteroids. Therefore, physicians who treat children with AIHA should be aware of this rational therapeutic tool, even from the early stages of non-responsive cases, in order to avoid other aggressive regimens such as splenectomy or immunomodulation.

Conflicts of Interest

The authors declare that they have no conflicts of interest.

References

[1] R. Naithani, N. Agrawal, M. Mahapatra, R. Kumar, H. P. Pati, and V. P. Choudhry, "Autoimmune hemolytic anemia in children," *Hematology and Oncology*, vol. 24, no. 4, pp. 309–315, 2007.

[2] S. Vaglio, M. C. Arista, M. P. Perrone et al., "Autoimmune hemolytic anemia in childhood: serologic features in 100 cases," *Transfusion*, vol. 47, no. 1, pp. 50–54, 2007.

[3] C. N. Branstetter, J. S. Hankins, D. Moreau, and K. A. Nottage, "Severe autoimmune hemolytic anemia in an infant caused by warm-reactive IGM and IGA autoantibodies: a case report and review of the literature," *Journal of Pediatric Hematology/Oncology*, vol. 37, no. 6, pp. 468–471, 2015.

[4] J. Sankaran, V. Rodriguez, E. K. Jacob, J. D. Kreuter, and R. S. Go, "Autoimmune hemolytic anemia in children: Mayo Clinic experience," *Journal of Pediatric Hematology/Oncology*, vol. 38, no. 3, pp. e120–e124, 2016.

[5] M. Michel, "Classification and therapeutic approaches in autoimmune hemolytic anemia: an update," *Expert Review of Hematology*, vol. 4, no. 6, pp. 607–618, 2011.

[6] N. Aladjidi, G. Leverger, T. Leblanc et al., "New insights into childhood autoimmune hemolytic anemia: a French national observational study of 265 children," *Haematologica*, vol. 96, no. 5, pp. 655–663, 2011.

[7] M. Zecca, P. De Stefano, B. Nobili, and F. Locatelli, "Anti-CD20 monoclonal antibody for the treatment of severe, immune-mediated, pure red cell aplasia and hemolytic anemia," *Blood*, vol. 97, no. 12, pp. 3995–3997, 2001.

[8] P. Quartier, B. Brethon, P. Philippet, J. Landman-Parker, F. Le Deist, and A. Fischer, "Treatment of childhood autoimmune haemolytic anaemia with rituximab," *The Lancet*, vol. 358, no. 9292, pp. 1511–1513, 2001.

[9] Q. Reynaud, I. Durieu, M. Dutertre et al., "Efficacy and safety of rituximab in auto-immune hemolytic anemia: a meta-analysis of 21 studies," *Autoimmunity Reviews*, vol. 14, no. 4, pp. 304–313, 2015.

[10] A. Rao, M. Kelly, M. Musselman et al., "Safety, efficacy, and immune reconstitution after rituximab therapy in pediatric patients with chronic or refractory hematologic autoimmune cytopenias," *Pediatric Blood and Cancer*, vol. 50, no. 4, pp. 822–825, 2008.

[11] J. Svahn, F. Fioredda, M. Calvillo et al., "Rituximab-based immunosuppression for autoimmune haemolytic anaemia in infants," *British Journal of Haematology*, vol. 145, no. 1, pp. 96–100, 2009.

[12] S. Ansari, M. Tashvighi, B. Darbandi, A. B. Salimi, and M. Golpaygani, "Rituximab for child with chronic relapsing autoimmune hemolytic anemia," *Pediatric Hematology and Oncology*, vol. 28, no. 2, pp. 164–166, 2011.

[13] N. Gupta, S. Sharma, T. Seth et al., "Rituximab in steroid refractory autoimmune hemolytic anemia," *Indian Journal of Pediatrics*, vol. 79, no. 6, pp. 803–805, 2012.

[14] H. Ajmi, S. Mabrouk, S. Hassayoun et al., "Success of anti-CD20 monoclonal antibody treatment for severe autoimmune hemolytic anemia caused by warm-reactive immunoglobulin A, immunoglobulin G, and immunoglobulin M autoantibodies in a child: a case report," *Journal of Medical Case Reports*, vol. 11, no. 1, p. 321, 2017.

[15] S. Ducassou, G. Leverger, H. Fernandes et al., "Benefits of rituximab as a second-line treatment for autoimmune haemolytic anaemia in children: a prospective French cohort study," *British Journal of Haematology*, vol. 177, no. 5, pp. 751–758, 2017.

[16] W. F. Rosse, "Quantitative immunology of immune hemolytic anemia: II. The relationship of cell-bound antibody to hemolysis and the effect of treatment," *Journal of Clinical Investigation*, vol. 50, no. 4, pp. 734–743, 1971.

[17] R. S. Go, J. L. Winters, and N. E. Kay, "How I treat autoimmune hemolytic anemia," *Blood*, vol. 129, no. 22, pp. 2971–2979, 2017.

[18] K. Dussadee, O. Taka, A. Thedsawad, and W. Wanachiwanawin, "Incidence and risk factors of relapses in idiopathic autoimmune hemolytic anemia," *Journal of the Medical Association of Thailand*, vol. 93, no. 1, pp. S165–S170, 2010.

[19] A. Zanella and W. Barcellini, "Treatment of autoimmune hemolytic anemias," *Haematologica*, vol. 99, no. 10, pp. 1547–1554, 2014.

[20] N. B. Sitkovskii, V. G. Bebeshko, V. D. Drozdova, S. S. Kireeva, and L. N. Kuz'minskii, "Splenectomy as an operation of desperation in children with blood diseases," *Klinichna khirurhiia*, vol. 6, no. 74, 1986.

[21] N. Y. Patel, A. M. Chilsen, M. A. Mathiason, K. J. Kallies, and W. A. Bottner, "Outcomes and complications after splenectomy for hematologic disorders," *American Journal of Surgery*, vol. 204, no. 6, pp. 1014–1020, 2012.

[22] F. Duru, A. Gurgey, M. Cetin, T. Kanra, and C. Altay, "Chronic autoimmune hemolytic anemia in children: a report of four patients," *Journal of Medicine*, vol. 25, no. 3-4, pp. 231–240, 1994.

[23] V. K. Rao, F. Dugan, J. K. Dale et al., "Use of mycophenolate mofetil for chronic, refractory immune cytopenias in children with autoimmune lymphoproliferative syndrome," *British Journal of Haematology*, vol. 129, no. 4, pp. 534–538, 2005.

[24] Y. Usta, F. Gurakan, Z. Akcoren, and S. Ozen, "An overlap syndrome involving autoimmune hepatitis and systemic lupus erythematosus in childhood," *World Journal of Gastroenterology*, vol. 13, no. 19, pp. 2764–2767, 2007.

[25] M. Miano, M. Calvillo, E. Palmisani et al., "Sirolimus for the treatment of multi-resistant autoimmune haemolytic anaemia in children," *British Journal of Haematology*, vol. 167, no. 4, pp. 571–574, 2014.

[26] A. M. Tan, J. Lou, and H. K. Cheng, "Danazol for treatment of refractory autoimmune hemolytic anaemia," *Annals of the Academy of Medicine, Singapore*, vol. 18, no. 6, pp. 707–709, 1989.

[27] N. Gombakis, M. Trahana, M. Athanassiou, and F. Kanakoudi-Tsakalidou, "Evans syndrome: successful management with multi-agent treatment including intermediate-dose intravenous cyclophosphamide," *Journal of Pediatric Hematology/Oncology*, vol. 21, no. 3, pp. 248-249, 1999.

[28] K. Ma and S. Caplan, "Refractory IgG warm autoimmune hemolytic anemia treated with eculizumab: a novel application of anticomplement therapy," *Case Reports in Hematology*, vol. 2016, Article ID 9181698, 3 pages, 2016.

[29] K. Halligan, L. Vasiljevic, P. Roehrs et al., "Use of eculizumab in a patient with refractory autoimmune hemolytic anemia with heterozygous *NFκB1* mutation," *Blood*, vol. 130, no. 1, p. 4743, 2017.

[30] V. K. Rao, S. Price, K. Perkins et al., "Use of rituximab for refractory cytopenias associated with autoimmune lymphoproliferative syndrome (ALPS)," *Pediatric Blood and Cancer*, vol. 52, no. 7, pp. 847–852, 2009.

[31] D. G. Motto, J. A. Williams, and L. A. Boxer, "Rituximab for refractory childhood autoimmune hemolytic anemia," *Israel Medical Association Journal*, vol. 4, no. 11, pp. 1006–1008, 2002.

[32] C. McMahon, L. Babu, A. Hodgson, A. Hayat, N. O. Connell, and O. P. Smith, "Childhood refractory autoimmune haemolytic anaemia: is there a role for anti-CD20 therapy (rituximab)?," *British Journal of Haematology*, vol. 117, no. 2, pp. 480–483, 2002.

[33] S. Hongeng, P. Tardtong, S. Worapongpaiboon, A. Ungkanont, and S. Jootar, "Successful treatment of refractory autoimmune haemolytic anaemia in a post-unrelated bone marrow transplant paediatric patient with rituximab," *Bone Marrow Transplantation*, vol. 29, no. 10, pp. 871-872, 2002.

[34] I. Kerridge, I. Hann, M. Ethel, M. Potter, and H. G. Prentice, "Anti-CD20 monoclonal antibody (rituximab) therapy in a child with refractory chronic autoimmune haemolytic anaemia," *Internal Medicine Journal*, vol. 33, no. 11, pp. 544-545, 2003.

[35] M. Zecca, B. Nobili, U. Ramenghi et al., "Rituximab for the treatment of refractory autoimmune hemolytic anemia in children," *Blood*, vol. 101, no. 10, pp. 3857–3861, 2003.

[36] N. G. Gottardo, D. L. Baker, and F. R. Willis, "Successful induction and maintenance of long-term remission in a child with chronic relapsing autoimmune hemolytic anemia using rituximab," *Pediatric Hematology and Oncology*, vol. 20, no. 7, pp. 557–561, 2003.

[37] M. Wakim, A. Shah, P. A. Arndt et al., "Successful anti-CD20 monoclonal antibody treatment of severe autoimmune hemolytic anemia due to warm reactive IgM autoantibody in a child with common variable immunodeficiency," *American Journal of Hematology*, vol. 76, no. 2, pp. 152–155, 2004.

[38] A. Raj, S. Bertolone, and A. Cheerva, "Successful treatment of refractory autoimmune hemolytic anemia with monthly rituximab following nonmyeloablative stem cell transplantation for sickle cell disease," *Journal of Pediatric Hematology/Oncology*, vol. 26, no. 5, pp. 312–314, 2004.

[39] S. T. van Daalen, P. J. van Dijken, R. Y. Tamminga, and P. P. Brons, "Rituximab instead of splenectomy in 4 children with chronic or refractory autoimmune haemolytic anaemia," *Nederlands Tijdschrift Voor Geneeskunde*, vol. 149, no. 42, pp. 2350–2354, 2005.

[40] M. Bonduel, M. Zelazko, C. Figueroa, G. Magaldi, J. Rossi, and A. del Pozo, "Successful treatment of autoimmune hemolytic anemia with rituximab in a child with severe combined immunodeficiency following nonidentical T-cell-depleted bone marrow transplantation," *Bone Marrow Transplantation*, vol. 35, no. 8, pp. 819–821, 2005.

[41] B. Silvana, L. M. Antonella, P. Basilia, D. Trombetta, A. Saija, and C. Salpietro, "Rituximab for the treatment of post-bone marrow transplantation refractory hemolytic anemia in a child with Omenn's syndrome," *Pediatric Transplantation*, vol. 11, no. 5, pp. 552–556, 2007.

[42] J. J. Kim, A. J. Thrasher, A. M. Jones, E. G. Davies, and C. M. Cale, "Rituximab for the treatment of autoimmune cytopenias in children with immune deficiency," *British Journal of Haematology*, vol. 138, no. 1, pp. 94–96, 2007.

[43] M. G. Schappi, H. Ozsahin, T. Peyrard et al., "Severe autoimmune hemolytic anemia in a liver transplanted child," *Pediatric Transplantation*, vol. 12, no. 7, pp. 809–812, 2008.

[44] C. Beretta, V. Leoni, M. R. Rossi et al., "Prolonged extracorporeal membrane oxygenation therapy for severe acute respiratory distress syndrome in a child affected by rituximab-resistant autoimmune hemolytic anemia: a case

report," *Journal of Medical Case Reports*, vol. 3, no. 1, p. 6443, 2009.

[45] T. Simms-Waldrip, A. Ikeda, D. Goldfinger, T. Moore, and S. Yuan, "Dramatic response to rituximab in a child with severe cold autoimmune hemolytic anemia arising after allogeneic hematopoietic SCT," *Bone Marrow Transplantation*, vol. 45, no. 1, pp. 201-202, 2010.

[46] G. Lucchini, N. Masera, G. Foti, G. Assali, P. Perseghin, and E. Biagi, "A life-threatening paediatric case of acute autoimmune haemolytic anaemia (AIHA) successfully cured by plasma-exchange and combined immunosuppressive treatment," *Transfusion and Apheresis Science*, vol. 40, no. 2, pp. 115–118, 2009.

[47] W. Haller, J. Hind, S. Height, R. Mitry, and A. Dhawan, "Successful treatment of mixed-type autoimmune hemolytic anemia with rituximab in a child following liver transplantation," *Pediatric Transplantation*, vol. 14, no. 3, pp. E20–E25, 2010.

[48] A. A. van der Linde, E. J. Schatorje, A. M. van der Weij, E. F. Gemen, and E. de Vries, "B-lymphocyte reconstitution after repeated rituximab treatment in a child with steroid-dependent autoimmune hemolytic anemia," *Pediatric Reports*, vol. 3, no. 4, p. e28, 2011.

[49] M. Kuzmanovic and V. Jurisic, "Rituximab for treatment of autoimmune hemolytic anemia," *Indian Pediatrics*, vol. 49, no. 8, pp. 672–674, 2012.

[50] K. Moriya, T. Matsuhashi, M. Onuma et al., "Successful treatment with rituximab of an infant with refractory autoimmune hemolytic anemia," *International Journal of Hematology*, vol. 98, no. 2, pp. 237–239, 2013.

[51] N. O'Connell, M. Goodyer, M. Gleeson et al., "Successful treatment with rituximab and mycophenolate mofetil of refractory autoimmune hemolytic anemia post-hematopoietic stem cell transplant for dyskeratosis congenita due to TINF2 mutation," *Pediatric Transplantation*, vol. 18, no. 1, pp. E22–E24, 2014.

[52] D. Makadia, S. R. Siddaiahgari, and M. S. Latha, "Anti B cell targeted therapy for autoimmune hemolytic anemia in an infant," *Indian Journal of Pharmacology*, vol. 45, no. 5, pp. 526-527, 2013.

[53] M. Faraci, M. Zecca, M. Pillon et al., "Autoimmune hematological diseases after allogeneic hematopoietic stem cell transplantation in children: an Italian multicenter experience," *Biology of Blood and Marrow Transplantation*, vol. 20, no. 2, pp. 272–278, 2014.

[54] M. Dev, N. Mushtaq, and A. Faisal, "A case of autoimmune haemolytic anaemia achieving complete response with rituximab," *Journal of the Pakistan Medical Association*, vol. 64, no. 6, pp. 700–702, 2014.

[55] M. Gonzalez-Vicent, J. Sanz, J. L. Fuster et al., "Autoimmune hemolytic anemia (AIHA) following allogeneic hematopoietic stem cell transplantation (HSCT): a retrospective analysis and a proposal of treatment on behalf of the Grupo Espanol De Trasplante de Medula Osea en Ninos (GETMON) and the Grupo Espanol de Trasplante Hematopoyetico (GETH)," *Transfusion Medicine Reviews*, vol. 12, no. 3, pp. 179–185, 2018.

Unusual Presentation of a Small-Cell Variant of Anaplastic Large-Cell Lymphoma Case: When a Septic Picture is not Sepsis

Zhou Yu,[1,2] Yifan Pang,[2,3] Linda Wang,[2,3] Daniel E. Ezekwudo,[1,2] Foluso Ogunleye,[1,2] Susanna S. Gaikazian,[1,2] Mark Micale,[2,4] James Huang,[2,4] Ann Marie Blenc,[2,4] and Ishmael Jaiyesimi[1,2]

[1]*Department of Hematology and Oncology, William Beaumont Hospital, Royal Oak, MI, USA*
[2]*Oakland University William Beaumont School of Medicine, Rochester, MI, USA*
[3]*Department of Internal Medicine, William Beaumont Hospital, Royal Oak, MI, USA*
[4]*Department of Pathology and Laboratory Medicine, William Beaumont Hospital, Royal Oak, MI, USA*

Correspondence should be addressed to Zhou Yu; zhou.yu@beaumont.edu

Academic Editor: Tatsuharu Ohno

We report a case of a small-cell variant of anaplastic large-cell lymphoma, with an unusual clinical presentation mimicking sepsis and a fulminant clinic course, in a 48-year-old Caucasian female. In this report, we discuss the diagnostic challenge, histopathologic features, and unique cytogenetic features of this case, in order to raise awareness of this rare presentation and emphasize the importance of meticulous peripheral smear examination and early bone marrow evaluation.

1. Introduction

Anaplastic large-cell lymphoma (ALCL) is a rare aggressive T-cell lymphoma, comprising 3% of adult-onset non-Hodgkin lymphomas. According to the 2016 WHO classification, ALCL consists of four major groups: primary systemic anaplastic lymphoma kinase-positive (ALK+) ALCL, primary systemic anaplastic lymphoma kinase-negative (ALK−) ALCL, primary cutaneous ALCL, and breast implant-associated ALCL [1]. ALK+ ALCLs exhibit a wide histologic spectrum, including classic type, small-cell, lymphohistiocytic, and sarcomatoid variants [2]. The small-cell variant of ALK+ ALCL comprises 5–10% of cases. Overall, the prognosis of ALK+ ALCL is remarkably better than of ALK− ALCL. However, even though all small-cell variant cases have been shown to be ALK+, the prognosis is very poor for this subgroup [3, 4]. Here, we present a case of ALK+ ALCL with small-cell variant morphology.

2. Case Presentation

A 48-year-old previously healthy Caucasian female presented with progressive shortness of breath on exertion, right upper quadrant abdominal pain, and left lower extremity pain and swelling. On presentation, the patient was afebrile; however, she was borderline hypotensive, tachycardic, and tachypneic. Laboratory results showed marked leukocytosis (37.3×10^9/L) with predominant neutrophilia and mild thrombocytopenia, as well as acute kidney injury, elevated transaminases with hyperbilirubinemia, and metabolic acidosis. Table 1 summarizes the relevant laboratory findings. Initial differential diagnosis included sepsis, cholecystitis, or pulmonary embolism. Empiric broad-spectrum antibiotics were initiated immediately. Imaging studies did not show any venous thromboembolism or cholecystitis but revealed hepatomegaly, small lung nodules, and mild axillary lymphadenopathy.

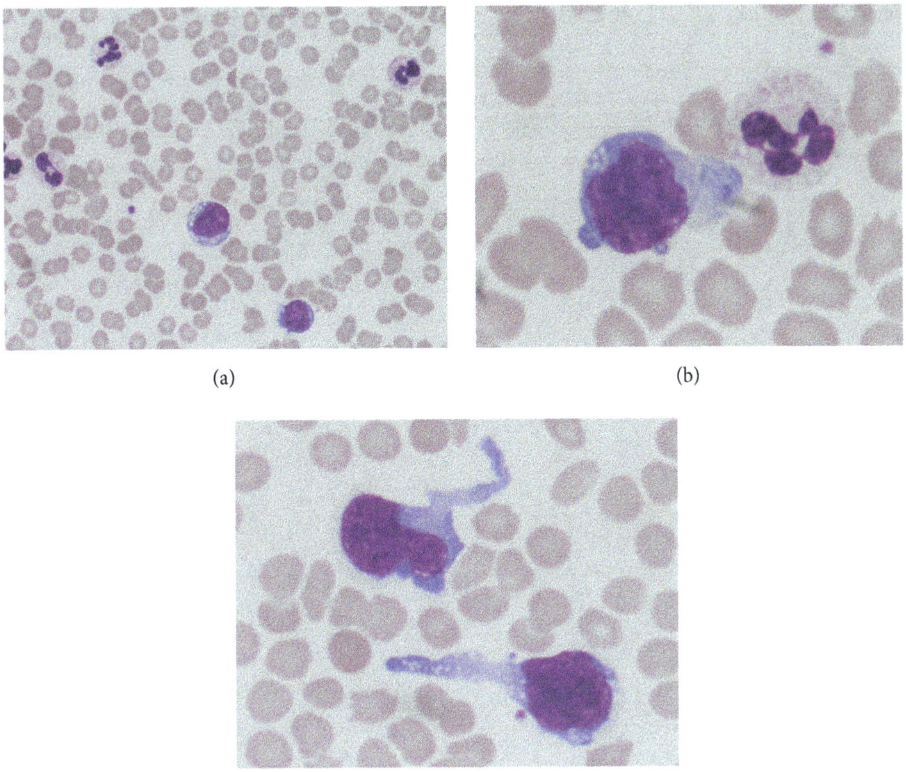

(a) (b) (c)

FIGURE 1: Peripheral blood examination. (a) The patient's peripheral blood smear shows leukocytosis with neutrophilia, left shift, and toxic granulation (Wright's stain, 40x). (b) Scattered medium size atypical cells are present. These cells feature prominent nuclear irregularities and vacuoles (Wright's stain, 100x oil). (c) Atypical cells have pseudopodial cytoplasmic projections (Wright's stain, 50x oil).

TABLE 1: Laboratory parameters on admission.

Laboratory tests	On admission	Reference range
Total WBC ($\times10^9$/L)	37.3	4–10
Hemoglobin (g/dL)	12.7	12–15
Platelet ($\times10^9$/L)	127	150–400
Neutrophil ($\times10^9$/L)	31.7	1.6–7.2
Lymphocyte ($\times10^9$/L)	1.8	1.1–4.0
Serum creatinine (mg/dL)	1.65	0.6–1.4
Serum BUN (mg/dL)	31	8–22
Alkaline phosphatase (U/L)	229	30–110
AST (U/L)	46	10–37
ALT (U/L)	29	8–37
Bilirubin (mg/dL)	2.3	0.3–1.2
Direct bilirubin (mg/dL)	1.2	0–0.3
Lactic acid (mmol/L)	6	0.5–2.2
LDH (U/L)	207	100–238

WBC: white blood cells; BUN: blood urea nitrogen; AST: aspartate aminotransferase; ALT: alanine aminotransferase; LDH: lactate dehydrogenase.

Extensive infectious workup studies including urine culture, blood culture, respiratory virus panel, hepatitis, and HIV were all negative. The peripheral blood smear showed severe neutrophilia with toxic granulation and a small number of atypical lymphocytes (Figure 1). These atypical cells have an irregular nuclear contour and prominent nucleoli and vacuoles. Hematolymphoid malignancies were added to the differential diagnosis list. Flow cytometric analysis of peripheral blood (Figure 2(a)) revealed a small population of abnormal T-cells, which was positive for CD45 and CD7, but negative for CD2, CD3, CD4, CD5, CD8, CD16, CD56, and CD57. In addition, aberrant CD13 expression was also detected (data not shown). These cells featured increased forward scatter and side scatter, when compared with immunophenotypically normal lymphocytes. While pathological evaluation of the bone marrow was in process, the patient's leukocytosis rapidly worsened and peaked at 110.6 billion/L. She developed multiorgan failure requiring ventilator support, continuous renal replacement therapy, and multiple vasopressors. Her laboratory parameters along her clinical course are shown in Figure 3. Despite maximum supportive therapy, her condition continued to decline. After extensive discussion, her family decided to pursue comfort care and she expired approximately 80 hours after initial presentation.

The flow cytometric analysis of the bone marrow aspirate (Figure 2(b)) showed a small T-cell population (3.7% of marrow nucleated cells) with identical immunophenotypic features to those in peripheral blood. Bone marrow core biopsy revealed hypercellularity with loose clusters of small to medium sized neoplastic cells, accounting for 5–10% of the

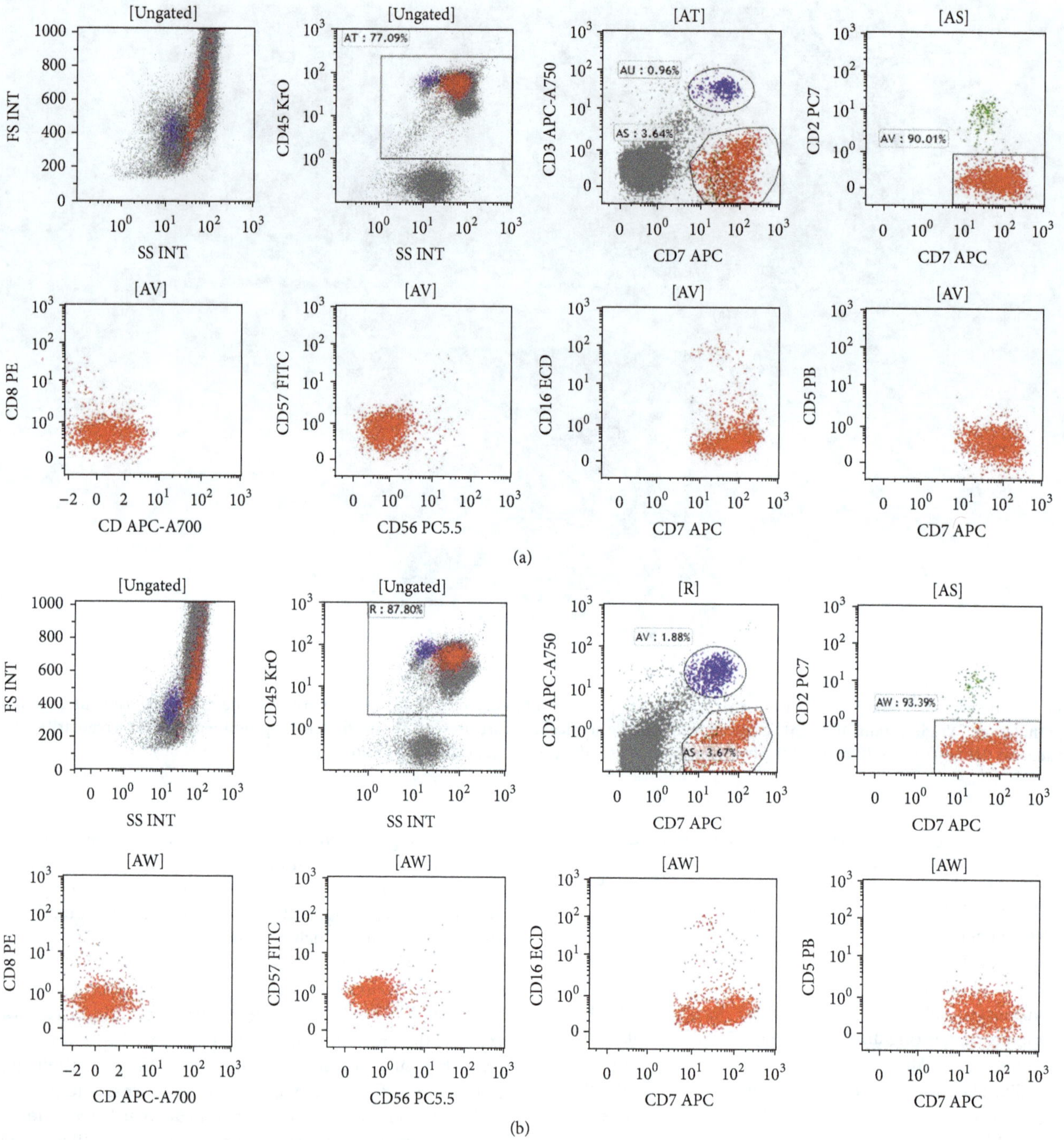

FIGURE 2: Peripheral blood and bone marrow aspiration analyzed by flow cytometry. Flow cytometry analysis of peripheral blood (a) and bone marrow (b) revealed a similar small population of atypical lymphocytes (red) which are positive for CD45 and CD7 and negative for CD2, CD3, CD4, CD5, CD8, CD16, CD56, and CD57. Normal T-cells are in blue and normal natural killer cells are in green.

marrow cellularity (Figures 4 and 5). The immunohistochemistry studies of the core biopsy revealed that lymphoma cells expressed CD30 (strong), CD7 (strong), and ALK (cytoplasmic) (Figure 5). The expression of epithelial membrane antigen (EMA) appeared to be equivocal. Autopsy showed diffuse microscopic lymphoma infiltration of the spleen (Figures 6(a) and 6(b)), lung (Figures 6(c) and 6(d)), and liver. Intravascular lymphoma involvement was present in both brain and lung (Figures 6(e) and 6(f)). Bone marrow cytogenetic evaluation identified an unusual chromosome 2 inversion [inv(2)(p23q22)] resulting in ALK gene rearrangement, as well as a translocation involving the inv(2) chromosome

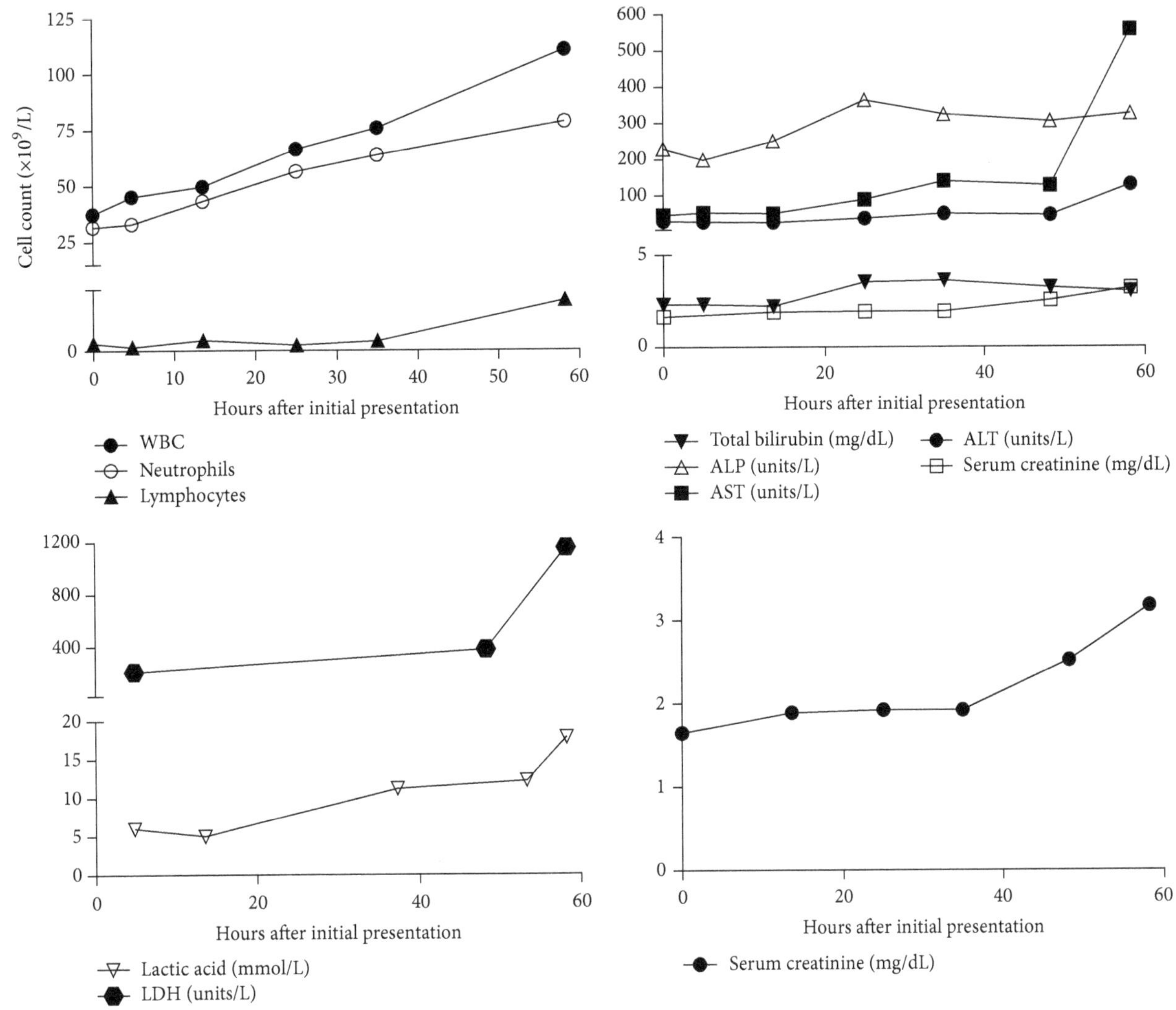

FIGURE 3: Laboratory parameters along the patient's clinical course. White blood cells (WBC), absolute neutrophil counts, lymphocyte counts, renal and liver function tests, and lactic acid and lactate dehydrogenase (LDH) levels are shown.

with chromosome 22q (Figure 7(a)); however, fluorescence in situ hybridization (FISH) studies demonstrated that the ALK gene was not involved in the translocation with chromosome 22 (Figure 7(b)). These findings are consistent with small-cell variant of ALCL.

3. Discussion

Prognosis in ALK+ ALCL is good overall, except for the small-cell variant [3, 5]. Correct clinical diagnosis of the small-cell variant of ALCL is often challenging as the scarce "hallmark cells" are scattered among inflammatory cells and may be difficult to recognize. Table 2 lists characteristics of small-cell and classic variants of ALCL. The extraordinary leukocytosis and "left shift" often prompt an extensive microbiology and serology workup in search for a cause of presumed infection or sepsis. Mosunjac et al. reviewed 23 autopsy cases of ALCL and reported a distinct subset of 5 fatal and premortem unrecognized ALCL cases [7]. Similar to our case, these cases were characterized by unusual presentations of fever of unknown origin (FUO), sepsis, hepatosplenomegaly, lactic acidosis, rapid clinical deterioration, and absence of significant peripheral lymphadenopathy. These characteristics are different than the classic presentation of ALCL, which includes night sweats, weight loss, and peripheral lymphadenopathy. Recognition of a combination of clinic pictures with markers of sepsis, lactic acidosis, hepatosplenomegaly, and a negative infectious workup should trigger suspicion to rule out ALCL. A meticulous examination of peripheral blood smears, comprehensive immunophenotypic studies, and early bone marrow and lymph node biopsy are needed to facilitate diagnosis. In our case, peripheral smear evaluation revealed atypical lymphocytes which raised suspicion for lymphoma and prompted early bone marrow evaluation. However, the patient's rapid deterioration precluded further lymph node biopsy.

About 60% of ALCL cases are associated with chromosomal translocations involving ALK on chromosome 2p23

TABLE 2: Comparison of classic and small-cell variant ALCL.

	Classic ALCL variant	Small-cell ALCL variant
Frequency	70% of ALCL	5%–10% of ALCL
ALK rearrangement	ALK-positive and ALK-negative	ALK-positive
Morphology	Characterized with numerous large round or pleomorphic cells with horseshoe-shaped nuclei with multiple (or single) prominent nucleoli; these cells are also called "hallmark" cells	The majorities of cells are small to medium in size and have clear cytoplasm and irregular nuclei; a minor population of "hallmark" cells can present singly or in cluster [5]
Peripheral leukemia involvement	Extremely rare	Very common [5, 6]
Bone marrow involvement	Relatively infrequent (10%–30% of cases)	Common; usually subtle bone marrow involvement with a small cluster of small lymphocytes and only rare scattered large tumor cells [5, 6]
Systemic involvement	Relatively less infrequent	Frequently associated with widespread disseminated disease [6]
Prognosis	2-year survival of 73%	2-year survival of 50% and 3-year disease-free survival of 25% [3, 5]

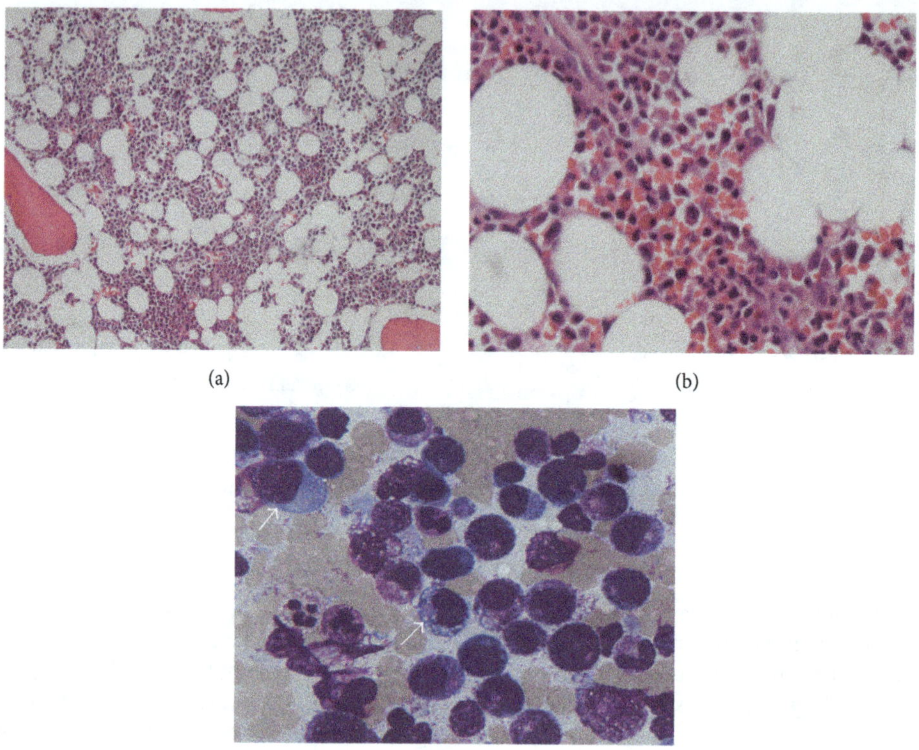

(a) (b) (c)

FIGURE 4: Morphological features of bone marrow core biopsy and aspiration. The H&E *section of* bone marrow core biopsy demonstrated hypercellularity for the patient's age with myeloid hyperplasia ((a) 100x magnification; (b) 400x magnification). Scattered lymphoma cells (pointed by the white arrows) were easily seen on aspirate smears ((c) Wright's stain, 1000x magnification) but not easily discernible on H&E sections.

[8], which encodes a transmembrane receptor tyrosine kinase that belongs to the insulin receptor superfamily. ALK signaling can be activated by the oncogenic fusion of the ALK gene with a variety of partner genes through translocation events. The constitutive activation of chimeric ALK fusion proteins leads to complex signaling transduction pathways including the JAK/STAT and PI3K/AKT pathways, which control cell proliferation, survival, and cell cycling [8].

Among ALK+ ALCLs, about 80% of cases contain the t(2;5) (p23;q35) translocation, resulting in the formation of an NPM-ALK fusion protein, a transmembrane tyrosine kinase receptor [9]. Variant translocations involving ALK and other

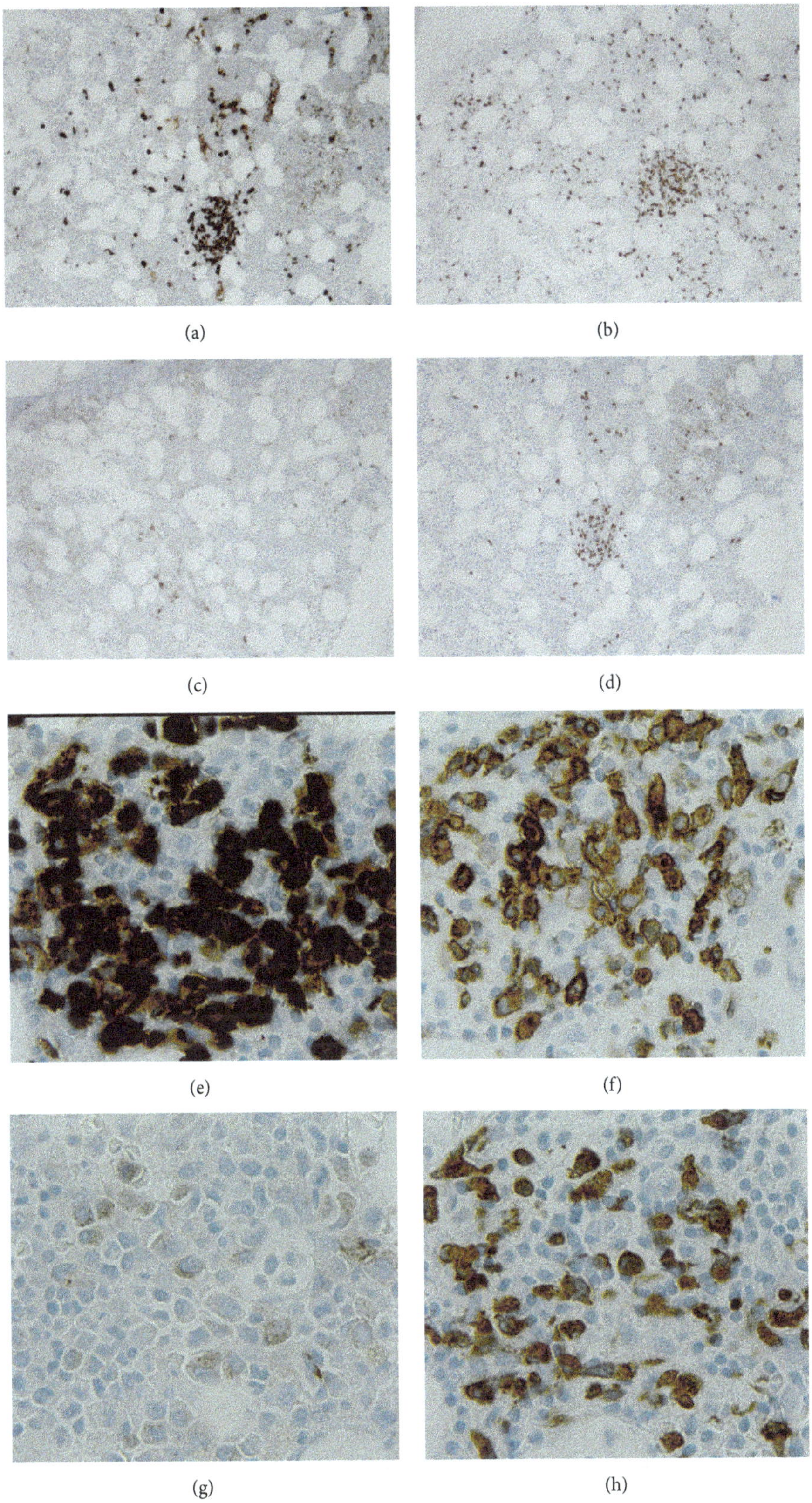

FIGURE 5: Immunohistochemistry staining of bone marrow core biopsy. Small to intermediate sized neoplastic cells form loose clusters and comprise 5–10% of marrow cellularity. These cells stain positive for CD30 (a, e), CD7 (b, f), EMA (equivocal) (c, g), and ALK (d, h). (a–d) 100x magnification; (e–h) 1000x magnification.

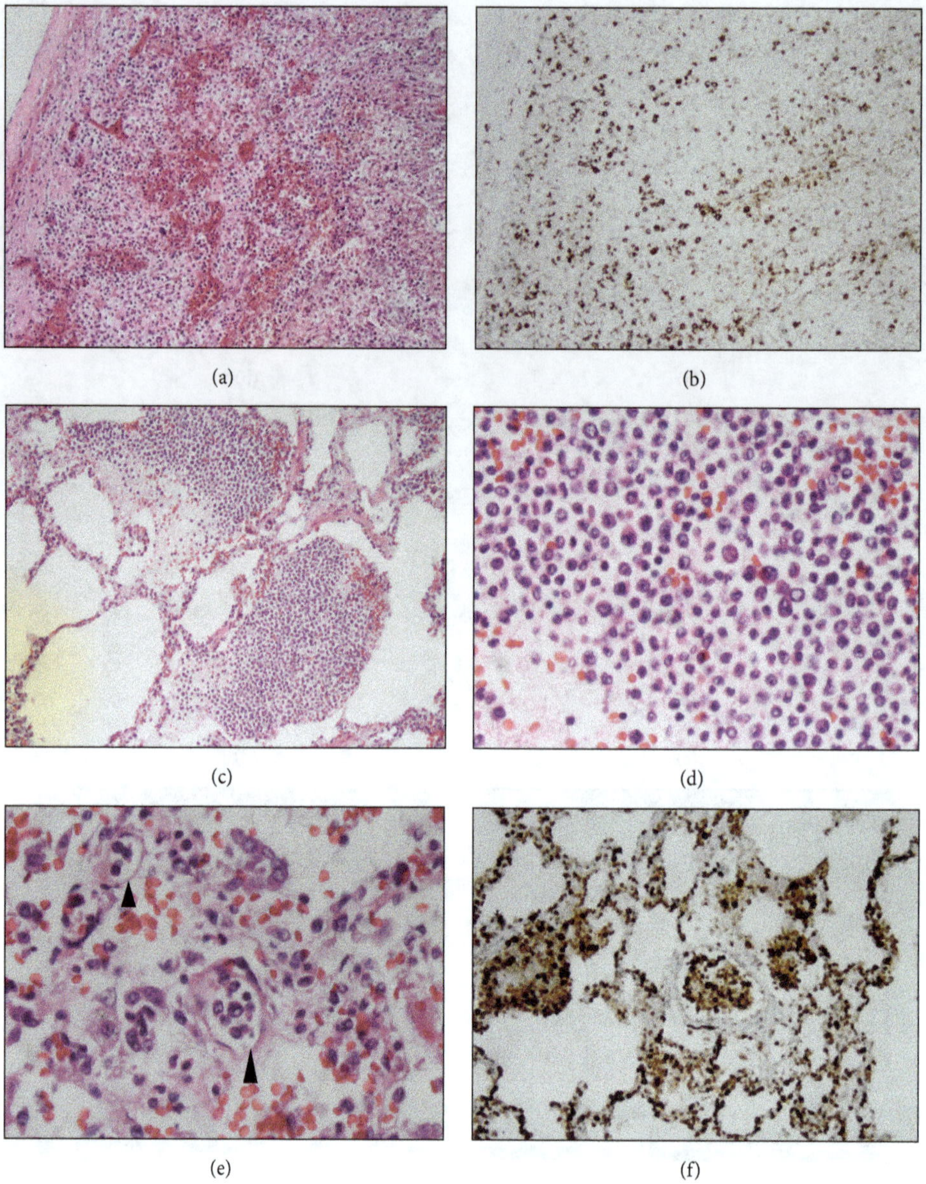

FIGURE 6: Representative autopsy sections from spleen and lung. Lymphoma cells were not overtly discernible on H&E section ((a) 100x magnification) but clearly identified by immunostains ((b) CD30 staining) in the spleen. In the lung parenchyma, lymphoid infiltrates were prominent with predominantly small to medium sized cells (H&E staining; (c) 100x magnification; (d) 400x magnification). Intravascular lymphoma involvement was evident morphologically ((e) H&E staining, 400x magnification) and confirmed by immunostains ((f) CD30, 200x magnification). Black arrowheads in (e) refer to intravascular lymphoma involvement.

partner genes on chromosomes 1, 2, 3, 17, 19, 22, and X also occur [9]. Rare ALK gene rearrangement variants involving inv(2)(p23;q35), resulting in ATIC-ALK fusion, have also been reported previously [10]. The cytogenetic abnormality in our patient with inv(2)(p23q22) has never been reported previously. Because FISH studies confirmed that ALK did not translocate to chromosome 22, the translocation in this patient appears to be dissimilar to the t(2;22) reported in the literature for ALCL. Therefore, ALK rearrangement in this case would appear to generate a novel ALK fusion gene.

While leukemic peripheral blood involvement is rare in ALCL, an association has been reported with small-cell variants [5, 6, 11], which may be a potential explanation for the poor prognosis and aggressive nature of small-cell variant ALCL. Extreme leukocytosis involving neutrophils and atypical lymphocytes is usually the feature noted in the peripheral blood. The neutrophils are often left shifted with toxic granulation features, whereas the lymphocytes are a mixture of small to medium size atypical cells, with an irregular nuclear contour and cytoplasmic azurophilic granules. Large basophilic vacuolated cells can occasionally be seen as well [5].

Another unique feature of our case is the rare intravascular pattern of lymphoma involvement in this presentation of

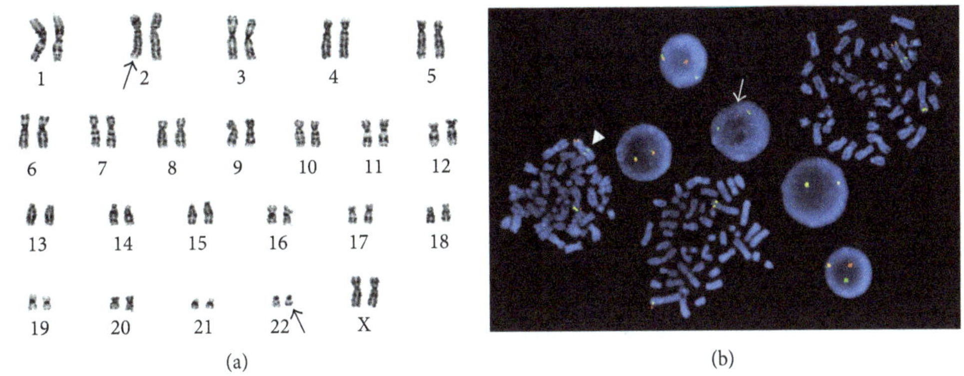

FIGURE 7: Cytogenetic analysis of bone marrow. (a) The G-banded metaphase cell demonstrates abnormalities involving chromosomes 2 and 22 (black arrows), interpreted to represent an initial chromosome 2 pericentric inversion that disrupts the ALK gene at band 2p23 and translocates the centromeric portion of the gene to band 2q22. This is followed by a translocation between the inverted chromosome 2 (with a breakpoint distal to the ALK gene) and chromosome 22q. The karyotype is designated as 46,XX,inv(2)(p23q22)t[inv(2);22)(p24;q12)]. (b) Fluorescence in situ hybridization (FISH) utilizing an ALK gene break-apart probe demonstrates disruption of the gene (white arrow) and relocation of the centromeric portion of the gene to the long arm of chromosome 2 (white arrow head) as a result of the chromosome 2 pericentric inversion.

ALK+ ALCL. The vast majority of reported cases are in B-cell lineage lymphomas, and intravascular lymphoma involvement is rarely seen in T-cell lymphoma. Among the small number of cases reported in T-cell lymphoma, the majority of these are peripheral T-cell lymphoma [12, 13]. A review of the literature demonstrated only 11 documented cases of CD30-positive T-cell lymphomas, suggestive of ALCL as the lymphoma type [7, 13–18]. Intravascular involvement was seen in all 5 autopsy cases reported by Mosunjac et al., all of which were ALK-negative, except one [7]. Other than this case described by Mosunjac et al. and our case, only one other ALK+ ALCL case, which mimicked inflammatory breast carcinoma, was reported to have intravascular involvement in the reported English literature [18]. It has been postulated that systemic symptoms and the aggressive course of the disease might be related to release of cytokines. Direct interaction of vascular endothelial cells and lymphoma cells may trigger the proinflammatory cytokine cascade and distort hemostatic balance. Intravascular involvement may be an indicator for poor prognosis as seen in our case and is also suggested by previously reported cases [7].

Despite the generally favorable prognosis of ALK + ALCL, cases with peripheral leukemic involvement often respond poorly to standard first-line anthracycline-based multiagent chemotherapy. Brentuximab vedotin (Adcetris), a CD30 antibody-drug conjugate, has been approved for relapsed or treatment refractory ALCL cases. A Phase III clinical trial is underway to evaluate brentuximab vedotin combined with chemotherapy in the first-line treatment of ALCL (clinical trial number NCT01777152). Crizotinib and ceritinib, ALK tyrosine kinase inhibitors, have shown encouraging activity in small case series [19, 20]. These agents are currently being explored in ongoing clinical trials. Hopefully, these novel therapies may improve the prognosis for ALK+ ALCL variants.

4. Conclusion

We report a case of ALK+ ALCL small-cell variant with a presentation mimicking sepsis. Small-cell variant, leukemic peripheral involvement, and intravascular involvement are associated with unfavorable prognosis.

Conflicts of Interest

The authors declare that they have no conflicts of interest.

References

[1] S. H. Swerdlow, E. Campo, S. A. Pileri et al., "The 2016 revision of the World Health Organization classification of lymphoid neoplasms," *Blood*, vol. 127, no. 20, pp. 2375–2390, 2016.

[2] H. Stein, H.-D. Foss, H. Durkop et al., "CD30^{+} anaplastic large cell lymphoma: a review of its histopathologic, genetic, and clinical features," *Blood*, vol. 96, no. 12, pp. 3681–3695, 2000.

[3] E. Youd, A. M. Boyde, R. L. Attanoos, and S. D. Dojcinov, "Small cell variant of anaplastic large cell lymphoma: A 10-year review of the All Wales Lymphoma Panel database: Correspondence," *Histopathology*, vol. 55, no. 3, pp. 355–358, 2009.

[4] L. Lamant, K. McCarthy, E. D'Amore et al., "Prognostic impact of morphologic and phenotypic features of childhood ALK-positive anaplastic large-cell lymphoma: results of the ALCL99 study," *Journal of Clinical Oncology*, vol. 29, no. 35, pp. 4669–4676, 2011.

[5] T. A. Summers and J. T. Moncur, "The small cell variant of anaplastic large cell lymphoma," *Archives of Pathology & Laboratory Medicine*, vol. 134, no. 11, pp. 1706–1710, 2010.

[6] M. C. Kinney, R. A. Higgins, and E. A. Medina, "Anaplastic large cell lymphoma: twenty-five years of discovery," *Archives of Pathology & Laboratory Medicine*, vol. 135, no. 1, pp. 19–43, 2011.

[7] M. B. Mosunjac, J. B. Sundstrom, and M. I. Mosunjac, "Unusual presentation of anaplastic large cell lymphoma with clinical course mimicking fever of unknown origin and sepsis: autopsy

study of five cases," *Croatian Medical Journal*, vol. 49, no. 5, pp. 660–668, 2008.

[8] H. M. Amin and R. Lai, "Pathobiology of ALK+ anaplastic large-cell lymphoma," *Blood*, vol. 110, no. 7, pp. 2259–2267, 2007.

[9] R. Chiarle, C. Voena, C. Ambrogio, R. Piva, and G. Inghirami, "The anaplastic lymphoma kinase in the pathogenesis of cancer," *Nature Reviews Cancer*, vol. 8, no. 1, pp. 11–23, 2008.

[10] G. W. B. Colleoni, J. A. Bridge, B. Garicochea, J. Liu, D. A. Filippa, and M. Ladanyi, "ATIC-ALK: A novel variant ALK gene fusion in anaplastic large cell lymphoma resulting from the recurrent cryptic chromosomal inversion, inv(2)(p23q35)," *American Journal of Pathology*, vol. 156, no. 3, pp. 781–789, 2000.

[11] J. T. Nguyen, M. R. Condron, N. D. Nguyen, J. De, L. J. Medeiros, and A. Padula, "Anaplastic large cell lymphoma in leukemic phase: Extraordinarily high white blood cell count," *Pathology International*, vol. 59, no. 5, pp. 345–353, 2009.

[12] B. C. Gleason, N. K. Brinster, S. R. Granter, G. S. Pinkus, N. I. Lindeman, and D. M. Miller, "Intravascular cytotoxic T-cell lymphoma: A case report and review of the literature," *Journal of the American Academy of Dermatology*, vol. 58, no. 2, pp. 290–294, 2008.

[13] L. Cerroni, C. Massone, H. Kutzner, T. Mentzel, P. Umbert, and H. Kerl, "Intravascular large T-cell or NK-cell lymphoma: A rare variant of intravascular large cell lymphoma with frequent cytotoxic phenotype and association with Epstein-Barr virus infection," *American Journal of Surgical Pathology*, vol. 32, no. 6, pp. 891–898, 2008.

[14] E. Takahashi, K. Kajimoto, T. Fukatsu, M. Yoshida, T. Eimoto, and S. Nakamura, "Intravascular large T-cell lymphoma: A case report of CD30-positive and ALK-negative anaplastic type with cytotoxic molecule expression," *Virchows Archiv*, vol. 447, no. 6, pp. 1000–1006, 2005.

[15] Y. H. Ko, J. H. Han, J. H. Go et al., "Intravascular lymphomatosis: A clinicopathological study of two cases presenting as an interstitial lung disease," *Histopathology*, vol. 31, no. 6, pp. 555–562, 1997.

[16] F. Lopez-Gil, M. Roura, I. Umbert, and P. Umbert, "Malignant proliferative angioendotheliomatosis or angiotropic lymphoma associated with a soft-tissue lymphoma," *Journal of the American Academy of Dermatology*, vol. 26, no. 1, pp. 101–104, 1992.

[17] N. Sepp, G. Schuler, N. Romani et al., ""Intravascular lymphomatosis" (angioendotheliomatosis): Evidence for a T-cell origin in two cases," *Human Pathology*, vol. 21, no. 10, pp. 1051–1058, 1990.

[18] C. Krishnan, S. Moline, K. Anders, and R. A. Warnke, "Intravascular ALK-positive anaplastic large-cell lymphoma mimicking inflammatory breast carcinoma," *Journal of Clinical Oncology*, vol. 27, no. 15, pp. 2563–2565, 2009.

[19] C. Gambacorti Passerini, F. Farina, A. Stasia et al., "Crizotinib in advanced, chemoresistant anaplastic lymphoma kinase-positive lymphoma patients," *Journal of the National Cancer Institute*, vol. 106, no. 2, p. djt378, 2014.

[20] V. Mak, J. Hamm, M. Chhanabhai et al., "Survival of patients with peripheral T-cell lymphoma after first relapse or progression: spectrum of disease and rare long-term survivors," *Journal of Clinical Oncology*, vol. 31, no. 16, pp. 1970–1976, 2013.

25

Chronic Lymphocytic Leukemia and Myelofibrosis

Fares Darawshy,[1] Arieh Ben-Yehuda,[1] Karine Atlan,[2] and Deborah Rund[3]

[1]*Internal Medicine Division, Internal Medicine C Department, Hebrew University-Hadassah Medical Organization, Jerusalem, Israel*
[2]*The Pathology Institute, Hebrew University-Hadassah Medical Organization, Jerusalem, Israel*
[3]*Hematology Department, Hebrew University-Hadassah Medical Organization, Jerusalem, Israel*

Correspondence should be addressed to Fares Darawshy; faresdarawshy@gmail.com

Academic Editor: Pier P. Piccaluga

Background. Chronic lymphocytic lymphoma (CLL) can be associated with several malignancies, but rarely with myelofibrosis. Only isolated case reports in the literature described the association between CLL and primary myelofibrosis (PMF) in the same patient. *Objectives.* We describe a case of CLL characterized by the development of PMF and a review of literature. *Methods.* We describe an 86-year-old female diagnosed as having CLL and followed by the development of splenomegaly and progressively rising LDH levels 27 months later. A bone marrow biopsy was consistent with the diagnosis of PMF, with positive JAK-2 V617F mutation. We also review the clinical and molecular characteristics of patients with CLL and PMF. *Results.* Patients with CLL and PMF are usually older. A lead diagnosis of CLL harbored by PMF is the most common clinical course, although concomitant diseases may occur in 31.7% of patients. JAK-2 V617F mutation can be found in 48.7% of patients. *Conclusion.* This case reported here constitutes an unusual situation of CLL characterized by the development of PMF. Etiologic and pathogenic associations—the role of *t* (1; 6) and JAK-2 V617F mutation—are discussed.

1. Introduction

Chronic lymphocytic leukemia (CLL) is a mature B-cell low-grade lymphoproliferative malignancy, characterized by monoclonal B lymphocytes expressing the CD5 antigen. This malignancy stems from mature lymphocytes in the germinal center of human lymph nodes, and bone marrow involvement in CLL is considered to be secondary. Chromosomal abnormalities that can be found in cytogenetic analysis include trisomy 12 and abnormalities in chromosome 13 [1, 2]. Primary myelofibrosis (PMF) is a disorder of a multipotent hematopoietic progenitor cell that causes clonal myeloproliferation accompanied by reactive bone marrow fibrosis and extramedullary hematopoiesis [3]. JAK-2 mutation can be found in 50% of PMF patients [4], and chromosomal abnormalities include trisomy 8, trisomy 9, and deletion 13, 9, or 20.

CLL has been associated with several malignancies, including transformation to diffuse large B-cell lymphoma and solid neoplasms [5], and any bone marrow involvement in CLL is assumed to be secondary. Usually, CLL is not associated with primary or secondary bone marrow fibrosis. The association between CLL and PMF and other myeloproliferative neoplasms (MPN) is unusual and has been reported [6–16]. Despite the growing number of reported patients with CLL and myeloproliferative disorders, the incidence of concomitant CLL and PMF is underreported and the clinical, molecular, and prognostic data are still lacking. The purpose of this report is to describe a patient diagnosed with CLL, and her clinical course was characterized by the development of myelofibrosis. A review of the literature and possible etiologic and pathogenic associations are discussed.

2. Case Report

An 86-year-old female, with a history of hypertension, type 2 diabetes mellitus, hiatus hernia, and diverticulosis, attended

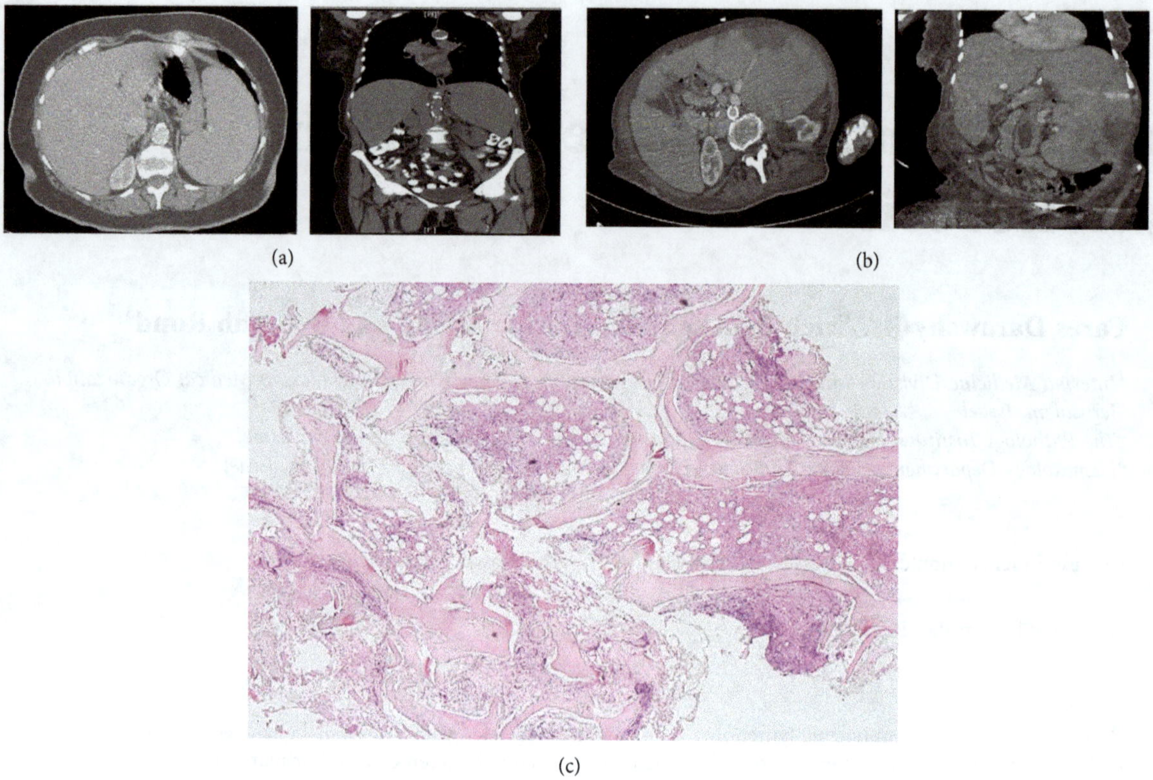

FIGURE 1: CT scan showing (a) 15 cm splenomegaly after CLL diagnosis in 2006. (b) CT scan in 2013 showing increased massive splenomegaly (28 cm) with splenic infarct and hepatomegaly, after PMF diagnosis. (c) Bone marrow biopsy showing hypercellular bone marrow with fibrosis, consistent with the diagnosis of myelofibrosis.

the hematology clinic in February 2003 for evaluation of lymphocytosis. Physical examination revealed neither lymphadenopathy nor organomegaly. The hemoglobin concentration was 11.4 g/dL, leukocyte count was 16.1×10^9/L with 60% lymphocytes, mean corpuscular volume (MCV) 88.4 fL, and platelet count 332×10^9/L. LDH was 569 units, mild IgG paraproteinemia (1130 mg/dL). Phenotypic analysis of blood lymphocytes by flow cytometry revealed CD5/19+ coexpression of 78% of the lymphocytes. No bone marrow biopsy was done. On abdominal ultrasound from June 2002, the spleen length was 9 cm. All these findings were suggestive for the diagnosis of CLL, Rai stage 0/Binet stage A.

The patient was followed up for 27 months, during which progressive disproportionate splenomegaly (15 cm) with progressive rise in serum LDH (999 units) developed. In addition, the patient complained of anorexia and 30 kg weight loss. Physical examination revealed an enlarged spleen approximately 6 cm below the costal margin, but no palpable lymphadenopathy or hepatomegaly. Complete blood count showed hemoglobin concentration of 11.3 g/dL, leukocyte count of 19.8×10^9/L with 58% lymphocytes, and platelet count of 240×10^9/L. Peripheral blood smear revealed teardrop-shaped and nucleated red blood cells and immature cells of the myeloid lineage. Bone marrow biopsy revealed a hypercellular bone marrow with increased reticulin stain and fibrosis (Figure 1). A karyotype from the bone marrow showed chromosomal abnormalities of

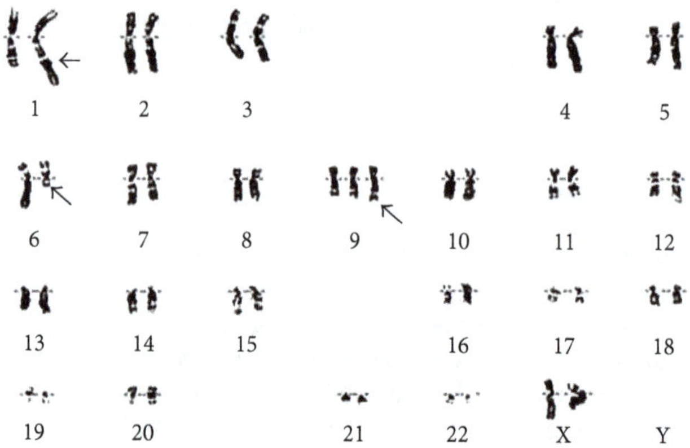

FIGURE 2: Karyotype showing trisomy 9, *t* (1; 6).

trisomy 9 (+9) and *t* (1; 6) (Figure 2). All findings were compatible with the diagnosis of myelofibrosis. The presence of the JAK-2 mutation was not examined at the time of diagnosis. Cytometric analysis of blood lymphocytes showed a majority of B cells (77% CD19+, 80% CD20+, and 42% CD22+). The patient was lost to follow-up for 2 years and admitted to the internal medicine department three times, two years later. Patient's last admission was due to anorexia, weight loss, dysphagia, and recurrent aspirations. Complete blood count showed normocytic anemia and stable lymphocytosis. Peripheral blood smear was compatible with bone marrow fibrosis. Imaging studies showed massive splenomegaly (Figure 1, about 28 cm on CT scan). With a diagnosis of suspected PMF presenting with massive splenomegaly, the patient was advised to be treated with ruxolitinib, a JAK-2 inhibitor. The patient refused to take any treatment and died due to infection. After her death, JAK-2 V617F mutation analysis was positive in the bone marrow biopsy that revealed bone marrow fibrosis, assuring the diagnosis of PMF.

3. Discussion

A variety of lymphoproliferative diseases can cause secondary bone marrow fibrosis, including Hodgkin's disease, multiple myeloma, hairy cell leukemia, and non-Hodgkin's lymphoma. In the patient described above, a diagnosis of myelofibrosis was made subsequent to CLL.

In the above reported patient, a diagnosis of CLL preceded PMF diagnosis by 27 months, based on phenotypic analysis and complete blood count only. Although bone marrow biopsy was not done at the time of CLL diagnosis, patient had no symptoms, signs, or laboratory criteria suggestive for myelofibrosis. The bone marrow biopsy done later, together with JAK-2 V617F mutation, confirms the diagnosis of PMF.

The association or coexistence of CLL with PMF in the same host is extremely unusual but was reported previously. Three cases of rapidly developing myelofibrosis after the diagnosis of CLL [5, 6, 12, 13] were reported, in addition to reports describing the coexistence of CLL and myelofibrosis [7, 8, 14]. In addition, a growing evidence from retrospective reviews revealed a clear association between lymphoproliferative disease and MPN, especially CLL and MPN. A retrospective review reported 46 cases suffering from concomitant CLL and myeloproliferative disorders, 4 of whom were PMF [10]. There was no association between the development of the myeloproliferative malignancy and the chemotherapy given for CLL. In addition, the course of CLL was not affected by the treatment of PMF and vice versa. Todisco et al. [15] retrospectively examined the clinical and biological characteristics of 13 patients with CLL and MPN, 8 of them with PMF which occurred in 1 patient who was followed and treated for CLL and in one patient concomitantly with CLL. JAK-2 mutation was found in 3 patients with CLL/PMF. These findings suggest that CLL and PMF pathological etiology and process and cooccurrence might not be random. Our patient's clinical course and findings are compatible with that reported by Todisco et al. Marchetti et al. [16] reviewed data from 50 papers reporting 214 individuals harboring both MPN and lymphoproliferative disease. Among 50 patients with myelofibrosis, 23 harbored CLL—7 were synchronous, 12 cases with prior CLL, and 4 with prior myelofibrosis. CLL was the most common lymphoproliferative disease particularly among patients with lymphoproliferative disease preceding MPN, and most of subsequent MPN developed by CLL patients were PMF. The median time between CLL and MPN diagnosis was 72 months.

Despite the number of reported patients with CLL and PMF getting larger, the clinical, molecular, and prognostic characteristics are still lacking. Tables 1 and 2 show the major clinical and molecular characteristics of available reported cases and series with CLL and PMF diagnosis in the same patient. Overall, 41 cases were reported, and average age was 61.75 years. Although some data are lacking, most of the reported patients with available data were males, and a finding by Marchetti et al. also reported that CLL and PMF can present concomitantly (in 13/41 (31.7%) of cases) or CLL can precede PMF diagnosis, with lead time varying between 2.3 and 13.6 years. Analysis of survival is limited due to lack of data, but previous reports [16] did not show any significant difference from the overall population except for higher age at MPN diagnosis. In addition, molecular data available are very limited, but it is worth mentioning that JAK-2 V617F mutation was present in 20/41 (48.7%) of reported cases, compared to 37.5% reported by Todisco et al.

The exact mechanism in which myelofibrosis develops in the presence of CLL is also still unclear. Kimura et al. reported a case of CLL with secondary myelofibrosis and confirmed the role of interleukin-1 alpha (IL-1α) in the pathogenesis, stating that CLL cells secrete IL-1 which stimulates the growth of fibroblasts, causing bone marrow fibrosis in vitro [11]. Several pathogenic mechanisms were suggested to explain the association between CLL and PMF, including independent proliferations of two separate clonal cells causing two unrelated diseases, chromosomal or molecular abnormality in a multipotent cell causing bilineage clonal proliferation and incidental association [6, 8].

In our case, the diagnosis of PMF was confirmed by the histological method. In our opinion, in the reported patient, CLL preceded the development of PMF, and JAK-2 V617F mutation contributed to PMF development. This hypothesis is supported by results of previous studies [10, 15, 16] showing that CLL is the most common lymphoproliferative disease preceding PMF, along with the development of JAK-2 V617F mutation which is known to increase the risk for lymphoma [17, 18]. Our patient did not have any therapy for CLL or other types of cancer, deferring therapy, and cancer-related myelofibrosis. Unfortunately, JAK-2 mutation and karyotype were not done at time of CLL diagnosis, but it was done later showing JAK-2 V617F mutation, trisomy 9 which was known to be associated with PMF, and *t* (1; 6) which was reported by L. Michaux et al. to be a novel cytogenetic aberration exclusively found in unmutated CLL [19]. This translocation was found to be associated with an aggressive clinical course but had no known association to myelofibrosis. We do notice the coexistence of *t* (1; 6) and trisomy 9, chromosomal abnormalities that appear in CLL and PMF, but no clear association can be found between both. We do suggest further evaluation of the role of *t* (1; 6) in bone marrow fibrosis in future studies.

4. Conclusion

In this case report, we reported a patient in whom a diagnosis of CLL and myelofibrosis was made. No clear association was found between these two diseases in past reports. Older patients tend to develop CLL and PMF, with the most common clinical course of CLL preceding PMF

TABLE 1: Clinical characteristics of reported patients with CLL and PMF.

Report	Patient's number	Age at CLL diagnosis, mean (years)	Sex, males/females (% males)	Time between CLL and PMF Dx, median (years)	Chemotherapy, n (%)	Simultaneous diagnosis of CLL and myelofibrosis, n (%)	Death after myelofibrosis diagnosis, n (%)	Survival, median (years)
Lennard et al. [6]	1	42	0/1 (0)	6.3	1 (100)	0 (0)	1 (100)	0.45
Nieto et al. [7]	1	70	0/1 (0)	2.3	Not given	0 (0)	Not available	Not available
Palta et al. [8]	1	60	1/0 (100)	0	Prednisolone	1 (100)	Not available	Not available
Burgstaller et al. [9]	1	61	0/1 (0)	0	Lenalidomide	1 (100)	No	Not available
Laurenti et al. [11]	4	69.75	4/0 (100)	Not available	1 (25)	2 (50)	Not available	Not available
Salama et al. [14]	2	68	2/0 (100)	4.5 (0–9)	Hydroxyurea	1 (50)	No	Not available
Todisco et al. [15]	8	60.3	Not available	6.05 (0–13.6)	5 (62.5)	1 (12.5)	4 (50)	8.9 (0.7–15.7)
Marchetti et al. [16]	23	66.5 (26–81)	Not available	6	Not available	7 (30.4)	Not available	Not available

TABLE 2: Molecular characteristics of reported patients with CLL and PMF.

Report	Karyotype at CLL diagnosis	IGHV mutation, n (%)	JAK-2 mutation, n (%)	Karyotype at myelofibrosis diagnosis
Lennard et al. [6]	Not available	Not available	Not available	Not available
Nieto et al. [7]	Not available	Not available	Not available	Not available
Palta et al. [8]	Not available	Not available	Negative	Not available
Burgstaller et al. [9]	Normal	Not available	Negative	Normal
Laurenti et al. [10]	Not available	1 (25)	2 (50)	Not available
Salama et al. [14]	Not available	Negative	Negative	Not available
Todisco et al. [15]	Normal (50%) t (3; 12) (12.5%) Del 20q11 (12.5%) Del 5q, del 13q (12.5%) Not available (12.5%)	4 (50)	3 (37.5)	Del 7 (12.5) Del 8q21, del 20q11 (12.5) Del 5q, del 13q (12.5) t (3; 12) (12.5)
Marchetti et al. [16]	Not available	Not available	15 (65.2)	Not available

diagnosis, and nearly 50% of patients have JAK-2 V617F mutation. Unfortunately, we could not find any new molecular or chromosomal abnormalities that explain the development or coexistence of myelofibrosis in CLL, but we do suggest the role of JAK-2 V617F mutation and t (1; 6) as main molecular abnormalities.

Conflicts of Interest

The authors declare that they have no conflicts of interest.

References

[1] D. L Longo, "Malignancies of lymphoid cells," in *Harrison's Principles of Internal Medicine*, D. Longo, A. Fauci, and D. Kasper, Eds., pp. 919–935, McGraw-Hill Medical Publishing Division, New York, NY, USA, 18th edition, 2012.

[2] G. Juliusson, D. G. Oscier, M. Fitchett et al., "Prognostic subgroups in B-cell chronic lymphocytic leukemia defined by specific chromosomal abnormalities," *New England Journal of Medicine*, vol. 323, no. 11, pp. 720–724, 1990.

[3] A. Tefferi, "Myelofibrosis with myeloid metaplasia," *New England Journal of Medicine*, vol. 342, no. 17, pp. 1255–1265, 2000.

[4] J. T. Reilly, "Idiopathic myelofibrosis: pathogenesis to treatment," *Hematological Oncology*, vol. 24, no. 2, pp. 56–63, 2006.

[5] D. Manusow and B. H. Weinerman, "Subsequent neoplasia in chronic lymphocytic leukemia," *Journal of the American Medical Association*, vol. 232, no. 3, pp. 267–269, 1975.

[6] A. L. Lennard and S. J. Proctor, "Chronic lymphocytic leukemia terminating in acute myelofibrosis," *Journal of Clinical Pathology*, vol. 37, no. 5, pp. 564–567, 1984.

[7] L. H. Nieto, J. M. Raya Sánchez, H. A. Arguelles, M. L. Brito Barroso, and B. G. González, "A case of chronic lymphocytic leukemia overwhelmed by rapidly progressing idiopathic myelofibrosis," *Haematologica*, vol. 85, no. 9, pp. 973–977, 2000.

[8] A. Palta, S. Garg, S. Chauhan, and N. Varma, "Simultaneous presence of two hematological malignancies: chronic lymphocytic leukemia and myelofibrosis in a patient," *Indian Journal of Hematology and Blood Transfusion*, vol. 27, no. 1, pp. 33-34, 2011.

[9] S. Burgstaller, S. Wimmer, B. Mayrbaeurl, W. Hoebling, and J. Thaler, "Coexistence of primary myelofibrosis and chronic lymphocytic leukemia: treatment of two different diseases with one agent," *Blood Cancer Journal*, vol. 1, no. 5, p. e20, 2011.
[10] L. Laurenti, M. Tarnani, I. Nichele et al., "The coexistence of chronic lymphocytic leukemia and myeloproliperative neoplasms: a retrospective multicentric GIMEMA experience," *American Journal of Hematology*, vol. 86, no. 12, pp. 1007–1012, 2011.
[11] A. Kimura, H. Hyodo, Y. Nakata, and A. Kuramoto, "Chronic lymphocytic leukemia associated with bone marrow fibrosis: possible role of interleukin 1 alpha in the pathogenesis," *American Journal of Hematology*, vol. 43, no. 1, pp. 47–50, 1993.
[12] S. Ristić, M. Radojković, T. Kostić, V. Spasovski, S. Pavlović, and V. Cemerikić-Martinović, "JAK2V617F mutation in a patient with B-cell chronic lymphocytic leukemia and prefibrotic primary myelofibrosis," *Srpski Arhiv za Celokupno Lekarstvo*, vol. 143, no. 11-12, pp. 739–743, 2015.
[13] J. Böhm, H. E. Schaefer, and P. Fisch, "Coincidence of chronic idiopathic myelofibrosis and chronic lymphocytic leukaemia. A rare phenomenon?," *Der Pathologe*, vol. 23, no. 6, pp. 480–485, 2002.
[14] M. E. Salama, S. I. Swierczek, T. Tashi, C. A. Warby, N. S. Reading, and J. T. Prchal, "Calreticulin mutated prefibrotic-stage myelofibrosis and PMF represent an independent clone from coexisting CLL," *Blood*, vol. 124, no. 10, pp. 1691-1692, 2014.
[15] G. Todisco, T. Manshouri, S. Verstovsek et al., "Chronic lymphocytic leukemia and myeloproliferative neoplasms concurrently diagnosed: clinical and biological characteristics," *Leukemia and Lymphoma*, vol. 57, no. 5, pp. 1054–1059, 2016.
[16] M. Marchetti, A. Carobbio, E. Capitoni, and T. Barbui, "Lymphoproliferative disorders in patients with chronic myeloproliferative neoplasms: a systematic review," *American Journal of Hematology*, vol. 93, no. 5, pp. 698–703, 2018.
[17] A. M. Vannucchi, G. Masala, E. Antonioli et al., "Increased risk of lymphoid neoplasms in patients with Philadelphia chromosome-negative myeloproliferative neoplasms," *Cancer Epidemiology Biomarkers and Prevention*, vol. 18, no. 7, pp. 2068–2073, 2009.
[18] C. Nielsen, H. S. Birgens, B. G. Nordestgaard, L. Kjaer, and S. E. Bojesen, "The JAK2 V617F somatic mutation, mortality and cancer risk in the general population," *Hamatologica*, vol. 96, no. 3, pp. 450–453, 2011.
[19] L. Michaux, I. Wlodarska, K. Rack et al., "Translocation t(1;6)(p35.3;p25.2): a new recurrent aberration in "unmutated" B CLL," *Leukemia*, vol. 19, no. 1, pp. 77–82, 2005.

26

West Nile Encephalitis, an Unusual Infection in a Chronic Lymphocytic Leukemia Patient

Manuel R. Espinoza-Gutarra,[1] Sherri L. Cervantez,[2] and Zohra Nooruddin[3]

[1] *Department of Internal Medicine, UT Health San Antonio, 7703 Floyd Curl Drive, San Antonio, TX 78229, USA*
[2] *Department of Hematology-Oncology, Mays Cancer Center, UT Health San Antonio, 7979 Wurzbach Rd., San Antonio, TX 78229, USA*
[3] *Department of Hematology-Oncology, South Texas VA, 7400 Merton Minter, San Antonio, TX 78229, USA*

Correspondence should be addressed to Manuel R. Espinoza-Gutarra; espinozaguta@uthscsa.edu

Academic Editor: Massimo Gentile

CNS involvement by CLL is a rare occurrence, usually happening in the context of a transformation to a more aggressive lymphoma in what is known as Richter's transformation. We report a patient with active CLL who developed confusion and was found to have West Nile encephalitis that initially mimicked CNS involvement by CLL. The patient recovered with supportive treatment and later restarted ibrutinib therapy. This case illustrates the importance of maintaining a broad differential among cancer patients with new onset confusion as well as that of questioning malignant infiltration of CNS when there is concomitant active CNS infection.

1. Introduction

Chronic lymphocytic leukemia (CLL) is the most common leukemia in adults; however, central nervous system (CNS) involvement is rare. CLL infiltration of the CNS is often seen with Richter's or prolymphocytoid transformation [1, 2] and is a known, albeit, infrequent complication of CLL with a reported rate of 1-2% [3] with clinically significant disease occurring in only 0.4–0.7% [1]. Higher rates of CNS involvement ranging from 20% to 50% [4, 5] have been reported in autopsy series, but this discrepancy can be explained by inclusion of data on involvement of the spinal cord, the most frequently affected part of the CNS. Far fewer data are available regarding transient CNS infiltration by CLL in the setting of an acute infection.

West Nile virus is a member of the single-stranded RNA Flavivirus family, a member of the Japanese encephalitis virus antigenic complex, which has peak incidence from late August to early September [6]. West Nile virus infection, particularly in its neuroinvasive presentation, is an emerging disease in North America, with increasing rates of morbidity and mortality since an initial outbreak in 1999 and with annual rates of over 1000 cases of neuroinvasive disease over the last decade [7]. Prompt clinical suspicion and recognition of this condition would benefit patients living in these new endemic areas, as migration and climate change will likely increase its incidence [8].

West Nile virus encephalitis is usually asymptomatic; however, it is known to cause clinically significant disease in immunocompromised hosts including severe persistent infection with fatal outcomes [9]. In rare instances, it has been shown to produce clinically significant CNS illness in patients with CLL with poor outcomes [10]. In the case reported by Hollander et al., a patient with known CLL developed acute altered mental status and proceeded to deteriorate clinically; serology studies were negative, but West Nile virus was found on brain tissue during autopsy without evidence of neoplastic infiltration or biologic transformation. Similar to other viral infections, it is characterized by lymphocytosis on CSF studies with normal or slightly elevated protein and normal glucose.

Table 1: Laboratory values.

	Normal range	13 years prior to admission	10 years prior to admission	5 years prior to admission	1 year prior to admission	On admission	On discharge
WBC	4.8–10.8 $10^3/\mu L$	30.4	196.9	113.7	91.9	13	4.3
HCT	42–50%	42.3	40.9	37.6	35.9	28.6	23.9
Hb	14–17 g/dL	14.9	13.3	12.6	11.8	10.1	8.4
RBC count	4.7–6.1	4.67	4.30	4.05	3.83	3.16	2.59
PLT	140–400 $10^3/\mu L$	223	238	150	143	49	36
MCV	80–99 fL	90.6	95.1	92.7	93.7	90.4	92.3
Differential count: percentage (absolute)							
Neutrophils	40–74% (1.9–8 $10^3/\mu L$)	19.3 (5.9)	8.3 (16.4)	10 (11.3)	6.9 (6.4)	50.8 (6.6)	54.5 (2.3)
Lymphocytes	19–48% (0.9–5.2 $10^3/\mu L$)	75 (22.8)	91.1 (179.4)	64 (72.7)	90.8 (83.4)	44.8 (5.8)	37.7 (1.6)
Atypical lymphocytes	0–10%	6% + smudge cells	22% + smudge cells	20% and 2% blasts	27%	2%	3.1%
Monocytes	3.4–9% (0.16-1 $10^3/\mu L$)	4.1 (1.2)	0.5 (0.9)	3 (3.4)	1.5 (1.3)	3 (0.4)	2.1 (0.1)
Eosinophils	0–7% (0–0.8 $10^3/\mu L$)	1.4 (0.4)	0 (0.1)	1 (1.1)	0.5 (0.5)	0.4 (0.1)	5.6 (0.2)
Basophils	0–1.5% (0–0.2 $10^3/\mu L$)	0.2 (0.1)	0.1 (0.2)	2 (2.2)	0.3 (0.3)	1 (0.1)	0.1 (0.0)
IgA	85–385 mg/dL	128			23		
IgG	564-1765 mg/dL	1130			489		
IgM	45–250 mg/dL	121			28		
LDH	98–192 IU/L		154	225	377	261	

2. Case Report

We present a 64-year-old Hispanic male with Rai Stage II, IgH mutated, and trisomy 12 positive CLL, diagnosed 13 years prior to admission. He was initially observed for 3 years and then received first-line fludarabine, cyclophosphamide, and rituximab (FCR) for 3 cycles with good response. He remained on observation for 4 additional years and then received an additional 4 cycles of FCR followed by 5 cycles of maintenance rituximab. Five years later, he was found to have 17p deleted recurrent disease and he was started on ibrutinib with good response. He presented to an outside facility with acute onset altered mental status after stopping ibrutinib 2 months earlier due to financial constraints. Cerebrospinal fluid (CSF) analysis was initially concerning for CLL infiltration of the CNS with neoplastic-appearing lymphocytes identified by cytomorphology; however, serological tests for West Nile virus indicated acute infection based on positive IgM and negative IgG; however, PCR could not be performed. The patient received therapy for presumed CNS involvement by CLL with intrathecal methotrexate along with intravenous rituximab and methylprednisolone before being transferred to our institution. On admission, his complete blood count revealed leukocytosis with a normal differential and thrombocytopenia, after reviewing the patients' historical trends, we could discern that the platelet count had been within normal limits in the past and had likely decreased due to the acute illness; additionally, we can appreciate the increasing trend in WBCs until the start of treatment around 10 years prior to this admission (Table 1). Peripheral blood smear showed normal platelet morphology and moderate leukocytosis with lymphocytosis with coarse, block-like chromatin pattern concerning for prolymphocytoid transformation which had not been present previously. Bone marrow biopsy revealed hypercellularity with diffuse infiltrate of the medium to large-sized mononuclear cells with irregular nuclear contours and prominent nucleoli similar to that seen in the peripheral blood smear (Figure 1). Repeat CSF studies at our hospital showed lymphocytes accounting for 49% of total events per flow cytometry, positive for CD19, CD20, CD5, and CD23, with lambda light chain restriction, and negative for CD10 and FMC-7 (Figure 2). The morphology of lymphocytes in CSF was consistent with neoplasia; however, given the admixture of reactive lymphocytes and the presence of known CNS infection, it was deemed that this most likely represented peripheral blood contamination and reactive infiltration of neoplastic lymphocytes.

He was treated supportively during his hospital stay and improved without any further CNS-directed therapy. Ibrutinib was later reinstated after the resolution of thrombocytopenia and BTK mutational testing proved negative. The patient continued to improve during outpatient follow-up, prolymphocitoid morphology disappeared from peripheral smear, and brain MRI showed no evidence of CNS disease.

3. Discussion

Previous reports have highlighted the fact that an infectious process can confound the diagnosis, with transmigration of clonal CLL cells being detected even by flow cytometry (FC) and detecting false positives [11, 12]. West Nile virus specifically has been known to cause significant disease in CLL patients, mimicking CNS infiltration, especially because active neoplasm and immunosuppression are the known risk

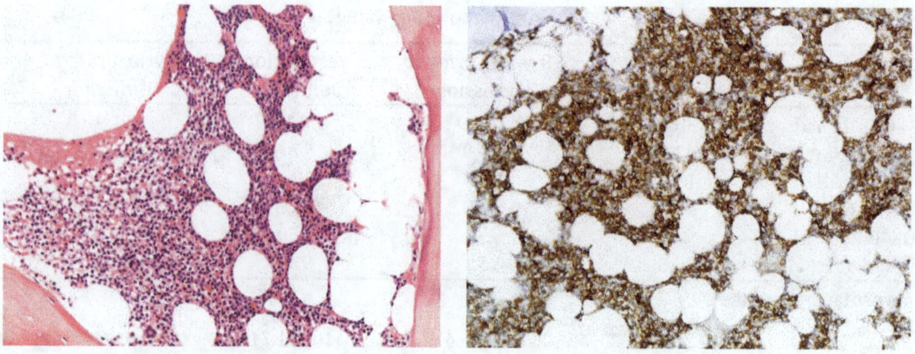

(a) (b)

FIGURE 1: (a) H&E shows infiltrate of small lymphocytes ×50. (b) Immunohistochemistry of CD20 highlighting the lymphocytes ×50.

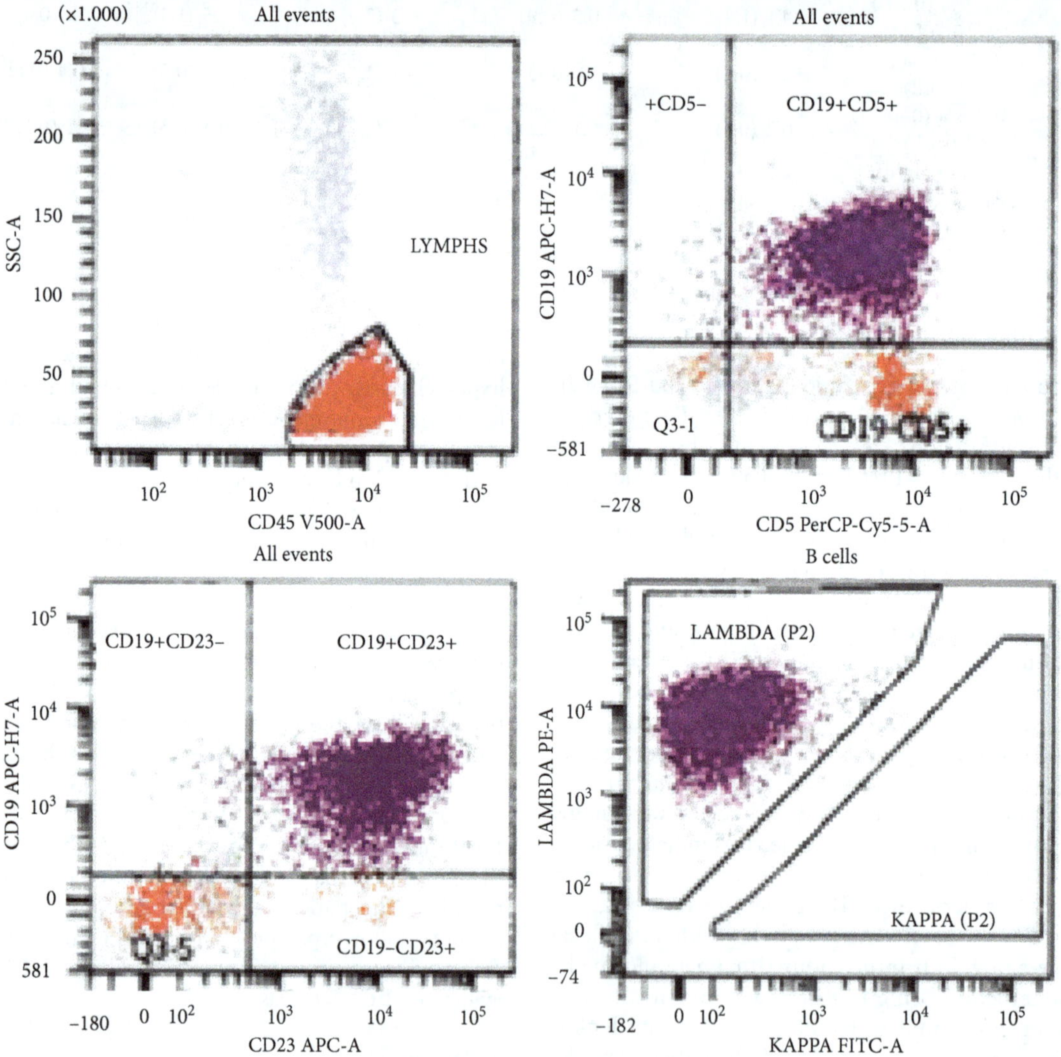

FIGURE 2: CSF flow cytometry.

factors for developing the disease as well as having poorer outcomes [13]. In our patient, prompt diagnosis was aided by the fact that he was not on chemotherapy since patients on active rituximab often have negative IgM titers [14].

The differentiation of true CNS infiltration by CLL and peripheral blood contamination or reactive lymphocyte infiltration is usually done through FC analysis. CD49d and CD82 have been proposed as biomarkers that predict CNS infiltration in CLL [15]; however, these studies were not done in our patient. A study by Wu et al. [16] showed that FC was superior to cytomorphology in diagnosing CNS infiltration; however, FC has been shown to be positive for monoclonal lines in the setting of purely nonmalignant conditions or underlying neoplasm without true CNS infiltration [12]. Therefore, cytomorphology still plays a crucial part in expedient clinical decision-making.

Several reports show that patients with true CNS infiltration by CLL have worse outcomes in the setting of prior CLL-directed therapy [1–3, 10]. A previous series identified the need for aggressive systemic and/or intrathecal treatment in the setting of true CLL involvement of CNS [17]. Additionally, presence of prolymphocytoid morphology has been associated with high-risk mutations, Richter's transformation, and overall more aggressive disease [18]. Although our patient received a single dose of chemotherapy, his continued clinical improvement with mere supportive therapy for West Nile encephalitis argued against active CNS infiltration by CLL.

4. Conclusion

Our case report highlights the complexities in differentiating West Nile virus encephalitis from CNS involvement by CLL due to the presence of reactive CLL cells in the CSF. This case further exemplifies the need for thorough evaluation with FC, cytopathology, and infectious markers prior to treatment of apparent CLL infiltration of the CNS as reversible infectious etiologies may mimic more serious leukemic transformations.

Conflicts of Interest

The authors declare that they have no conflicts of interest.

References

[1] P. Strati, J. H. Uhm, T. J. Kaufmann et al., "Prevalence and characteristics of central nervous system involvement by chronic lymphocytic leukemia," *Haematologica*, vol. 101, no. 4, pp. 458–465, 2016.

[2] H. Kuwabara, H. Kanamori, H. Takasaki et al., "Involvement of central nervous system in prolymphocytoid transformation of chronic lymphocytic leukemia," *Leukemia & Lymphoma*, vol. 44, no. 7, pp. 1235–1237, 2003.

[3] M. C. J. Hanse, M. B. van't Veer, K. van Lom, and M. J. van den Bent, "Incidence of central nervous system involvement in chronic lymphocytic leukemia and outcome to treatment," *Journal of Neurology*, vol. 255, no. 6, pp. 828–830, 2008.

[4] M. Barcos, W. Lane, G. A. Gomez et al., "An autopsy study of 1206 acute and chronic leukemias (1958 to 1982)," *Cancer*, vol. 60, no. 4, pp. 827–837, 1987.

[5] M. B. MøLler and J. L. Nielsen, "CNS involvement in leukemia," *Acta Pathologica Microbiologica Scandinavica Series A: Pathology*, vol. 91, no. 1–6, pp. 209–216, 1983.

[6] W. N. Virus, "Information for healthcare providers," 2015, http://www.cdc.gov/westnile.

[7] C. Chancey, A. Grinev, E. Volkova, and M. Rios, "The global ecology and epidemiology of West Nile virus," *BioMed Research International*, vol. 2015, Article ID 376230, 20 pages, 2015.

[8] K. C. Hoover and C. M. Baker, "West Nile virus, climate change and circumpolar vulnerability," *Wiley Interdisciplinary Reviews: Climate Change*, vol. 7, no. 2, pp. 283–300, 2016.

[9] R. G. Penn, J. Guarner, J. J. Sejvar et al., "Persistent neuroinvasive West Nile virus infection in an immunocompromised patient," *Clinical Infectious Diseases*, vol. 42, no. 5, pp. 680–683, 2006.

[10] H. Hollander, P. W. Schaefer, and E. Tessa Hedley-Whyte, "Case 22-2005: an 81-year-old man with cough, fever, and altered mental status," *New England Journal of Medicine*, vol. 353, no. 3, pp. 287–295, 2005.

[11] C. D. Schweighofer, G. Fätkenheuer, P. Staib, M. Hallek, and M. Reiser, "Lyme disease in a patient with chronic lymphocytic leukemia mimics leukemic meningeosis," *Oncology Research and Treatment*, vol. 30, no. 11, pp. 564–566, 2007.

[12] G. S. Nowakowski, T. G. Call, W. G. Morice, P. J. Kurtin, R. J. Cook, and C. S. Zent, "Clinical significance of monoclonal B cells in cerebrospinal fluid," *Cytometry Part B: Clinical Cytometry*, vol. 63, no. 1, pp. 23–27, 2005.

[13] N. P. Lindsey, J. E. Staples, J. A. Lehman, and M. Fischer, "Medical risk factors for severe West Nile virus disease, United States, 2008–2010," *American Journal of Tropical Medicine and Hygiene*, vol. 87, no. 1, pp. 179–184, 2012.

[14] S. D. Mawhorter, A. Sierk, S. M. Staugaitis et al., "Fatal West Nile virus infection after rituximab/fludarabine-induced remission for non-hodgkin's lymphoma," *Clinical Lymphoma and Myeloma*, vol. 6, no. 3, pp. 248–250, 2005.

[15] C. M. Rojas-Hernandez, J. Nemunaitis, K. D. Marjon, D. Bustamante, Q. Y. Zhang, and J. M. Gillette, "Chronic lymphocytic leukemia with clinical debut as neurological involvement: a rare phenomenon and the need for better predictive markers," *BMC Hematology*, vol. 17, no. 1, p. 3, 2017.

[16] J. M. Wu, M. F. Georgy, F. H. Burroughs, E. G. Weir, D. L. Rosenthal, and S. Z. Ali, "Lymphoma, leukemia, and pleiocytosis in cerebrospinal fluid: is accurate cytopathologic diagnosis possible based on morphology alone?," *Diagnostic Cytopathology*, vol. 37, no. 11, pp. 820–824, 2009.

[17] A. Wanquet, R. Birsen, C. Bonnet et al., "Management of central nervous system involvement in chronic lymphocytic leukemia: a retrospective cohort of 30 patients," *British Journal of Haematology*, vol. 176, no. 1, pp. 37–49, 2017.

[18] D. Oscier, M. Else, E. Matutes, R. Morilla, J. C. Strefford, and D. Catovsky, "The morphology of CLL revisited: the clinical significance of prolymphocytes and correlations with prognostic/molecular markers in the LRF CLL4 trial," *British Journal of Haematology*, vol. 174, no. 5, pp. 767–775, 2016.

Treatment Sequencing in a Chronic Lymphocytic Leukemia Patient with Central Nervous System Involvement

Filipa Mousinho,[1] Tatiana Mendes,[1] Paula Sousa e Santos,[1] Maria João Acosta,[2] José Pereira,[2] Maria Arroz,[2] Cândido Silva,[3] Ana Paula Azevedo,[3] Rita Oliveira,[4] Martinha Chorão,[4] and Fernando Lima[1]

[1]*Clinical Hematology Department, Hospital de São Francisco Xavier, Centro Hospitalar de Lisboa Ocidental, Lisbon, Portugal*
[2]*Clinical Pathology Department, Flow Cytometry Laboratory, Hospital de São Francisco Xavier, Centro Hospitalar de Lisboa Ocidental, Lisbon, Portugal*
[3]*Clinical Pathology Department, Hematology Laboratory, Hospital de São Francisco Xavier, Centro Hospitalar de Lisboa Ocidental, Lisbon, Portugal*
[4]*Pathology Department, Hospital de Egas Moniz, Centro Hospitalar de Lisboa Ocidental, Lisbon, Portugal*

Correspondence should be addressed to Paula Sousa e Santos; pcsslx@gmail.com

Academic Editor: Yusuke Shiozawa

Early-stage chronic lymphocytic leukemia (CLL) with neurologic involvement is a rare condition and should require a careful follow-up. Although no standard protocol exists for this condition, intrathecal chemotherapy, combined with systemic chemoimmunotherapy, has been used previously. This case describes the treatment of a patient with CLL and symptomatic compromise of the central nervous system. Our results suggest that a combination of chemotherapy, radiotherapy, and ibrutinib, administered sequentially over a 2-year period, led to a near-complete resolution of the cerebral spinal fluid neoplastic infiltration. Importantly, this response has been maintained with ibrutinib monotherapy for more than 12 months.

1. Introduction

B-cell chronic lymphocytic leukemia (B-CLL) is a chronic, long-term, and slowly developing leukemia characterized by a progressive accumulation of functionally incompetent monoclonal B lymphocytes. It is the most common form of leukemia found in adults of Western countries, but neurologic complications, arising from direct leukemic involvement of the central nervous system (CNS), are reported in only 1% of patients with B-CLL [1–3]. Although neurological symptoms can occur in patients with CLL, clinically significant CNS involvement (iCNS) by CLL cells is a rare condition [4]. The clinical manifestations of CLL with iCNS are heterogeneous and include headache, cranial nerve palsies, cerebellar signs, visual problems, and motor and/or sensory deficits. Imaging studies are neither specific nor sensitive in the detection of CLL involvement of the CNS, and the diagnosis is usually confirmed by flow cytometry (FC) analysis of the CSF.

Here, we describe the case of a patient with diagnosis of B-CLL who developed a neurologic impairment because of iCNS. The patient underwent treatment with schemes that included intrathecal chemotherapy, high-dose methotrexate, radiotherapy and ibrutinib, a Bruton tyrosine kinase (BTK) inhibitor. After nearly 26 months of follow-up, he had an almost complete response, with near-complete resolution of his neurologic symptoms.

2. Case Presentation

The 65-year-old man was diagnosed in 2006, with a B-CLL, with stage Rai 0/Binet A, and 13q deletion. He was kept under standard surveillance until significant disease progression with associated lymphocytosis. In January

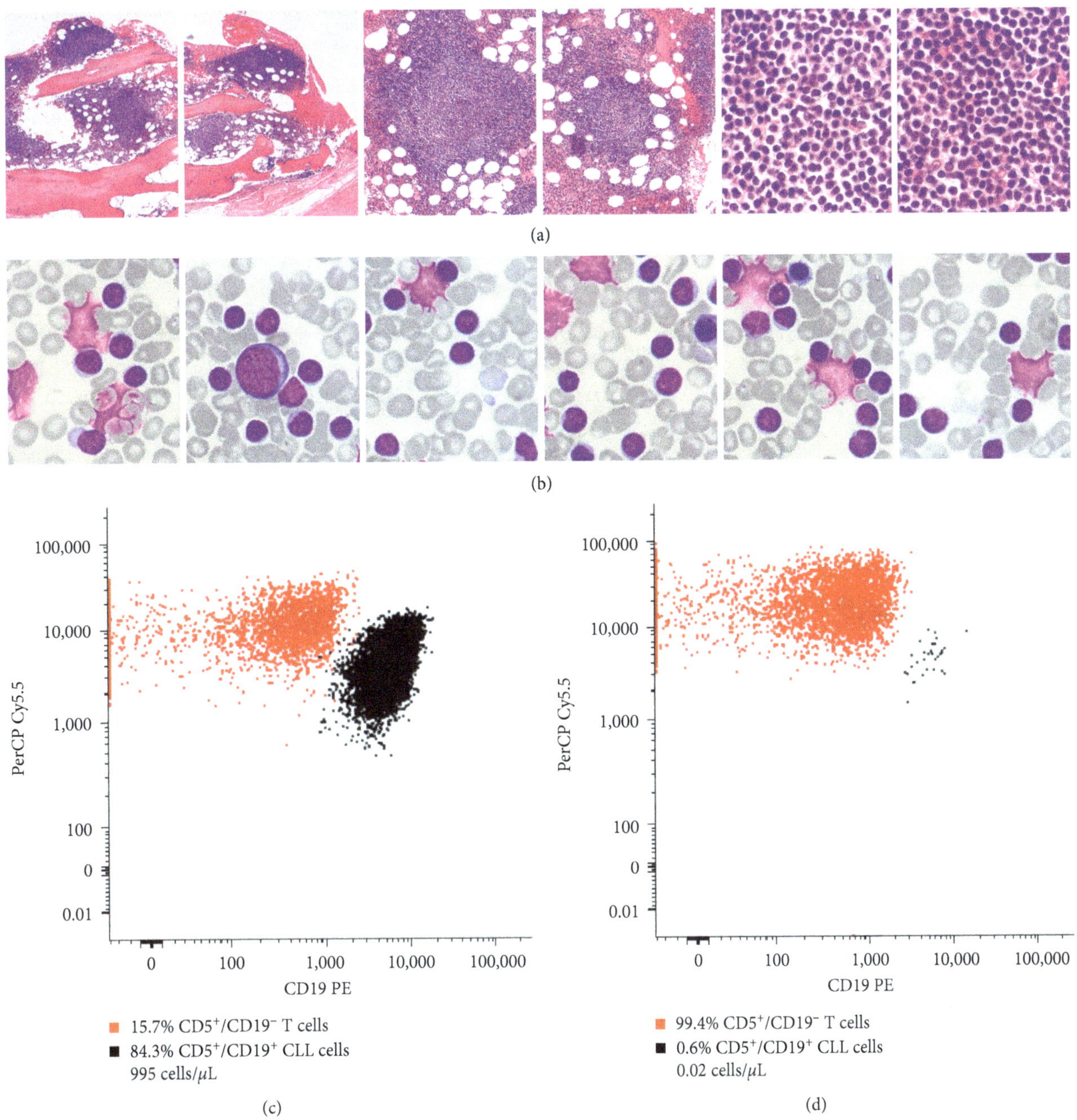

Figure 1: B-CLL characterization. (a) Bone marrow biopsy (HE): in September 2015, there was a 70% nodular and interstitial infiltration of small lymphocytes. (b) Bone marrow smear (MGG): in January 2016, numerous small lymphocytes, with clumped chromatin and scanty cytoplasm, smudge cells, and a few erythroblasts were detected. Dot plots illustrating cerebral spinal fluid (CSF), immunophenotyping $CD5^{+}/CD19^{-}$ T cells (red dots) and $CD19^{+}/CD5^{+}$ B-CLL cells (black dots) in October 2015 (c) and in August 2017 (d). Magnification: (a) ×40 (left), ×100 (center), and ×600 (right) and (b) ×100.

2007, he started chlorambucil monotherapy as first-line treatment. This patient was treated for one year (12 cycles), achieving partial remission. In May 2015, this patient evidenced worsening of preexisting lymphocytosis, and later, on August 2015, it was also associated with palpable inguinal adenopathies. In September 2015, he was observed at the emergency hospital because of headache complaints, photophobia, vertigo, and extensive pain (from the cervical spine down to the inferior limbs). This pain led to an ataxic march that mimicked that of a cerebrovascular event, but the remaining neurologic examination was unremarkable.

At that time, he was admitted to the hematology ward for characterization and management of the sudden neurologic impairment. We re-evaluated the disease, and a bone marrow study revealed a 70% CLL involvement, confirmed by FC, biopsy analysis (Figure 1(a)), and aspirate analysis (Figure 1(b)). In addition, cytogenetic evaluation using FISH confirmed the presence of a CLL clone with a 13q deletion, but no other anomalies were detected. In the

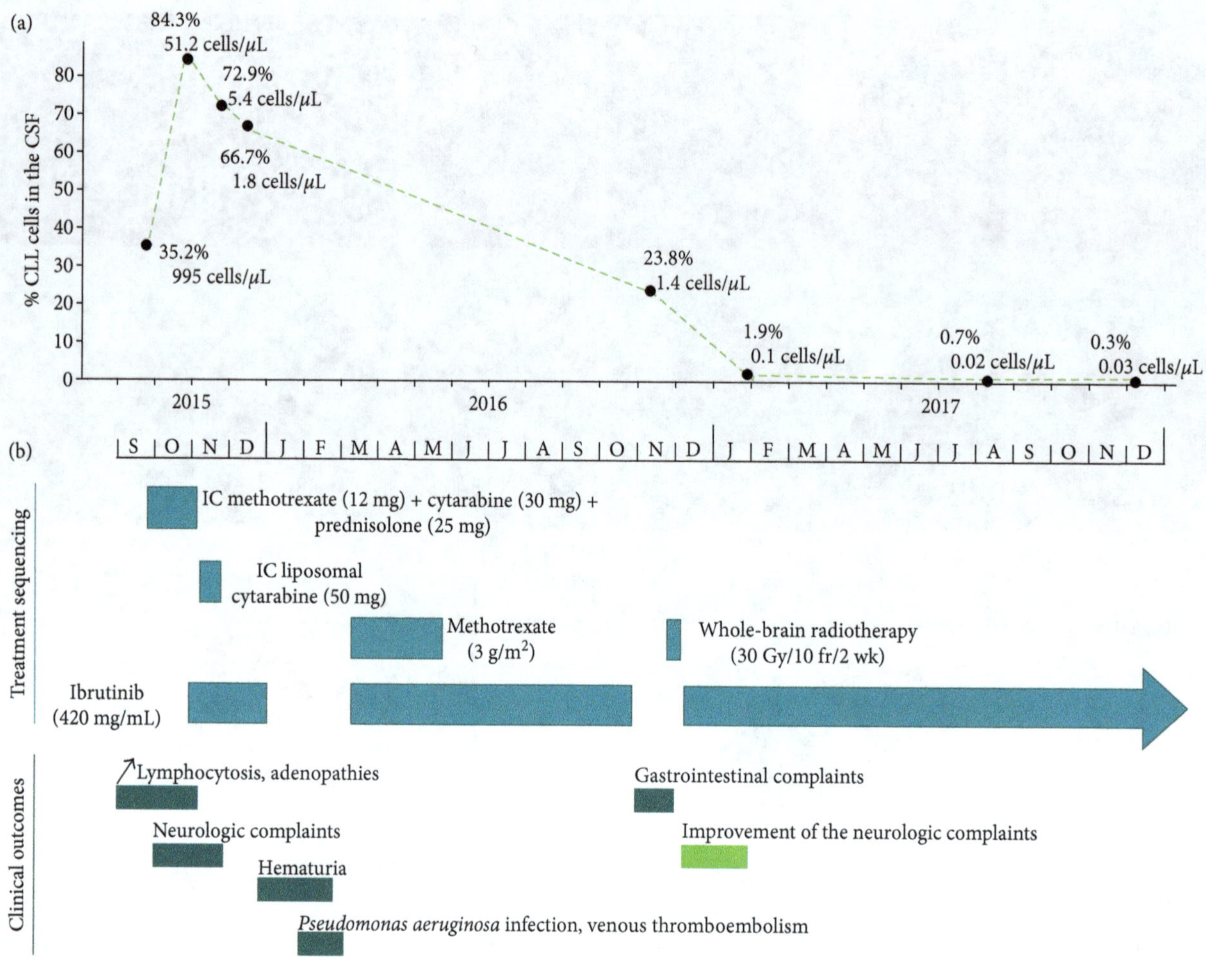

FIGURE 2: Evaluation of the CNS response and the clinical outcomes over time. (a) Flow cytometry analysis of the CSF over time, illustrating the % of CLL cells detected. The absolute number of counted CLL cells present in the diluted sample is shown underneath the percentage of cells detected, in dark grey. (b) Treatment course followed, illustrating therapy combinations and ibrutinib interruptions as well as the patient's clinical outcomes. Triple IC with methotrexate, cytarabine, and prednisone was administered 15 times, biweekly, but did not result in a positive response. Liposomal cytarabine was given 2 times (on the 10th and on the 24th of November 2015) but led to no response and might have led to the worsening of the neurologic symptoms due to a toxic myelitis. After resolution of the first toxicity (grade-2 hematuria), systemic high-dose methotrexate was administered together with ibrutinib. Whole-brain radiotherapy was administered (30 Gy/10 fr, in a regimen of 3 Gy/cycle/day, from the 24th of November until the 9th of December 2016) to decrease the CSF infiltration. After the first interruption, ibrutinib was restarted at 140 mg/day and then weekly increased to 280 mg/day and to 420 mg/day. After the second interruption, it was restarted at full dose (420 mg/day).

context of CNS evaluation, the cerebral CT scan did not reveal any focal or diffuse lesions on the cerebral parenchyma. Further evaluation with magnetic resonance imaging (MRI) of the brain and spine was conducted with no evidence of acute signs to account for the symptoms. A diagnostic lumbar puncture was performed, and the cerebral spinal fluid (CSF) had normal glucose and protein levels. However, there was an elevated white blood cell count of 2.828 cells/μL, with predominance of mononucleated cells. The FC analysis of the CSF revealed the presence of 35.2% of monoclonal B cells, 995 cells/μL, compatible with B-CLL infiltration (Figure 2(a)). The cytogenetic analysis of the CSF was made using fluorescence in situ hybridization (FISH) and was also positive for del (13q14.3) in 88% of the analyzed nuclei. These findings were suggestive of CLL involvement of the CNS, and we started a second-line therapy consisting of a BTK inhibitor combined with intrathecal chemotherapy (IC).

While awaiting approval for the targeted oral therapy, ibrutinib, the patient started IC. From September to November 2015, a total of 17 IC administrations were performed (15 administrations of methotrexate, cytarabine, and prednisolone, twice a week followed by 2 doses of liposomal cytarabine every 2 weeks). Nevertheless, no response was achieved, and there was a progressive worsening of the neurological deficits, with the development of paraplegia. We suspect that, at that stage, the worsening of the neurological condition was, at least in part, due to an eventual toxic myelitis related to IC administrations.

During IC treatment, in October 2015, CSF re-evaluation by FC revealed an infiltration degree of 84.3% (Figures 1(c) and 2(a)). By the end of October 2015, the patient started ibrutinib, at 420 mg/day, and after the first week of treatment, the adenopathies disappeared. Nonetheless, two months later, ibrutinib had to be temporarily suspended due to the onset of grade-2 hematuria. This adverse event was resolved within two months, and therapy was re-introduced in a safe way.

On December 2015, the FC analysis of the CSF showed persistent neoplastic infiltration of about 66.7% and motivated the association of high-dose methotrexate, every 15 days, which was administered for a total of 6 cycles, until May 2016. Treatment with methotrexate plus ibrutinib was delayed until the beginning of March because of the onset of a *Pseudomonas aeruginosa* infection and because of an episode of venous thromboembolism. The combination of high-dose methotrexate with ibrutinib seems to have led to a decrease in the % of CNS infiltrating CLL cells from 66.7% to 23.8% (Figure 2(a)).

Later that year, due to gastrointestinal complaints (related with intestinal pseudo-occlusion), ibrutinib treatment was suspended for another month. These complaints were not attributable to other etiologies, and after resolution, ibrutinib was re-introduced at full dose in December 2016. Meanwhile, because there was still a 23.8% CLL infiltration of the CSF, CNS radiotherapy was delivered, in November 2016, as denoted in Figure 2. Since then, ibrutinib therapy has been maintained, without further interruptions or dose reductions, and CSF analysis by FC has shown a continuous decrease in the number of infiltrated CLL cells (towards a minimum of 0.3% on the last analysis, Figure 1 (d)).

Over the follow-up of 26-month treatment, there was almost a complete improvement of all neurologic deficits, and at the time of the last lumbar puncture, the patient presented only a small degree of paraparesis. Physical rehabilitation was commenced and has been contributing to an improvement of the paraparesis. Finally, there is still no evidence of splenomegaly or adenopathies, and the patient is continued to be treated daily with ibrutinib.

3. Discussion

Patients with early-stage, long-standing, or advanced CLL disease may experience localized leptomeningeal disease. However, a leptomeningeal dissemination of CLL cells in patients with early-stage disease is extremely rare [5], making it difficult to distinguish between CLL involvement and other etiologies [6]. The optimal treatment course for patients who have CLL with iCNS is unclear. The majority of them undergo treatment regimens that include IC with or without radiation therapy or receive systemic chemotherapy. For IC, common systemic drugs, that penetrate the blood-brain barrier (BBB), such as methotrexate, cytarabine, and corticosteroids, can be administered alone or in combination [7]. Also, several studies have demonstrated that ibrutinib crosses the BBB in patients with B-cell malignancies [8, 9] and can achieve a response in sensitive cases with iCNS. Nevertheless, because there are not many cases described, no treatment protocols have been established for CLL with iCNS.

In this case, aggressive regimens, such as those including fludarabine, have been excluded due to the patient's age and, especially, due to other comorbidities (severe pulmonary tuberculosis, in 2008, submitted to right upper lobectomy, with mixed ventilatory sequelae and a hypertensive cardiomyopathy). Hence, it seemed to us that IC with ibrutinib was an option with lower toxicity, with a lower risk of pulmonary infections, and easier to handle without delays between cycles, thus providing greater comfort to the patient.

After more than 2 years of combined treatment with chemotherapy, radiotherapy, and ibrutinib, the patient had a near-complete resolution of the CSF infiltration, which has been maintained with ibrutinib monotherapy for 12 months. This suggests that this treatment sequencing may benefit patients in similar cases when there is a neoplastic CLL infiltration of the CNS. Lastly, we believe that continuous treatment with ibrutinib may progressively improve the clinical outcomes of this patient and help to maintain a durable CNS response.

Conflicts of Interest

The authors declare no conflicts of interest.

Authors' Contributions

Filipa Mousinho drafted and wrote the manuscript. Tatiana Mendes collected and analyzed the data. Paula Sousa e Santos conducted diagnostic and therapeutic management of the patient, analyzed the data, and revised the manuscript. Maria João Acosta, José Pereira, and Maria Arroz performed immunophenotypic analysis of peripheral blood, bone marrow aspirate, and CSF samples. Cândido Silva provided the bone marrow aspirate images and revised the manuscript. Rita Oliveira and Martinha Chorão provided the bone marrow biopsy images and revised the manuscript. Maria Arroz, Ana Paula Azevedo, and Fernando Lima revised the manuscript. All authors approved the final manuscript.

References

[1] T. Elter, M. Hallek, and A. Engert, "Fludarabine in chronic lymphocytic leukaemia," *Expert Opinion on Pharmacotherapy*, vol. 7, no. 12, pp. 1641–1651, 2006.

[2] M. C. J. Hanse, M. B. van't Veer, K. van Lom, and M. J. van den Bent, "Incidence of central nervous system involvement in chronic lymphocytic leukemia and outcome to treatment," *Journal of Neurology*, vol. 255, no. 6, pp. 828–830, 2008.

[3] R. Lopes da Silva, "Spectrum of neurologic complications in chronic lymphocytic leukemia," *Clinical Lymphoma Myeloma and Leukemia*, vol. 12, no. 3, pp. 164–179, 2012.

[4] P. Strati, J. H. Uhm, T. J. Kaufmann et al., "Prevalence and characteristics of central nervous system involvement by chronic lymphocytic leukemia," *Haematologica*, vol. 101, no. 4, pp. 458–465, 2016.

[5] S. Pohar, C. deMetz, S. Poppema, and J. Hugh, "Chronic lymphocytic leukemia with CNS involvement," *Journal of Neuro-Oncology*, vol. 16, no. 1, pp. 35–37, 1993.

[6] P. Strati, J. Uhm, T. Kaufmann et al., "Central nervous system involvement by chronic lymphocytic leukemia," *Blood*, vol. 126, no. 23, p. 2919, 2015.

[7] O. Benjamini, P. Jain, E. Schlette, J. S. Sciffman, Z. Estrov, and M. Keating, "Chronic lymphocytic leukemia with central nervous system involvement: a high-risk disease?," *Clinical Lymphoma Myeloma and Leukemia*, vol. 13, no. 3, pp. 338–341, 2013.

[8] C. Mason, S. Savona, J. N. Rini et al., "Ibrutinib penetrates the blood brain barrier and shows efficacy in the therapy of Bing Neel syndrome," *British Journal of Haematology*, vol. 179, no. 2, pp. 339–341, 2017.

[9] S. Bernard, L. Goldwirt, S. Amorim et al., "Activity of ibrutinib in mantle cell lymphoma patients with central nervous system relapse," *Blood*, vol. 126, no. 14, pp. 1695–1698, 2015.

An Unprecedented Case of p190 *BCR-ABL* Chronic Myeloid Leukemia Diagnosed during Treatment for Multiple Myeloma

Kosuke Miki,[1] Naoshi Obara,[2] Kenichi Makishima,[2] Tatsuhiro Sakamoto,[2] Manabu Kusakabe,[2] Takayasu Kato,[2] Naoki Kurita,[2] Hidekazu Nishikii,[2] Yasuhisa Yokoyama,[2] Mamiko Sakata-Yanagimoto,[2] Yuichi Hasegawa,[2] and Shigeru Chiba[2]

[1]*School of Medicine, University of Tsukuba, Tsukuba, Japan*
[2]*Department of Hematology, Faculty of Medicine, University of Tsukuba, Tsukuba, Japan*

Correspondence should be addressed to Naoshi Obara; n-obara@md.tsukuba.ac.jp

Academic Editor: Massimo Breccia

We report the case of a 76-year-old man who was diagnosed as having chronic myeloid leukemia (CML) with p190 *BCR-ABL* while receiving treatment for symptomatic multiple myeloma (MM). The diagnosis of MM was based on the presence of serum M-protein, abnormal plasma cells in the bone marrow, and lytic bone lesions. The patient achieved a partial response to lenalidomide and dexamethasone treatment. However, 2 years after the diagnosis of MM, the patient developed leukocytosis with granulocytosis, anemia, and thrombocytopenia. Bone marrow examination revealed Philadelphia chromosomes and chimeric p190 *BCR-ABL* mRNA. Fluorescence in situ hybridization also revealed *BCR-ABL*-positive neutrophils in the peripheral blood, which suggested the emergence of CML with p190 *BCR-ABL*. The codevelopment of MM and CML is very rare, and this is the first report describing p190 *BCR-ABL*-type CML coexisting with MM. Moreover, we have reviewed the literature regarding the coexistence of these diseases.

1. Introduction

Multiple myeloma (MM) is a lymphoid cancer that is characterized by monoclonal proliferation of malignant plasma cells in the bone marrow, monoclonal protein in the serum, and organ dysfunction [1]. Chronic myeloid leukemia (CML) is a clonal disorder of myeloid origin that is characterized by the Philadelphia chromosome, t(9; 22) (q34; q11), in which the *BCR-ABL* fusion gene is created. Several types of *BCR-ABL* are known, with the p210 and p190 types being the most common, distinguished by the break point in the *BCR* gene. The vast majority of CML cases result from the p210-type of *BCR-ABL*, while the p190-type is rarely found in CML [2]. The coexistence of MM and CML in the same patient is rare, with only 22 reported cases [3–23], all involving p210 *BCR-ABL*. Therefore, we report a case of coexisting MM and CML with p190 *BCR-ABL*. Given the rarity of this case, we also discuss the origins of these hematologic malignancies and review the relevant literature.

2. Case Report

A 76-year-old man was referred to our hospital in September 201X, because of right leg pain, lower back pain, and weight loss of 3 kg. Lumbar magnetic resonance imaging and computed tomography (CT) suggested the presence of lumbar spinal canal stenosis and a sacral tumor (Figure 1(a)). Laboratory testing revealed a markedly elevated serum IgG level (5,436 mg/dL, normal: 800–1,800 mg/dL) and an elevated serum beta-2 microglobulin level (4.1 μg/mL, normal: 0–3 μg/mL), although there were

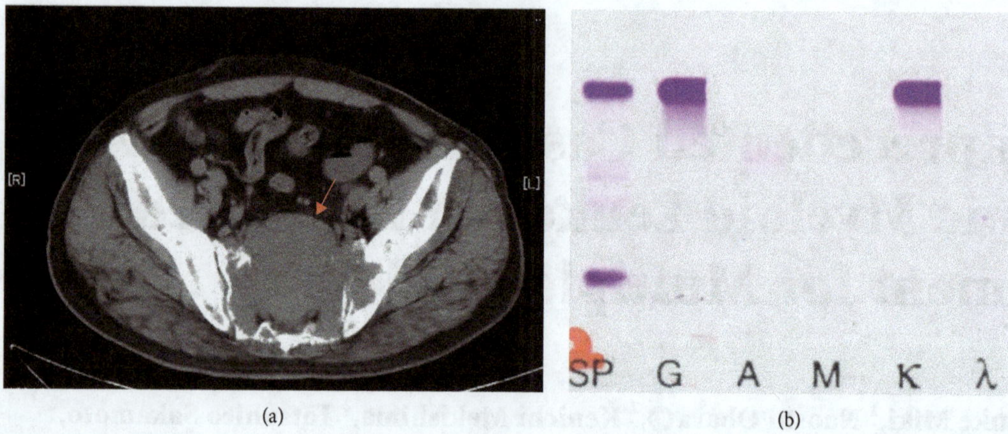

FIGURE 1: (a) Computed tomography (CT) at the time of multiple myeloma (MM) diagnosis. Sacral tumor and lytic bone involvement in the lumbar spine are shown (arrow). (b) Serum immunofixation at the time of MM diagnosis. SP, size marker; G IgG; A IgA; M IgM; κ, kappa chain; λ, lambda chain.

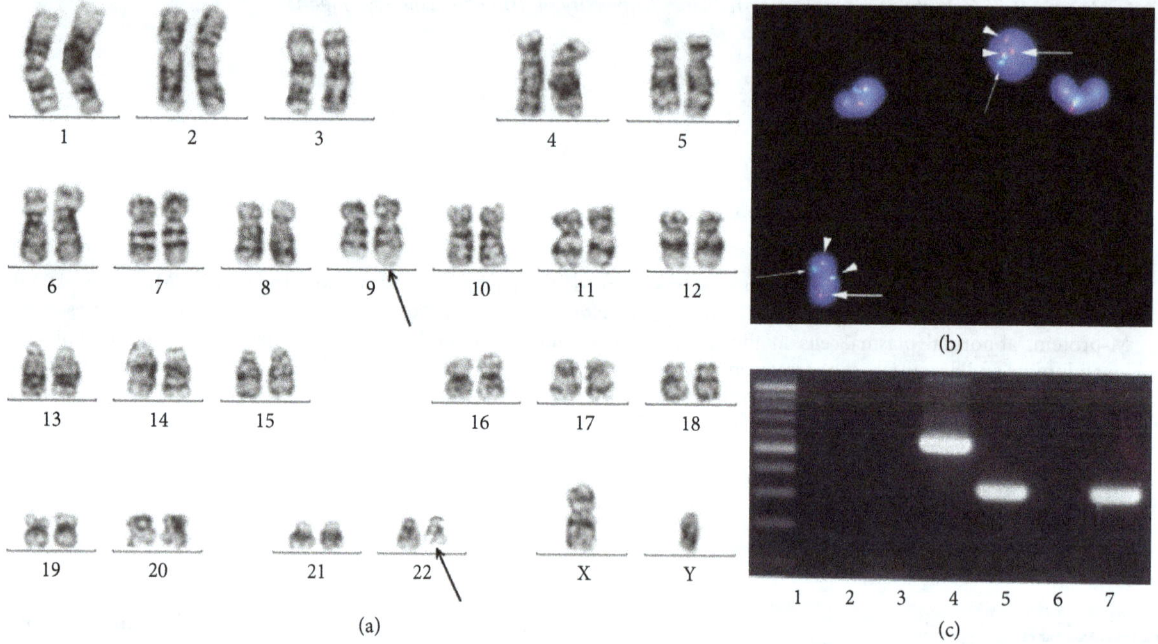

FIGURE 2: (a) Karyotype from a bone marrow specimen at the time of chronic myeloid leukemia (CML) diagnosis. t(9; 22) is shown by using arrows. (b) Fluorescence in situ hybridization for peripheral blood cells. Arrowheads, *BCR-ABL* fusion gene (yellow); large arrows, *ABL* signal (red); small arrows, *BCR* signal (green). (c) Polymerase chain reaction (PCR) amplification analysis from the bone marrow specimen taken at the time of CML diagnosis. Lane 1, size marker; lane 2, p210 negative control; lane 3, p190 negative control; lane 4, p210 positive control; lane 5, p190 positive control; lane 6, p210 patient's sample; lane 7, p190 patient's sample.

no signs of anemia, renal dysfunction, or proteinuria. Serum immunofixation revealed IgGκ-type M-protein, with an estimated serum-free κ and λ chain ratio of 21.5 : 1 (Figure 1(b)). Microscopic examination and flow cytometric analysis of bone marrow aspirate revealed elevated numbers of CD138-positive abnormal plasma cells. Cytogenetic analysis of the bone marrow revealed 46XY, and the patient was diagnosed as having MM (R-ISS, stage II). Chimeric p190 *BCR-ABL* mRNA was not detected in the bone marrow sample at this point. The patient underwent two cycles of bortezomib plus dexamethasone and two cycles of cyclophosphamide, bortezomib, and dexamethasone (CBD) but did not respond to either treatment regimen. The treatment was switched to lenalidomide (25 mg/day) plus dexamethasone (20 mg/week; Ld therapy), and there was a marked response, with a substantial decrease in the M-protein and disappearance of the sacral tumor on CT. After 24 cycles of Ld therapy, the patient achieved a partial response based on the International Myeloma Working Group criteria.

In December 201X+2, the patient developed leukocytosis (white blood cell count: 35.8×10^9/L) and thrombocytopenia

Table 1: Concomitant multiple myeloma and chronic myeloid leukemia cases.

Pt	Age/Sex	Year	First disease	Diagnosis interval (month)	Type of M-protein	Therapy for MM	Therapy for CML	Confirmation method of Ph+	Type of Ph	Reference
1	77M	1972	MM	33	BJP	No treatment	No treatment	Chr		MacSween and Langley [3]
2	65/F	1974	CML	113	IgG-κ	No treatment	Busulfan	Chr		Derghazarian and Whittemore [4]
3	58/M	1982	MM and CML	Simultaneous	IgG-κ	MP, RT	HU, Busulfan,	Chr		Boots and Pegrum [5]
4	71/M	1993	MM	24	IgG-κ	MP, RT	HU	Chr		Klenn et al. [6]
5	72/F	1998	MM and CML	Simultaneous	IgG-κ	VP	IFN-α	Chr, PCR, FISH	P210	Tanaka et al. [7]
6	70/M	1999	MM	33	IgG-κ	Not reported	Not reported	Chr		Nitta et al. [8]
7	81/M	2001	MM and CML	Simultaneous	IgA-κ	MP	No treatment	Chr, PCR		Alvarez-Larrán et al. [9]
8	66/M	2003	MM and CML	Simultaneous	IgG-κ	MP	INF-α, HU, Busulfan	Chr, PCR, FISH	P210	Schwarzmeier et al. [10]
9	47/M	2003	MM	33	BJP	LOAD-IN	Not reported	Chr		Nakagawa [11]
10	68/M	2005	CML	20	IgG-λ	MP	IFN-α, imatinib	Chr, PCR	P210	Garipidou et al. [12]
11	85/F	2005	MM and CML	Simultaneous	IgG-λ	Not reported	Not reported	Chr, PCR	P210	Wakayama et al. [13]
12	76/M	2009	CML	14	IgA-κ	MP	IFN-α, imatinib	Chr, PCR, FISH	P210	Galanopoulos et al. [14]
13	57/F	2009	CML	65	IgA-κ	TD, VAD	Imatinib	Chr, PCR	P210	Michael et al. [15]
14	72/F	2010	CML	3	IgG-κ	No treatment	Imatinib	Chr, PCR	P210	Ide et al. [16]
15	71/F	2012	MM and CML	Simultaneous	IgG-κ	MP, Bd, Ld	Imatinib	Chr		Offiah et al. [17]
16	64/F	2013	MM and CML	Simultaneous	IgA-κ	BD	Imatinib	Chr		Romanenko et al. [18]
17	62/F	2013	MM	17	IgG-κ	RT, VCD, VCDD, VRD	Dasatinib	Chr, PCR	P210	Ragupathi et al. [19]
18	77/M	2014	MM and CML	Simultaneous	IgG-κ	RT, BD	No treatment	Chr, PCR	P210	Maerki et al. [20]
19	60/M	2014	MM	48	IgG-κ	RT, Ld	HU, dasatinib	Chr, FISH		Alsidawi et al. [21]
20	63/F	2012	CML	120	IgG-κ	BD, Ld	Imatinib	Chr, PCR	P210	Pessach et al. [22]
21	68/M	2012	MM	54	IgG-λ	VAD	Imatinib	Chr, PCR	P210	Pessach et al. [22]
22	76/M	2015	CML	38	IgA-λ	No treatment	Imatinib	Chr, PCR		Ahn et al. [23]
23	51/F	2016	MM	Unknown	IgG	BD	Imatinib	Chr, PCR		Wolleschak and Heidel [24]
24	88/M	2016	MM and CML	Simultaneous	IgD-κ	VRD	Imatinib	Chr		Ali et al. [25]
25	76/M	2018	MM	28	IgG-κ	Ld	Dasatinib, bosutinib	Chr, PCR, FISH	P190	Our case

BJP, Bence Jones protein; MP, melphalan, prednisolone; RT, radiation therapy; HU, hydroxyurea; LOAD-IN, melphalan, ranimustine, vincristine, IFN-α; PSL, prednisolone; VCD, bortezomib, cyclophosphamide, dexamethasone; VCDD, VCD plus doxorubicin; VRD, bortezomib, lenalidomide, dexamethasone; Ld, lenalidomide, dexamethasone; VAD, vincristine, doxorubicin, dexamethasone; BD, bortezomib, dexamethasone; CBD, BD plus cyclophosphamide; Rd, lenalidomide, dexamethasone; TD, thalidomide, dexamethasone; Chr, chromosome; PCR, polymerase chain reaction; FISH, fluorescence in situ hybridization.

(platelet count: 3×10^9/L). Bone marrow biopsy and aspiration revealed hypercellularity with a marked increase in myeloid lineage cells but without an increase in blast cells (4%). Cytogenetic analysis revealed 46XY t(9; 22) (q34; q11.2) in 20 of 20 cells, and fluorescence in situ hybridization (FISH) analysis revealed that 99.5% of the cells were positive for *BCR-ABL*. Peripheral blood neutrophils were also positive for *BCR-ABL* (98.8%) (Figures 2(a)–2(b)). Chimeric p190, but not p210, *BCR-ABL* mRNA was detected by using polymerase chain reaction (Figure 2(c)). The diagnosis was confirmed to be CML with p190 *BCR-ABL* in the accelerated phase (AP), which coexisted with MM (a maintained partial response). Dasatinib treatment (100 mg/day) was started immediately. The dose was subsequently decreased to 50 mg/day, due to the persistence of thrombocytopenia. In April 201X+3, a bone marrow examination indicated that the patient had achieved a second chronic phase, with 31% of this cells being positive for *BCR-ABL* upon FISH analysis, and that his peripheral blood count had normalized. However, 5 months later, FISH analysis revealed that 85.8% of his bone marrow cells were positive for *BCR-ABL*, and subsequently, his treatment was changed from dasatinib to bosutinib. This switch appeared to be ineffective, as no decrease in the *BCR-ABL*-positive bone marrow cells was detected after 2 months.

3. Discussion

There have only been 24 cases of coexisting MM and CML reported (Table 1) [3–25]. MM and CML were diagnosed simultaneously in 9 cases, and the diagnoses were sequential in the remaining cases, with MM being diagnosed first in 8 cases and CML being diagnosed first in 7 cases. Among the previous reports, all genotypes confirmed by PCR were p210-CML in patients with coexisting MM and CML. Our case is the first reported of MM coexisting with p190-CML in the same patient. The intervals between the sequential diagnoses ranged from 3 months to 120 months. Multiple possibilities could be considered regarding the association between MM and CML. First, these two malignancies could occur independently, and their coexistence, while very rare, could be simply coincidence. Second, common precursors, referred to as "clonal hematopoiesis of indeterminate potential (CHIP)," give rise to both MM and CML cells in a patient. Given our patient's relatively advanced age, it is possible that CHIP had a common origin, although we have no direct evidence to support this possibility. A third possible explanation is that the second disease might be a therapy-related malignancy that develops after treatment for the first disease. In the present case, the diagnosis of MM was followed by that of CML. The frequency of secondary carcinogenesis in patients with MM was evaluated for cohorts participating in clinical trials with lenalidomide, which were conducted from 2000 through 2012 [24]. This report showed that the incidence of secondary hematologic malignancies was increased in patients who concurrently received melphalan and lenalidomide, while it did not increase in those receiving other treatment protocols, regardless of whether lenalidomide was included [26]. There is no clear evidence that lenalidomide is carcinogenic, and there has only been one reported case of CML that developed after lenalidomide treatment. Therefore, the increased incidence of hematologic malignancies has been attributed to melphalan, because alkylating agents such as melphalan are known to cause therapy-related myelodysplastic syndromes. According to previous case reports of MM coexisting with CML, many patients received alkylating agents as treatment for MM (Table 1). In the present case, a small dose of an alkylating agent (cyclophosphamide; total: 2,400 mg/m^2) was administered during two cycles of CBD therapy. We, therefore, needed to consider the possibility that the cyclophosphamide treatment caused the CML. However, an accumulation of case reports and further investigations are required to draw definitive conclusions.

Although p190 *BCR-ABL* CML has been reported in 1% of CML cases, there have been several clinical observations suggesting that CML with p190 *BCR-ABL* is difficult to treat [27]. Furthermore, p190 *BCR-ABL* has been identified as a marker for high-risk disease, and early stem cell transplantation has been recommended if the patient is eligible [26]. Our patient received initial treatment of dasatinib for his CML in AP with p190 *BCR-ABL*, which provided a partial cytogenetic response at 4 months after the diagnosis. Although the long-term effects of dasatinib treatment in patients with p190 *BCR-ABL* CML are unknown, in the present case, the duration of response to dasatinib was relatively short.

Consent

Informed consent was obtained from the patient.

Conflicts of Interest

The authors declare that they have no conflicts of interest.

References

[1] A. Palumbo and K. Anderson, "Multiple myeloma," *New England Journal of Medicine*, vol. 364, pp. 1046–1060, 2011.

[2] W. Al Achkar, A. Wafa, H. Mkrtchyan, F. Moassass, and T. Liehr, "A rare case of chronic myeloid leukemia with secondary chromosomal changes including partial trisomy 17q21 to 17qter and partial monosomy of 16p13.3," *Molecular Cytogenetics*, vol. 3, no. 1, 2010.

[3] J. M. MacSween and G. R. Langley, "Light-chain disease (hypogammaglobulinemia and Bence Jones proteinuria) and sideroblastic anemia-preleukemic chronic granulocytic leukemia," *Canadian Medical Association Journal*, vol. 106, no. 9, pp. 995–998, 1972.

[4] C. Derghazarian and N. B. Whittemore, "Multiple myeloma superimposed on chronic myelocytic leukemia," *Canadian Medical Association Journal*, vol. 110, no. 9, pp. 1047–1050, 1974.

[5] M. A. Boots and G. D. Pegrum, "Simultaneous presentation of chronic granulocytic leukaemia and multiple myeloma," *Journal of Clinical Pathology*, vol. 35, no. 3, pp. 364-365, 1982.

[6] P. J. Klenn, B. H. Hyun, Y. H. Lee, and W. Y. Zheng, "Multiple myeloma and chronic myelogenous leukemia--a case report with literature review," *Yonsei Medical Journal*, vol. 34, no. 3, pp. 293–300, 1993.

[7] M. Tanaka, R. Kimura, A. Matsutani et al., "Coexistence of chronic myelogenous leukemia and multiple myeloma. Case report and review of the literature," *Acta Haematologica*, vol. 99, no. 4, pp. 221–223, 1998.

[8] M. Nitta, K. Tsuboi, S. Yamashita et al., "Multiple myeloma preceding the development of chronic myelogenous leukemia," *International Journal of Hematology*, vol. 69, no. 3, pp. 170–173, 1999.

[9] A. Alvarez-Larrán, M. Rozman, and F. Cervantes, "Simultaneous occurrence of multiple myeloma and chronic myeloid leukemia," *Haematologica*, vol. 86, no. 8, p. 894, 2001.

[10] J. D. Schwarzmeier, M. Shehata, J. Ackermann, M. Hilgarth, H. Kaufmann, and J. Drach, "Simultaneous occurrence of chronic myeloid leukemia and multiple myeloma: evaluation by FISH analysis and in vitro expansion of bone marrow cells," *Leukemia*, vol. 17, no. 7, pp. 1426–1428, 2003.

[11] M. Nakagawa, "A case of a 47-year-old man who developed chronic myelogenous leukemia after therapy for multiple myeloma," *Ja Hokkaido Koseiren Obihiro Kosei Hospital*, vol. 6, pp. 101–106, 2003.

[12] V. Garipidou, S. Vakalopoulou, and K. Tziomalos, "Development of multiple myeloma in a patient with chronic myeloid leukemia after treatment with imatinib mesylate," *Oncologist*, vol. 10, no. 6, pp. 457-458, 2005.

[13] T. Wakayama, S. Fujita, and H. Ago, "An elder patient coexisted with multiple myeloma and chronic myeloid leukemia before treatments," *Medical Journal of Shimane Prefectural Central Hospital*, vol. 29, pp. 63–67, 2005.

[14] A. Galanopoulos, S. I. Papadhimitriou, E. Kritikou-Griva, M. Georgiakaki, and N. I. Anagnostopoulos, "Multiple myeloma developing after imatinib mesylate therapy for chronic myeloid leukemia," *Annals of Hematology*, vol. 88, no. 3, pp. 281-282, 2009.

[15] M. Michael, M. Antoniades, E. Lemesiou, N. Papaminas, and F. Melanthiou, "Development of multiple myeloma in a patient with chronic myeloid leukemia while on treatment with imatinib mesylate for 65 months," *Oncologist*, vol. 14, no. 12, pp. 1198–1200, 2009.

[16] M. Ide, N. Kuwahara, E. Matsuishi, S. Kimura, and H. Gondo, "Uncommon case of chronic myeloid leukemia with multiple myeloma," *International Journal of Hematology*, vol. 91, no. 4, pp. 699–704, 2010.

[17] C. Offiah, J. P. Quinn, P. Thornton, and P. T. Murphy, "Coexisting chronic myeloid leukaemia and multiple myeloma: rapid response to lenalidomide during imatinib treatment," *International Journal of Hematology*, vol. 95, no. 4, pp. 451-452, 2012.

[18] N. A. Romanenko, S. S. Bessmel'tsev, U.'eva VIu et al., "The combination of chronic myeloid leukemia and multiple myeloma in one patient," *Voprosy Onkologii*, vol. 59, no. 2, pp. 103–110, 2013, in Russian.

[19] L. Ragupathi, V. Najfeld, A. Chari, B. Petersen, S. Jagannath, and J. Mascarenhas, "A case report of chronic myelogenous leukemia in a patient with multiple myeloma and a review of the literature," *Clinical Lymphoma Myeloma and Leukemia*, vol. 13, no. 2, pp. 175–179, 2013.

[20] J. Maerki, G. Katava, D. Siegel, J. Silberberg, and P. K. Bhattacharyya, "Unusual case of simultaneous presentation of plasma cell myeloma, chronic myelogenenous leukemia, and Jak2 positive myeloproliferative disorder," *Case Reports in Hematology*, vol. 2014, Article ID 738428, 6 pages, 2014.

[21] S. Alsidawi, A. Ghose, J. Qualtieri, and N. Radhakrishnan, "A case of multiple myeloma with metachronous chronic myeloid leukemia treated successfully with bortezomib, dexamethasone, and dasatinib," *Case Reports in Oncological Medicine*, vol. 2014, Article ID 962526, 4 pages, 2014.

[22] I. Pessach, V. Bartzis, T. Tzenou et al., "Multiple myeloma and chronic myelogenous leukemia; an uncommon coexistence in 2 patients, with literature review," *Annals of Hematology and Oncology*, vol. 2, p. 1030, 2015.

[23] S. Ahn, J. S. Park, J. H. Han et al., "A rare case of chronic myelogenous leukemia and plasma cell myeloma in the same patient," *Annals of Laboratory Medicine*, vol. 35, no. 3, pp. 370–372, 2015.

[24] D. Wolleschak and F. H. Heidel, "Chronic myelogenous leukemia evolving after treatment of multiple myeloma," *Blood*, vol. 128, no. 1, p. 146, 2016.

[25] N. Ali, P. V. Pickens, and H. E. Auerbach, "Immunoglobulin D multiple myeloma, plasma cell leukemia and chronic myelogenous leukemia in a single patient treated simultaneously with lenalidomide, bortezomib, dexamethasone and imatinib," *Hematology Reports*, vol. 8, no. 1, p. 6295, 2016.

[26] A. Palumbo, S. Bringhen, S. K. Kumar et al., "Second primary malignancies with lenalidomide therapy for newly diagnosed myeloma: a meta-analysis of individual patient data," *The Lancet Oncology*, vol. 15, no. 3, pp. 333–342, 2014.

[27] D. Verma, H. M. Kantarjian, D. Jones et al., "Chronic myeloid leukemia (CML) with P190BCR-ABL: analysis of characteristics, outcomes, and prognostic significance," *Blood*, vol. 114, no. 11, pp. 2232–2235, 2009.

Successful Antimicrobial Treatment of Phlegmonous Gastritis

Madiha Iqbal,[1] Rabia Saleem,[2] Salman Ahmed,[1] Prachi Jani,[1] Salvador Alvarez,[1] and Han W. Tun[1]

[1]*Department of Hematology and Oncology, Mayo Clinic, Jacksonville, FL, USA*
[2]*University of Oklahoma, Oklahoma City, OK, USA*

Correspondence should be addressed to Madiha Iqbal; iqbal.madiha@mayo.edu

Academic Editor: Massimo Breccia

Phlegmonous gastritis is an uncommon acute bacterial infection of the stomach that carries a fatal prognosis in spite of the advent of antibiotics. A high index of suspicion is required in patients with risk factors. An immunocompromised state is identified as one of the most important risk factors. We hereby report a case of successful antimicrobial treatment of phlegmonous gastritis in a patient who was receiving intensive chemotherapy for acute myelogenous leukemia. We have also carried out a review of literature over the past ten years. *Streptococcus pyogenes* is identified as the most common causative organism, and patient presentation is usually nonspecific. Conservative treatment with prompt institution of antibiotics can lead to rapid resolution in the majority of patients.

1. Introduction

Phlegmonous gastritis (PG) is a rare acute bacterial infection, which primarily involves the submucosal layer of the stomach wall, but can also involve the muscularis layer and rarely the mucosa [1–3]. It is rapidly fatal if untreated and thus requires prompt diagnosis and management. Even with the correct diagnosis and antimicrobial therapy, the mortality rate remains high at 27–40% [2, 3]. PG primarily affects the middle-aged population of 45–74 years, with a 65% male predominance [4]. The underlying etiology is largely unknown, although an immunocompromised state associated with malignancy, chemotherapy-induced neutropenia, acquired immunodeficiency syndrome (AIDS), alcoholism, and immunosuppressive drugs is considered an important risk factor [5]. We herein report a patient who developed PG in the setting of prolonged neutropenia related to relapsed acute myeloid leukemia (AML) and intensive chemotherapy and was successfully treated with systemic antimicrobial therapy.

2. Case Presentation

The patient reported is a 56-year-old woman who was diagnosed with acute myeloid leukemia (AML) with cytogenetic abnormality of inversion 16 in 2013. She achieved a complete remission (CR) after standard induction chemotherapy with 7 + 3 regimen consisting of ara-C and daunorubicin followed by consolidation with high-dose ara-C (HiDAC). She relapsed a year later and was re-induced with a salvage chemotherapy regimen MEC (mitoxantrone, etoposide, and cytarabine) achieving a second CR, which was followed by a matched unrelated allogeneic stem cell transplant (allo-SCT). Her posttransplant course was uneventful without significant graft versus host disease and prolonged requirement for immunosuppression. Two years after allo-SCT, she had a central nervous system (CNS) relapse of her original leukemia and presented with an infiltrating lesion in the lumbosacral spine; her CSF cytology was positive for myeloblasts. She was admitted to the hospital to receive reinduction chemotherapy; her vitals

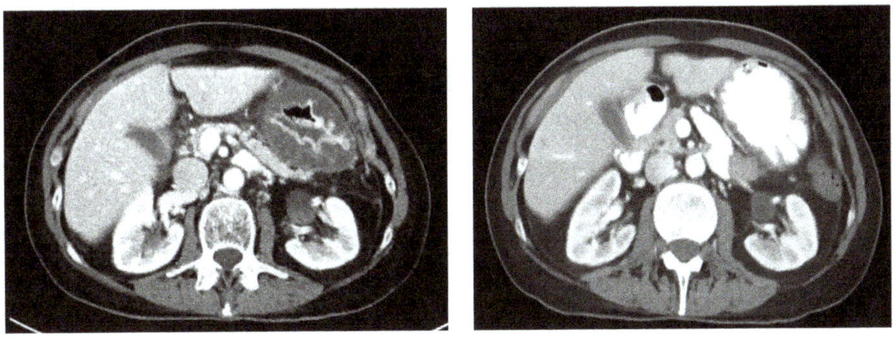

(a) (b)

Figure 1: (a) Diffuse thickening of the stomach wall with mucosal hyperenhancement and marked submucosal edema. (b) Marked interval improvement in gastric wall thickening and greater curvature intramural hypodensity after two weeks of antibiotic treatment.

upon admission were as follows: temperature 37.7 °C, blood pressure (BP) 129/65 mmHg, heart rate (HR) 72/min, and respiratory rate (RR) 14/min. She was started on intrathecal chemotherapy with ara-C and systemic chemotherapy with the salvage chemotherapy regimen FLAG-IDA (fludarabine, ara-C, and idarubicin). The day chemotherapy started for the patient was noted as day 1. On day 10, the patient developed neutropenic fever, and the white blood count (WBC) noted to be $<0.1 \times 10^9$/L with absolute neutrophil count (ANC) of 0. She was started on intravenous (IV) cefepime 2 g every 8 hour after evaluation for underlying infectious etiology was done. The work up did not isolate any organism and included blood culture, urine culture, and chest X-ray. On day 16, the patient developed left upper quadrant abdominal pain. Vital signs then were as follows: maximum temperature (T_{max}) 37.5°C, along with HR of 80–94/min, RR 16–18/min, and BP SBP 105–126/DBP 55–71 mmHg. Her blood tests then were as follows: WBC $<0.1 \times 10^9$/L, ANC 0, hemoglobin 8.0 g/dl, platelet 12×10^9/L, and serum blood chemistry and liver function tests were noted to be without significant derangements. A CT scan of the abdomen was performed that showed diffuse thickening of stomach wall (Figure 1(a)), concerning for infectious or infiltrative malignant process. Her absolute neutrophil count had been at the nadir for 10 days prior to this development. Her antimicrobial coverage was increased to include anaerobic coverage by changing her antibiotic regimen from IV cefepime 2 g every 8 hour to IV piperacillin/tazobactam 3.375 g every 6 hour, leading to short-lived symptomatic improvement for roughly two weeks. Upon symptom recurrence, the patient was noted to be febrile with T_{max} of 39.5°C, along with HR of 109–139/min, RR 18–20/min, and BP SBP 94–124/DBP 55–71. Two sets of peripheral blood cultures were drawn which did not show growth of any organism after 5 days of incubation. The patient continued to remain hemodynamically stable.

An upper gastrointestinal (GI) endoscopy was performed which showed a large ulcerative lesion with purulent discharge and inflammatory changes (Figure 2). *Citrobacter freundii*, *Enterococcus faecalis*, and *Bacillus cereus* were isolated from culture on gastric biopsies. Imaging, endoscopic, and microbiological findings were consistent with phlegmonous gastritis.

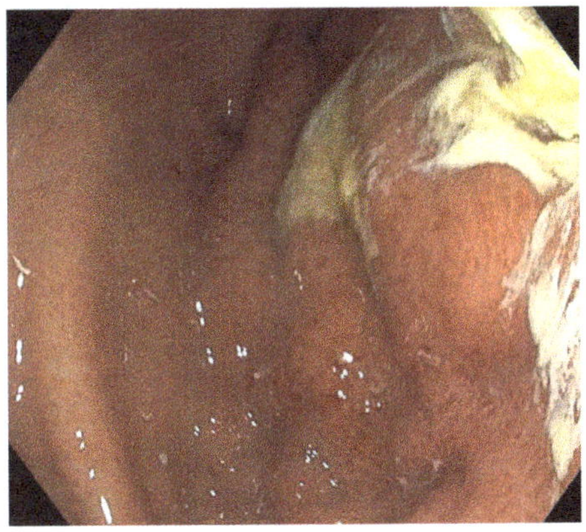

Figure 2: Upper endoscopy showing large nonobstructing nonbleeding gastric deep ulcerations with exudate material.

Infectious disease service was consulted, IV piperacillin/tazobactam 3.375 g every 6 hour was stopped, and the antibiotic regimen was changed to IV vancomycin (managed per pharmacy protocol based on weight and renal function) and IV meropenem 1 g IV every 8 hour. The recommendation for broad coverage of microorganisms was made by infectious disease service, given the high risk of mortality associated with phlegmonous gastritis. Prophylactic antifungal and antiviral for neutropenia were continued. Organism susceptibilities were carried out for *Citrobacter freundii* and *Enterococcus faecalis*, which revealed *Citrobacter freundii* to be resistant to ampicillin, cefazolin, and cefuroxime, while *Enterococcus faecalis* was noted to be pansensitive. Per organism susceptibility and with the help of infectious disease service, her antibiotic regimen was changed to IV cefepime 2 g every 8 hour, IV metronidazole 500 mg IV every 8 hour, and IV vancomycin per pharmacy protocol. This antibiotic regimen was continued for a total of two weeks. The patient's gastrointestinal symptoms resolved quickly, and she was able to resume normal diet. Follow-up CT scan a month later showed marked improvement in gastric thickening (Figure 1(b)). She is currently doing well with her AML in remission and no recurrence of her GI symptoms.

Table 1: Pertinent findings from our review of 25 case reports.

Author/Year	Sex	Age	Cause/risk factor	Symptoms	Pathogen/s	Diagnosis	Intervention/management	Complications	Result
Ajibe H, 2008	M	74	Endoscopic submucosal dissection for gastric adenocarcinoma	Epigastric pain, fever	*Citrobacter freundii, Enterobacter cloacae, and Streptococcus*	CT, EGD, EUS	Antibiotics, total gastrectomy	Nil	Discharge
Alonso et al., 2013 [7]	F	55	None	Chest pain	*Streptococcus pyogenes*	CT	Antibiotics, endoscopic abscess drainage	Nil	Discharge
Fan JQ, 2013	M	65	Esophagectomy for esophageal adenocarcinoma	Fever, dyspnea	Nil	CT, EGD	Antibiotics	Nil	Discharge
Flor-de-Lima F, 2015	M	7	Acute tonsillitis	Epigastric pain, nausea, vomiting	*Streptococcus pneumoniae*, EBV	CT, EGD with biopsy	Antibiotics	Nil	Discharge
Guo et al., 2009 [3]	M	57	CML, myeloid sarcoma	Dyspnea, chest pain, abdominal pain, fatigue	VRE	CT, EGD with biopsy, autopsy	Antibiotics	Upper GI bleed	Death
Huang et al., 2017 [5]	F	60	Uncontrolled DM	Fever, fatigue, chest pain	*Pseudomonas, Klebsiella*	CT, EGD	Antibiotics, surgery (not gastrectomy)	Hypopharyngeal abscess, esophageal perforation	Discharge
Ishigami T, 2008	M	70	None	Fever, abdominal pain	MDR *Streptococcus*	EGD	Antibiotics	Nil	Discharge
Itonaga M, 2012	F	70	EUS-FNA for pancreatic tumor	Fever, abdominal pain	Alpha-hemolytic *Streptococcus*	Ct, EGD, EUS	Antibiotics	Nil	Discharge
Kato et al., 2015 [1]	M	64	DM, chronic pancreatitis	Epigastric pain, nausea	*Peptostreptococcus*	CT, EGD with biopsy	Antibiotics, EUS-guided pseudocyst drainage	Nil	Discharge
Kim BY, 2017	M	51	Ankylosing spondylitis	Nausea, vomiting	Nil	CT, EGD	Antibiotics	Nil	Discharge
Kim et al., 2010 [9]	M	48	Alcoholism, uncontrolled DM	Fever, chest pain, abdominal pain, dyspnea	*Klebsiella* spp.	EGD	Antibiotics, surgery (not gastrectomy)	Bilateral pleural effusions	Discharge
Kim et al., 2016 [2]	M	74	Alcoholic cirrhosis, DM, recent EGD, gastric adenocarcinoma	Abdominal pain, vomiting	Nil	CT, EGD with biopsy	Antibiotics	Nil	Discharge
Kim NY, 2011	M	66	None	Epigastric pain, nausea, vomiting	*Klebsiella, Acinetobacter*	CT, EGD with biopsy	Antibiotics	Nil	Discharge
Liu YJ, 2013	M	84	Colon cancer, prostate cancer	Fever, nausea, vomiting	Polymicrobial (gram positive and gram negative organisms)	CT, exploratory laparotomy gastric biopsy	Antibiotics, gastrectomy	Nil	Discharge
Matsumoto H, 2015	M	74	Myelofibrosis, multiple myeloma, neutropenia	Epigastric pain, nausea	*Bacillus* spp.	CT, EGD	Antibiotics	Sepsis, disseminated intravascular coagulation	Death
Min et al., 2014 [6]	F	51	Gastric ulcer	Abdominal pain	*Streptococcus pyogenes*	CT, exploratory laparotomy	Antibiotics, total gastrectomy	Gastric submucosal dissection	Discharge
Morimoto et al., 2014 [4]	M	77	DM, gastric ulcers	Fever, nausea, vomiting	Group A *Streptococcus*	CT	Antibiotics		Death
Nomura K, 2015	F	80	None	Epigastric pain, vomiting	*Enterobacter cloacae and Enterococcus faecium*	CT, EGD with biopsy	Antibiotics, total gastrectomy (worsening gastric strictures)	Nil	Discharge

TABLE 1: Continued.

Author/Year	Sex	Age	Cause/risk factor	Symptoms	Pathogen/s	Diagnosis	Intervention/management	Complications	Result
Paik DC, 2010	M	45	Recent paranasal sinus surgery	Abdominal pain, nausea, vomiting	*Streptococcus pyogenes*	CT, exploratory laparotomy EGD	Antibiotics	Respiratory failure, renal failure, coagulopathy	Discharge
Park CW, 2010	F	73	Gastric outlet narrowing	Epigastric pain, abdominal distension	*E. coli*, *Acinetobacter*	CT, EGD with biopsy	Antibiotics, pyloric stent	Nil	Discharge
Rada-Palomino et al., 2014 [8]	M	62	HIV	Epigastric pain, hematemesis, diarrhea	*Streptococcus pyogenes*	CT, EGD with biopsy	Antibiotics	Nil	Discharge
Saito M, 2012	F	55	ALL	Neutropenia	*Bacillus* spp.	CT, EGD with biopsy	Antibiotics	Nil	Discharge
Sakata T, 2011	F	63	None	Fever	None reported	CT, EGD with biopsy	Antibiotics, drainage	Nil	Discharge
Shiozawa K, 2009	M	62	Uncontrolled DM	Epigastric pain	None reported	CT	Antibiotics, drainage	Nil	Discharge
Munroe CA, 2010	M	58	Chronic hepatitis B	Epigastric pain, nausea, fever	Alpha-hemolytic *Streptococcus*	CT, EGD, EUS with biopsy	Antibiotics, aspiration	Nil	Discharge

CML: chronic myeloid leukemia; DM: diabetes mellitus; HIV: human immunodeficiency virus; ALL: acute lymphoblastic leukemia; EBV: Epstein-Barr virus, VRE: vancomycin-resistant *Enterococcus*; MDR: multidrug resistance; Strep: *Streptococcus*; EUS: endoscopic ultrasound; CT: computed tomography; EGD: esophagogastroduodenoscopy; FNA: fine needle aspiration.

3. Discussion and Literature Review

Phlegmonous gastritis is a rare infection with less than 500 cases reported in literature [3]. We have carried out a bibliographical search using PubMed from 2007 to 2017 using the keyword "Phlegmonous Gastritis" and found 36 articles, in English, Spanish, and Japanese, of which we reviewed 25.

Our limited data review showed that there have been only 4 cases reported in the USA and 3 in Europe in the last 10 years, whereas the bulk was reported in Southeast Asia, namely Japan (13) and Korea (8). In addition to an immunocompromised state, the other reported risk factors are increased age, gastric mucosal injury from chronic gastritis, peptic ulcer, endoscopic procedures, gastric cancer, achlorhydria, infection, and malnutrition [6, 7]. Our review found malignancy to be a risk factor in 32% of the cases (8/25). The mortality rate has been reported to be higher in groups with an identified risk factor as compared to those without one [8]. PG has been further classified into primary and secondary types [1]. The primary type is usually idiopathic or occurs after direct damage to the gastric mucosa due to trauma, cancer, and endoscopic interventions, thereby leading to direct microbial invasion. The secondary type is either associated with infection of neighboring organs, such as infection due to pancreatitis, hepatic abscess, and cholecystitis, or hematogenous/lymphogenous spread from other organs.

PG is a rare infection that usually presents with nonspecific gastrointestinal symptoms. A high index of suspicion is necessary, especially in immunocompromised individuals. Epigastric/abdominal pain is the most common symptom, with other symptoms including but not limited to being fever, nausea, vomiting, and, less often, diarrhea and hematemesis [6]. PG should be highly suspected if a CT scan shows diffuse thickening of the stomach wall. The upper GI endoscopy should be performed as visual and microbiologic findings help establish the diagnosis and guide antimicrobial therapy. Although, *Streptococcus pyogenes* is the most frequently reported isolated organism in about 70% of cases, polymicrobial infection as seen in our patient is also quite common [2, 8, 9]. Our review of cases followed a similar pattern, wherein *Streptococcus* spp. was the most common pathogen identified in 44% of cases, but there were also other uncommon pathogens isolated such as *Citrobacter*, *Acinetobacter*, *Enterobacter* spp., and *Bacillus* spp., and even resistant pathogens like MDR (multidrug-resistant) *Streptococcus* and VRE (vancomycin-resistant enterococcus) (Table 1).

It is imperative to initiate empiric broad-spectrum antimicrobial coverage as soon as there is the clinical suspicion of possible phlegmonous gastritis, followed by adjustments as per microbiological culture results and clinical course. Early diagnosis and prompt institution of antibiotics has been shown to prevent patient mortality and defer the need of a surgical intervention [7]. All of the patients in our review received antibiotics, with resolution seen in 22/25 (88%) of the cases and death in 3/25 of the cases (12% mortality). This illustrates that prompt recognition and awareness of phlegmonous gastritis as possible complication of prolonged neutropenia in patients with hematological malignancies can clearly impact outcomes.

Invasive modality for management includes surgical gastrectomy and is mainly reserved for those with impending local complications such as perforation or sepsis [6, 7]. As mentioned above if promptly recognized, majority of the patients can be treated via conservative measures. Patients with hematologic malignancies are a unique population that is extremely susceptible to this complication due to prolonged neutropenia, secondary to intensive chemotherapy regimens. Prompt intervention and assistance from multiple medical specialties is needed to prevent fatality from this aggressive infection. Our case highlights the need for awareness of this rare infectious complication amongst health care professionals who take care of immunocompromised patients especially those suffering from hematological malignancies as knowledge of this rare complication can clearly impact patient mortality. Table 1 shows the major clinical characteristics, imaging findings, microbiology results, treatment, and survival outcomes from our literature review.

Conflicts of Interest

The authors declare that that there are no conflicts of interest regarding the publication of this paper.

References

[1] K. Kato, K. Tominaga, S. Sugimori et al., "Successful treatment of early-diagnosed primary phlegmonous gastritis," *Internal Medicine*, vol. 54, no. 22, pp. 2863–2866, 2015.

[2] K. H. Kim, C. G. Kim, Y. W. Kim et al., "Phlegmonous gastritis with early gastric cancer," *Journal of Gastric Cancer*, vol. 16, no. 3, pp. 195–199, 2016.

[3] J. Guo, S. K. Young, C. R. Lorenzo et al., "Phlegmonous gastritis in a patient with myeloid sarcoma: a case report," *Applied Immunohistochemistry & Molecular Morphology*, vol. 17, no. 5, pp. 458–462, 2009.

[4] M. Morimoto, S. Tamura, T. Hayakawa et al., "Phlegmonous gastritis associated with group A streptococcal toxic shock syndrome," *Internal Medicine*, vol. 53, no. 22, pp. 2639–2642, 2014.

[5] Y. C. Huang, C. Y. Cheng, C. Y. Liao, C. Hsueh, Y. S. Tyan, and S. Y. Ho, "A rare case of acute phlegmonous esophagogastritis complicated with hypopharyngeal abscess and esophageal perforation," *American Journal of Case Reports*, vol. 18, pp. 125–130, 2017.

[6] S. Y. Min, Y. H. Kim, and W. S. Park, "Acute phlegmonous gastritis complicated by delayed perforation," *World Journal of Gastroenterology*, vol. 20, no. 12, pp. 3383–3387, 2014.

[7] J. V. Alonso, J. J. de la Fuente Carillo, M. A. Gutierrez Solis, F. J. Vara Morate, and D. J. Lopez Ruiz, "Gastric wall abscess presenting as thoracic pain: rare presentation of an old disease," *Annals of Gastroenterology*, vol. 26, no. 4, pp. 360–362, 2013.

[8] A. Rada-Palomino, A. Munoz-Duyos, N. Perez-Romero et al., "Phlegmonous gastritis: a rare entity as a differential diagnostic of an acute abdomen. Description of a case and a bibliographic review," *Revista Española de Enfermedades Digestivas*, vol. 106, no. 6, pp. 418–424, 2014.

[9] H. S. Kim, J. H. Hwang, S. S. Hong et al., "Acute diffuse phlegmonous esophagogastritis: a case report," *Journal of Korean medical science*, vol. 25, no. 10, pp. 1532–1535, 2010.

A Case of Bing–Neel Syndrome Successfully Treated with Ibrutinib

Daniel S. O'Neil,[1] Mark A. Francescone,[2] Karen Khan,[3] Alobeid Bachir,[4] Owen A. O'Connor,[3] and Ahmed Sawas[3]

[1]*Herbert Irving Comprehensive Cancer Center, Columbia University Medical Center-College of Physicians and Surgeons, New York, NY, USA*
[2]*Department of Radiology, Columbia University Medical Center-College of Physicians and Surgeons, New York, NY, USA*
[3]*Center for Lymphoid Malignancies, Columbia University Medical Center-College of Physicians and Surgeons, New York, NY, USA*
[4]*Department of Pathology and Cell Biology, Columbia University Medical Center-College of Physicians and Surgeons, New York, NY, USA*

Correspondence should be addressed to Daniel S. O'Neil; dso2116@cumc.columbia.edu

Academic Editor: Maria K. Angelopoulou

Bing–Neel syndrome is a rare manifestation of Waldenström macroglobulinemia characterized by lymphoplasmacytic cells' infiltration into the central nervous system. We present a case of a 74-year-old patient with a known diagnosis of Waldenström macroglobulinemia and newly depressed consciousness. Flow cytology of his cerebral spinal fluid demonstrated a lambda light chain-restricted population of B-cells consistent with a CD5+ CD10+ B-cell lymphoma. Magnetic resonance imaging suggested involvement of the left optic nerve sheath and the bilateral orbital and parietal parenchyma and leptomeninges. He was diagnosed with Bing–Neel syndrome and treated with intrathecal liposomal cytarabine, intravenous high-dose methotrexate, and rituximab without improvement. Subsequently, he started treatment with ibrutinib 560 mg daily and concurrent rituximab. Within three months, he showed clinical and radiologic improvement. The patient has continued on ibrutinib and has now been stable for over 36 months. This represents the longest reported period of successful treatment of Bing–Neel syndrome with ibrutinib.

1. Introduction

Waldenström macroglobulinemia (WM) is a rare B-cell lymphoma, with an incidence of just 0.3 per 100,000 person-years [1]. While most neurologic complications of WM are neuropathies secondary to IgM activity, direct central nervous system (CNS) infiltration by malignant lymphoplasmacytic cells (LPCs) is a recognized complication known as the Bing–Neel syndrome (BNS).

We present a case of a patient with BNS refractory to chemoimmunotherapy achieving a complete response to ibrutinib and maintenance of response for 3 years.

2. Case Presentation

The patient presented in November 2010 at the age of 74 years with several splotchy, hyperpigmented lesions across his forehead. He reported that the lesions had been present for two years but were now growing in size. A skin punch biopsy showed scattered dense lymphocytic nodules and follicles in the dermis composed of large centroblast-like and smaller centrocyte-like cells with the appearance of germinal centers. Follicular B-cells expressed CD10 and Bcl-6, were equivocal for Bcl-2, and lacked MUM1 expression. CD21-positive follicular dendritic cell meshworks were associated with the follicles, and the Ki-67 staining index was 20–30%. Plasma cells were appreciated in the center of a few follicles and the interfollicular areas. Flow cytometry identified a population of B cells (3.6% of nucleated cells) with the following phenotypes: CD19+, CD20+, CD79a+, CD5−, CD10−, FMC-7+ (moderately bright), CD43−, CD103−, surface IgM−, surface IgD−, and CD52+. No IGH/BCL2 translocation was detected in the skin biopsy.

Bone marrow biopsy in December 2010 showed diffuse infiltration of small lymphocytes and mature-appearing plasma cells. CD20 staining identified B cells (CD23+/−, bcl2+, CD5−, CD10−, and CD43−) accounting for >50% of total cellularity, and CD138 showed lambda-restricted plasma cells (IgM+) accounting for 20–30% of cellularity. Serum protein electrophoresis performed at the same time detected a monoclonal IgM lambda protein at 2.6 g/dL concentration. Positron emission tomography-computed tomography (PET-CT) imaging showed hypermetabolic left axillary lymphadenopathy and osseous lesions within the T5 vertebral body and left iliac wing; splenomegaly and right axillary lymphadenopathy were also appreciated. At the time of bone marrow biopsy, the patient was anemic, with a hemoglobin of 6.0 g/dL and a mean corpuscular volume of 92.8 fL, and leukopenic, with a white blood cell count of $3.2 \times 103/\mu L$ and an absolute neutrophil count of $2.2 \times 103/\mu L$. Lactate dehydrogenase was elevated at 264 U/L. Laboratory testing of renal and liver function was normal. The diagnosis of WM was made.

Treatment was planned with rituximab and fludarabine for six cycles. The patient completed five cycles with the planned sixth cycle held after he developed a pneumonia.

His disease was quiescent until April 2014, when he presented back to clinic with a mass adjacent to the right brachial plexus causing upper extremity weakness, swelling, and pain. Cytology from fine-needle aspiration of the mass demonstrated clonal intermediate and large lymphoid cells with plasmacytoid features. A clonal IgH rearrangement was present, and the predominant B-cell phenotype on flow cytometry was CD19+, CD79a+, CD20+, CD10+, CD5+, CD23−, CD38+/−, FMC7−, CD43−/+, CD25+, CD103−, HLA-DR+, surface IgM+, and surface IgD+. Molecular testing of the soft tissue sample detected an *MYD88* L265P mutation. Bone marrow biopsy only showed a tiny population (<0.5%) of atypical plasma cells without a detectable clonal IgH rearrangement. He received a single cycle of rituximab-bendamustine combination therapy at an outside institution.

Unfortunately, over the course of July 2014, he developed progressive, intermittent confusion. Brain imaging was difficult to obtain, but cerebrospinal fluid (CSF) contained 420 nucleated cells/μL and protein at 296 mg/dL. CSF cytology was highly cellular with cells cytomorphologically consistent with non-Hodgkin's lymphoma, and flow cytometry showed a predominant population of lambda light chain-restricted B-cell phenotype CD19+, CD79a+, CD20+, CD10+, CD5+, CD23−, CD38+/1, FMC7−, CD43+, CD103−, surface IgM+, and surface IgD+. Again, an *MYD88* L265P mutation was detected. Serum IgM was 942 mg/dL; monoclonal protein concentration was 0.8 g/dL. He was treated with intrathecal liposomal cytarabine, intravenous high-dose methotrexate, and rituximab 750 mg every 4 weeks. His mental status improved initially, but he subsequently developed bacterial meningitis. His meningitis led to a prolonged hospitalization complicated by recurrent fevers of idiopathic etiology, aspiration pneumonia, balanitis, *Clostridium difficile* colitis, and declining mental status. Treatment was continued as permitted by recurrent infections. By October 2010, CSF studies still showed few lymphocytes suspicious for refractory disease, and the patient's mental status remained poor.

Magnetic resonance imaging (MRI) of the brain and orbits from December 2014 showed subcutaneous ependymal enhancement within the atria of both lateral ventricles with extensive bilateral adjacent periventricular parenchymal FLAIR hyperintensity, evidence of leptomeningeal spread in the parasagittal portion of both occipital and parietal lobes, and enhancement of the bilateral optic nerves and the left optic nerve sheath concerning for lymphomatous involvement (Figure 1).

In the late December 2014, our patient was started on ibrutinib 560 mg daily and continued rituximab. By February 2015, his mental status was clear, and he was reporting improvements in his vision and hearing. MRI brain was repeated in March 2015, showing interval improvement with decreased signal abnormality adjoining the atrium of the lateral ventricle and only mild persistent left optic nerve sheath enhancement (Figure 1). By that time, serum IgM was 738 mg/dL and monoclonal protein was 0.5 g/dL. By July 2015, MRI showed no abnormal enhancement in the brain at all. He has continued ibrutinib and periodic rituximab infusion through December 2016 with persistently normal MRI. Treatment has been complicated by hypogammaglobulinemia requiring occasional intravenous immunoglobulin administration and a hospital admission for methicillin-sensitive *Staphylococcus aureus* bacteremia. Otherwise, as of March 2018, he is doing well with minimal cytopenias or adverse effects.

3. Discussion

The clinical manifestations of BNS are diverse and, often, nonspecific. Patients may present with focal complaints, such as visual and auditory defects, or global manifestations, such as seizures or reduced consciousness. Per recently published expert consensus guidelines, the diagnosis is confirmed with biopsy of the involved parenchyma or leptomeninges and demonstration of LPC infiltration. In the absence of CNS biopsy, CSF can be examined for the presence of LPCs via cytology, flow cytometry, and molecular testing for clonal IgG gene rearrangement and *MYD88* L265P mutations. Immunofixation and electrophoresis may also identify IgM monoclonal proteins in the CSF [2]. Magnetic resonance imaging enhancement may be diffuse or localized. At the time of initial presentation, our patient met the Second International Workshop on Waldenstrom's Macroglobulinemia clinical criteria for the diagnosis of WM; the value of *MYD88* in the diagnosis of WM was not well described until 2012 [3, 4]. Soft tissue samples and CSF from 2014 did show *MYD88* L265P mutations, and the development of a CD5+ CD10+ phenotype does not exclude WM [5].

BNS is usually diagnosed in patients already known to have WM, but it has been reported as the first clinical manifestation of WM in 15% to 36% of cases [2]. A case series of 34 patients suggest that those with BNS as the initial presentation of WM have a better prognosis than those with a secondary presentation [6]. That same series report a median overall survival of just 59% at 3 years following diagnosis with BNS. While therapy typically includes intrathecal chemotherapy, high-dose methotrexate, systemic

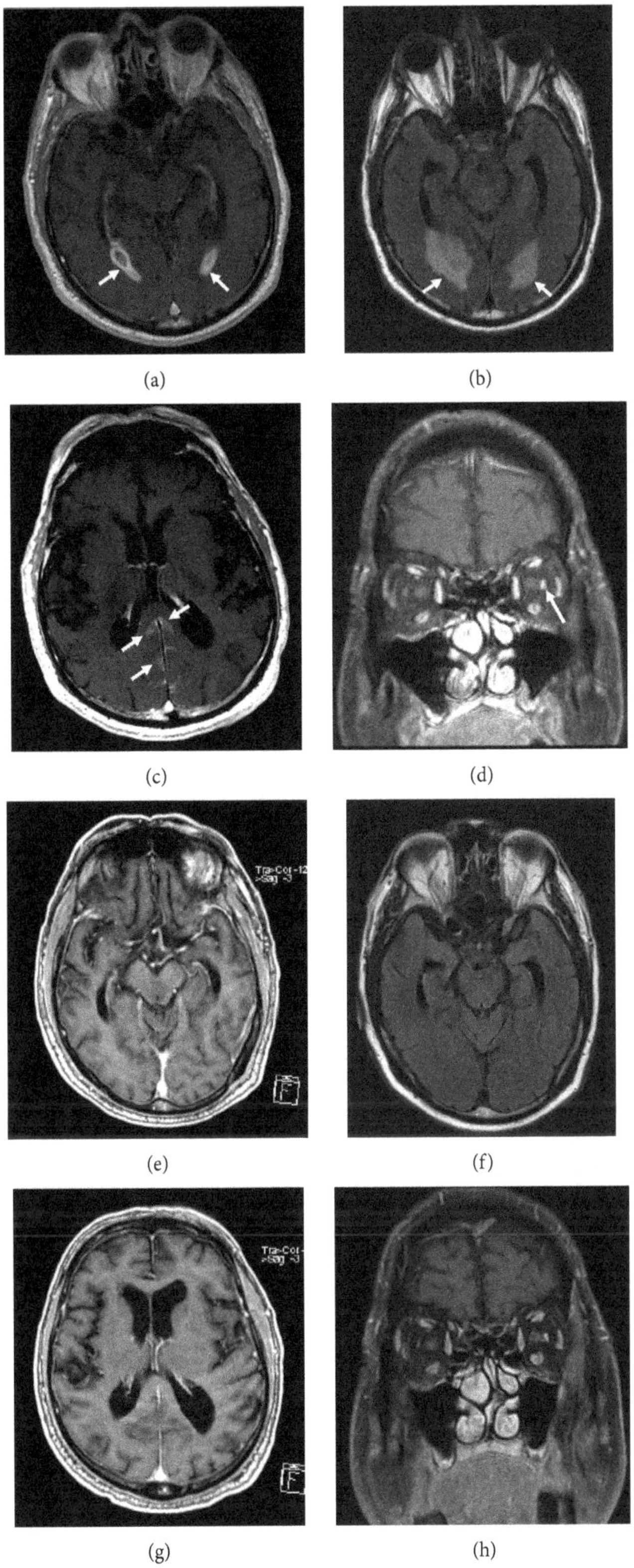

FIGURE 1: Magnetic resonance imaging of patient's brain obtained before and after initiation of ibrutinib. (a) Subependymal enhancement in December 2014 (T1 postcontrast). (b) Periventricular hyperintensity in December 2014 (FLAIR). (c) Leptomeningeal enhancement in December 2014 (postcontrast). (d) Left optic sheath enhancement in January 2015 (postcontrast). (e) Subependymal enhancement resolved in March 2015 (T1 postcontrast). (f) Periventricular hyperintensity resolved in March 2015 (FLAIR). (g) Leptomeningeal enhancement resolved in March 2015 (postcontrast). (h) Left optic sheath enhancement decreased in March 2015 (postcontrast).

Table 1: Summary of previously reported cases of ibrutinib use for the treatment of Bing–Neel syndrome.

Case report	Number of patients	Prior diagnosis of WM	Earlier BNS therapies	Ibrutinib dose	Length of response to ibrutinib
Cabannes-Hamy et al. [13]	2	Yes, yes	R/HD-MTX/L-AC → HDAC, R-DHAC → R	420 mg daily, 420 mg daily	6 months, 6 months
Mason et al. [14]	1	Yes	R/HD-MTX → B → L-AC	560 mg daily	23 months
Varettoni et al. [15]	1	No	BR/IT-MTX	Not reported	Not reported
Boudin et al. [16]	1	No	None	420 mg daily	11 months

BNS = Bing–Neel syndrome; WM = Waldenström macroglobulinemia; R = rituximab; HD-MTX = high-dose methotrexate; L-AC = intrathecal liposomal cytarabine; HDAC = high-dose cytarabine; R-DHAC = rituximab, dexamethasone, high-dose cytarabine, and carboplatin; B = bendamustine; BR = bendamustine and rituximab; IT-MTX = intrathecal methotrexate.

chemotherapy with fludarabine or bendamustine, or immunotherapy with rituximab, only rituximab use is associated with improved survival [6].

Ibrutinib is a potent inhibitor of Bruton's tyrosine kinase, a B-cell receptor involved in several signaling pathways essential to B-cell development and survival [7]. In previously treated patients with WM, ibrutinib monotherapy has an excellent overall response rate, exceeding 90%. Mutations to *MYD88* or *CXCR4* seem to improve the likelihood of response [8].

Ibrutinib is presently granted US Federal Drug Administration approval for use in chronic lymphocytic leukemia (CLL), mantle cell leukemia (MCL), marginal zone lymphoma, chronic graft-versus-host disease, and WM [9]. Activity against central nervous system lesions has been described in several of these diagnoses. Six patients in a series of 30 CLL patients with CNS disease confirmed by cerebral spinal fluid (CSF) analysis were treated with ibrutinib; four patients had received at least 2 prior lines of therapy. All patients showed some response, with three complete responses, and five were still alive at a median follow-up of 8 months [10]. For MCL, a small case series of three patients with intracerebral lesions all demonstrated clinical examination improvement within 3 to 8 days of initiating single-agent ibrutinib at the standard dose. Two of three showed complete response by MRI and PET-CT, with ongoing response at 1 year and 9 months of follow-up [11]. Similar results were reported among five MCL patients from the United Kingdom. All five patients achieved a response in CNS disease with ibrutinib, with a median length of 4 months (range 4 days–5 months), although two patients received concurrent systemic chemotherapy [12].

Individual case reports describe five patients with WM and CNS involvement undergoing treatment with ibrutinib, either as first-line therapy or after progressing on rituximab and systemic and intrathecal chemotherapy (Table 1). Response was reported for four, with the length of measured response lasting from 6 to 23 months [13–16]. CSF concentrations of ibrutinib were measured in several of these cases. In two MCL patients, they were 4.5 and 113.5 nmol/L, and one WM patient peaked at 34 nmol/L [11, 14]. These concentrations demonstrate ibrutinib's capacity to cross the blood-brain barrier and were all greater than its half maximal inhibitory concentration (0.5 nmol/L).

This case represents another instance of rapid, dramatic, and durable improvement of BNS upon initiation of ibrutinib. His response has now been maintained for over 36 months, the longest yet reported. The multiple instances of durable improvement of CNS infiltrates in CLL and MCL with ibrutinib and the growing number of similar responses in BNS suggest that ibrutinib should be routinely considered among the therapeutic options for these challenging patients.

Conflicts of Interest

The authors have no conflicts of interest to declare.

Acknowledgments

This work was funded by a T32 postdoctoral fellowship to Dr. O'Neil (T32 CA094061).

References

[1] J. Sekhar, K. Sanfilippo, Q. Zhang, K. Trinkaus, R. Vij, and D. Morgensztern, "Waldenström macroglobulinemia: a surveillance, epidemiology, and end results database review from 1988 to 2005," *Leukemia & Lymphoma*, vol. 53, no. 8, pp. 1625-1626, 2012.

[2] M. C. Minnema, E. Kimby, S. D'Sa et al., "Guideline for the diagnosis, treatment and response criteria for Bing-Neel syndrome," *Haematologica*, vol. 102, no. 1, pp. 43–51, 2017.

[3] R. G. Owen, S. P. Treon, A. Al-Katib et al., "Clinicopathological definition of Waldenstrom's macroglobulinemia: consensus panel recommendations from the Second International Workshop on Waldenstrom's Macroglobulinemia," *Seminars in Oncology*, vol. 30, no. 2, pp. 110–115, 2003.

[4] S. P. Treon, L. Xu, G. Yang et al., "MYD88 L265P somatic mutation in Waldenström's macroglobulinemia," *New England Journal of Medicine*, vol. 367, no. 9, pp. 826–833, 2012.

[5] Z. R. Hunter, A. R. Branagan, R. Manning et al., "CD5, CD10, and CD23 expression in Waldenstrom's macroglobulinemia," *Clinical Lymphoma*, vol. 5, no. 4, pp. 246–249, 2005.

[6] J. J. Castillo, S. D'Sa, M. P. Lunn et al., "Central nervous system involvement by Waldenström macroglobulinaemia (Bing-Neel syndrome): a multi-institutional retrospective study," *British Journal of Haematology*, vol. 172, no. 5, pp. 709–715, 2016.

[7] J. C. Byrd, R. R. Furman, S. E. Coutre et al., "Targeting BTK with ibrutinib in relapsed chronic lymphocytic leukemia," *New England Journal of Medicine*, vol. 369, no. 1, pp. 32–42, 2013.

[8] S. P. Treon, C. K. Tripsas, K. Meid et al., "Ibrutinib in previously treated Waldenström's macroglobulinemia," *New England Journal of Medicine*, vol. 372, no. 15, pp. 1430–1440, 2015.

[9] Drugs@FDA: FDA Approved Drug Products, December 2016, http://www.accessdata.fda.gov/scripts/cder/daf/index.cfm?event=overview.process&varApplNo=205552.

[10] A. Wanquet, R. Birsen, C. Bonnet et al., "Management of central nervous system involvement in chronic lymphocytic leukaemia: a retrospective cohort of 30 patients," *British Journal of Haematology*, vol. 176, no. 1, pp. 37–49, 2016.

[11] S. Bernard, L. Goldwirt, S. Amorim et al., "Activity of ibrutinib in mantle cell lymphoma patients with central nervous system relapse," *Blood*, vol. 126, no. 14, pp. 1695–1698, 2015.

[12] D. L. Tucker, G. Naylor, A. Kruger, M. S. Hamilton, G. Follows, and S. A. Rule, "Ibrutinib is a safe and effective therapy for systemic mantle cell lymphoma with central nervous system involvement-a multi-centre case series from the United Kingdom," *British Journal of Haematology*, vol. 178, no. 2, pp. 327–329, 2016.

[13] A. Cabannes-Hamy, R. Lemal, L. Goldwirt et al., "Efficacy of ibrutinib in the treatment of Bing-Neel syndrome," *American Journal of Hematology*, vol. 91, no. 3, pp. E17–E19, 2016.

[14] C. Mason, S. Savona, J. N. Rini et al., "Ibrutinib penetrates the blood brain barrier and shows efficacy in the therapy of Bing Neel syndrome," *British Journal of Haematology*, vol. 179, no. 2, pp. 339–341, 2016.

[15] M. Varettoni, I. Defrancesco, L. Diamanti, E. Marchioni, L. M. Farina, and A. Pichiecchio, "Bing-Neel syndrome: illustrative cases and comprehensive review of the literature," *Mediterranean Journal of Hematology and Infectious Diseases*, vol. 9, no. 1, article e2017061, 2017.

[16] L. Boudin, M. Patient, E. Roméo, J.-S. Bladé, and J.-P. de Jauréguiberry, "Efficacy of ibrutinib as first-line treatment of tumoral Bing-Neel syndrome," *Leukemia & Lymphoma*, pp. 1–3, 2018.

Suspected Pericardial Tuberculosis Revealed as an Amyloid Pericardial Mass

Sebastiano Cicco, Antonio G. Solimando, Patrizia Leone, Stefano Battaglia, Roberto Ria, Angelo Vacca, and Vito Racanelli

Department of Biomedical Sciences and Human Oncology, Section of Internal Medicine "G. Baccelli", University of Bari Aldo Moro Medical School, Bari, Italy

Correspondence should be addressed to Sebastiano Cicco; sebacicco@gmail.com

Academic Editor: Marie-Christine Kyrtsonis

Primary systemic amyloidosis is not easily diagnosed. The immunoglobulin deposits are usually localized in the kidney, heart, and liver. We describe an unusual case of a patient suffering from a pericardial amyloidoma with internal calcifications and air bubbles that compressed the right ventricle and shifted the heart to the left. Since the patient was in shock, urgent pericardiotomy was performed. This site showed PET uptake. A monoclonal component was present. On these findings, differential diagnoses included multiple myeloma and atypical pericardial tuberculosis, whereas a periumbilical fat tissue biopsy demonstrated amyloidosis. A previous *Salmonella* species infection had most likely stimulated the production of amyloid. The patient received bortezomib/dexamethasone treatment and achieved a good response.

1. Introduction

Primary systemic amyloidosis (or AL amyloidosis) is a rare disorder in which misfolded parts of immunoglobulins (usually a monoclonal light-chain fragment) form insoluble fibrillar deposits in organs and tissues [1–6]. Amyloidosis should be suspected in any patient with monoclonal gammopathy and unexplained shortness of breath, fatigue, edema, weight loss, or paresthesias. However, the clinician needs to be well aware of this rare condition because various different symptoms may be present, mimicking more common disorders.

2. Case Presentation

A 69-year-old Caucasian man was admitted to our Unit from the Emergency Department. He had been suffering from fever, dyspnea, fatigue, and dizziness for 10 days. He had no relevant medical history until the previous month, when he developed intermittent fever with chills. Ceftriaxone was administered at home without benefit. A few days before hospitalization, the patient's clinical condition worsened. On admission, the patient was confused, jaundiced, and had lower-limb edema.

Physical examination revealed jugular turgor, thready pulse with tachycardia, and hypotension (heart rate, 110 beats/minute; blood pressure, 90/60 mmHg) (Beck's triad). Chest auscultation revealed tachypnea (respiratory rate, 28 breaths/minute) and bilateral basal crepitations. Abdominal palpation disclosed hepatomegaly, splenomegaly, and a dull percussion sound in the lower abdominal quadrants.

Routine blood tests showed elevated white blood cells ($2146 \times 10^3/\mu L$; neutrophils, 91.1%), normal Hb and PLTs, hyperglycemia, hyperbilirubinemia (bilirubin 5.50 mg/dl; 53% direct), and signs of hepatic dysfunction (aspartate aminotransferase (AST) 93 units/L, alanine aminotransferase (ALT) 119 units/L, gamma glutamyl transferase-GGT 285 units/L, serum albumin 2.9 g/dl, and INR 1.81). NT-pro-BNP was increased (2901 pg/ml), whereas cardiac-specific troponin was in the normal range (Table 1).

Since the electrocardiogram (ECG) identified high frequency sites during atrial fibrillation, digoxin and

Table 1: Routine laboratory investigations.

Value	Admission	After surgery	
Hb	13.4	8.0	g/dl
MCV	60.0	62.3	fl
RBC	7.31	4.36	$\times 10^6/\mu l$
WBC	21.46	11.12	$\times 10^3/\mu l$
Neutrophils	91.1	91.6	%
Leucocytes	3.6	3.7	%
Monocytes	4.6	4.1	%
Eosinophils	0.3	0.3	%
Basophils	0.5	0.3	%
Platelets	132	80	$\times 10^3/\mu l$
Creatinine	1.44	1.85	mg/dl
BUN	46	68	mg/dl
Na^+	148	135	mmol/l
K^+	4.0	3.4	mmol/l
Cl^-	112		mmol/l
Ca^{++}	8.4		mg/dl
Glucose	152		mg/dl
Tot. bil.	5.5	9.10	mg/dl
Direct	3.5	5.20	mg/dl
AST	93 (×3.1)	Norm	Units/l
ALT	119 (×1.6)	Norm	Units/l
GGT	285 (×3.3)	Norm	Units/l
Tot. prot.	6.7		g/dl
Albumin	2.9	1.8	g/dl
Amylase	23		U/l
Lipase	190		U/l
CRP	132	195	mg/l
PT INR	1.81	1.79	
aPTT	1.05		
Fibrinogen	368	405	Mg/dl
cTnI	<0.01		ng/ml
NT-pro-BNP	2901	1430	pg/ml
Quantiferon	Negative	Negative	
Blood cultures	Negative	Negative	

low-molecular-weight heparin (LMWH) were administered. Abdominal ultrasonography (US) revealed signs of hepatic disease (parenchymal inhomogeneity and increased diameters), splenomegaly (longitudinal diameter = 20 cm), and ascites. Heart US showed a difficult contraction and reduced diameter of the right ventricle with right atrium diastolic collapse and no inspiratory changes in the vena cava diameter. Chest CT scan demonstrated a retrosternal mediastinal mass containing calcifications and air bubbles. This mass did not show a cleavage plane over the heart but compressed it and shifted it to the left. Bilateral pleural effusion was also observed (Figure 1). Within a few hours, the blood pressure progressively decreased to 70/40 mmHg; dopamine (7 μg/kg/min) and oxygen (12 L/min) were given, and ECG monitoring was instituted. Urgent pericardiotomy was performed. Constrictive purulent-like pericardium and a firm mass with calcifications were removed. The patient rapidly improved: alertness, arterial pressure, and pulse rate normalized but he still had edema. NT-pro-BNP decreased in a couple of weeks (1430 pg/dl).

Because of the fever, antibiotic treatment was started, and insulin was administered for persistent hyperglycemia. A good response to the therapy was observed and paralleled a reduction of the WBC ($11 \times 10^3/\mu l$) and an improvement of

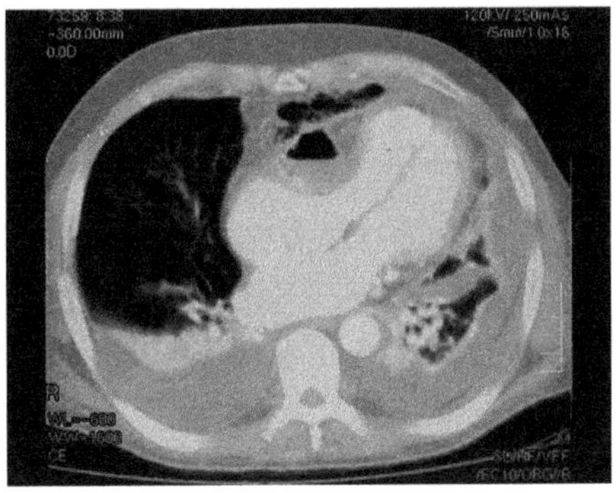

Figure 1: Chest CT scan. The mass is compressing the right ventricle and shifting the heart. Pleural effusion is present, with compression of the left lung.

liver function, as indicated by a decrease of AST, ALT, and GGT. However, the Hb value (8 g/dl) and PLT count ($80 \times 10^3/\mu l$) also decreased, with 3.1% of reticulocytes. Simultaneously, the albumin value was reduced (1.8 g/dl), whereas total bilirubin increased (9.1 mg/dl, 67% indirect), with a positive Coombs test for direct IgG. Therefore, albumin was administered.

One of the possible causes of effusive-constrictive pericarditis is tuberculosis (TBC) [7]. Since negative QuantiFERON ruled out classic TBC, we hypothesized atypical pericardial TBC or a fungal pericarditis. However, all viral (included HIV), microbiological, and cultural tests performed failed to reveal any infections.

Gamma-proteins were increased (30.8% vs 10–20% normal values) on serum protein electrophoresis and contained a monoclonal component (M component) accounting for 23.3% (1.64 g/dl) (Figure 2). Serum immunofixation demonstrated that the M component was IgG-λ. Mild renal failure was present with proteins in the urine (1.56 g/24 h) that contained the Bence Jones as free lambda chains. Our analysis showed that the patient had had previous hepatitis A and B infections but not hepatitis C. No bacteria were demonstrated at blood cultures.

The culture test of the pericardial effusion demonstrated the *Salmonella* species (*Salmonella suinis*), so imipenem and ciprofloxacin were given. A sample of periumbilical fat was taken and histologically analyzed: amyloid AL deposits were found as positive Congo red and apple-green birefringent areas under polarized light (Figure 3).

Bone marrow (BM) biopsy showed 4% plasma cells (CD138 and lambda light chain positive) but not amyloid deposits. Skeleton radiological analysis was negative for bone lesions.

PET-CT with 18 fluorodeoxyglucose (FDG) showed a low uptake only in the mediastinum behind the sternum close to the heart. Optical microscope histological examination of the mediastinal mass showed hematoxylin-eosin pink amorphous material which was Congo-red positive and apple-green birefringent and included some granulocytes and few plasma cells (CD138 and lambda light chain positive) near the vessels.

We decided to start treatment according to the chemotherapy scheme VEL/DEX (bortezomib 1.3 mg/m^2 i.v. on

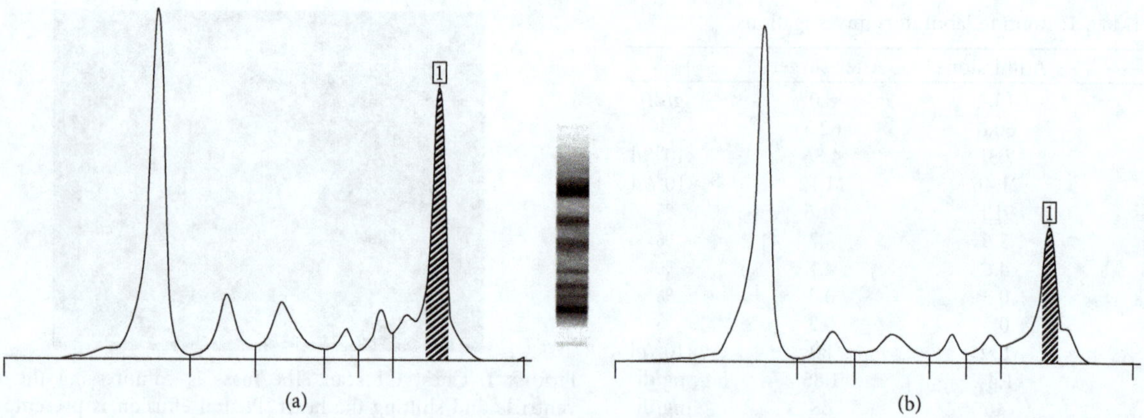

FIGURE 2: Serum protein electrophoresis before (a) and after (b) therapy. After therapy, there was a reduction of the monoclonal component (1).

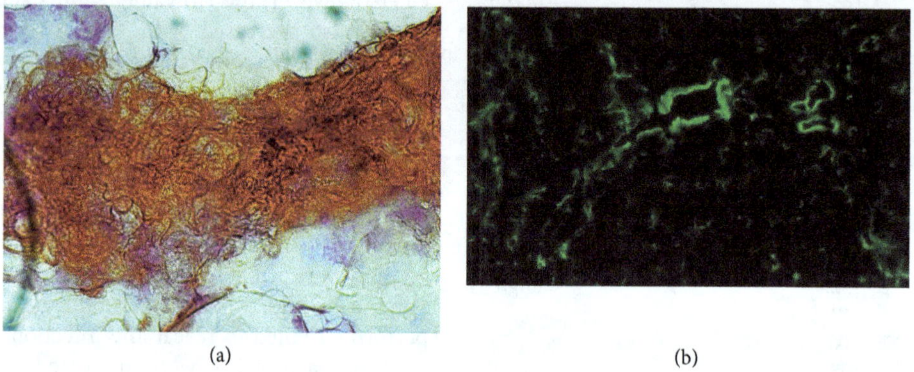

FIGURE 3: Amyloid deposition in periumbilical fat ((a)-Congo red) with apple-green birefringence (b) at polarized microscope analysis.

days 1, 4, 8, and 11; dexamethasone 40 mg i.v. on days 1, 2, 4, 5, 8, 9, 11, and 12).

The patient demonstrated good compliance and had a good response. The M component progressively lowered (12.2%, 0.67 g/dl), renal function improved, and urine proteins reduced. Epoetin A treatment was started to prevent a further decrease of Hb values.

At discharge, Hb, PLT, and serum bilirubin were stable; AST and ALT levels were normal; the pleural effusion, dyspnea, tachypnea, and edema had disappeared.

The patient underwent 4 cycles of Vel/Dex yielding a good clinical response. He slowly went back to work, with a good performance status.

3. Discussion

Amyloidosis is due to extracellular deposition of insoluble fibrils with a β-pleated sheet structure that are formed by the polymerization of misfolded proteins [1–4]. Regardless of the protein type, all amyloid proteins intercalate Congo red dye and show apple-green birefringence under polarized light because they share similar ultrastructural characteristics as seen on electron microscopy [1–6].

Amyloid deposition inside organs progressively interferes with structure and function and results in death. Commonly affected organs include the heart, kidneys, gastrointestinal tract, liver, and peripheral or autonomic nervous system [1–4]. Loss of heart function is the main cause of poor prognosis [5–7]. However, a pericardial extracardiac nodule, as described here, is rare. The amyloidosis deposits may be due to AL amyloidosis or sometimes due to lymphoproliferative disorders such as MALT lymphoma, multiple myeloma (MM), or diseases that involve chronic inflammation [8–16]. Therefore, our patient was subjected to BM biopsy.

Many reports show that the most common site of localized AL amyloidosis is the mucous membranes in contact with the environment [8]. Accordingly, it has been deduced that amyloidogenic plasma cell clones may be triggered by antigenic stimulation. In our patient, the amyloid deposition occurred in a serous membrane: one may tentatively hypothesize that the *Salmonella suinis* infection could have stimulated inflammation and consequent polyclonal immunoglobulin production as well the growth of a plasma cell clone producing the amyloidogenic IgG.

In clinical practice, several diagnostic problems may present. No imaging technique is able to characterize a mass as amyloid deposition. Many authors have described amyloid masses with an uptake activity that can be detected by FDG-PET. This finding could be due to the presence of a tumor and inflammatory cells inside the mass that are detected by FDG because of their increased metabolic activity. Although everyone agrees on the low rate of false positives, these can occur in cases of TBC, aspergillosis, histoplasmosis and inflammatory disorders. Moreover, FDG as a radiotracer may not be sensitive enough to detect amyloid, despite a few reports on the possible utility of FDG in AL amyloidosis, in patients with large masses [17–19].

Amyloid deposits are usually observed within a strictly limited but not encapsulated area. Involvement of vessel walls is common and occurs when vessels lie very close to the main deposit. Abdominal fat biopsy is the advisable choice for the examination of histopathological samples. It is highly informative for AL amyloidosis, featuring 73% sensitivity and 90% specificity, and a low risk of bleeding [20]. AL amyloid can localize in virtually any body site. However, soft tissue deposition is unusual [20–25]. In literature, only few cases of localization of an amyloidoma in the mediastinum, retroperitoneum, or pericardium have been described [25–27]. Those cases were mostly due either to tumor masses or to a previous history of autoimmune disorders, such as rheumatoid arthritis. In all cases, the deposits were in the thymus or in mediastinal lymph nodes [28]. In our patient, none of these previous pathologic conditions were described and the massive amyloid deposits on the pericardium were the only damage triggering the acute symptoms.

AL amyloidosis has a dismal prognosis, with a mean survival of one to two years after diagnosis, and only four months in cases of clinical heart failure if no treatment was performed [2, 3]. Although survival in AL amyloidosis has improved, with a 5-year overall survival rate of 28% of patients, it still remains poor compared to the survival rate of patients with MM (about 40% 5-year survival) [29]. The heart involvement usually determines the prognosis: death often occurs as a result of refractory heart failure or sudden arrhythmic death [1–4]. Cappelli et al. [30] demonstrated that right ventricle damage is of late onset in already known amyloidosis. Conversely, in our case, the right heart was involved at presentation: it was directly compressed by the pericardial amyloid mass. Perhaps, an overall myocardial deposition was also present, which could explain the onset of atrial fibrillation.

Because the pathogenesis of AL amyloidosis overlaps that of other plasma cell dyscrasias, such as MM, the treatment is the same. In our patient, a stem cell transplant was not feasible due to the bad clinical situation and to the high risk related to the procedure [2]. The choice of Vel/Dex therapy, already used in MM, seemed the most suitable. Many studies have demonstrated a good response to this regimen: 71% hematological response and 25% complete response [2–7, 31].

Initial clinical data showed the presence of constrictive pericarditis. One possible cause could be TBC: clinical symptoms in our patient were similar to those usually found in TBC. Pericardial tuberculosis is a rare condition in developed countries, affecting less than 4% of patients with TBC [32]. However, many new cases are arising in our latitude, mostly in HIV patients, immigrants, or in those who work with them [33]. The presence of calcification sustained this idea because it is mostly related to a long-term inflammation and it suggests a dry/adsorptive stage of tuberculous pericarditis [32]. Other infective conditions leading to a constructive purulent pericarditis are even rarer (<1%) [32].

On the other hand, the presence of the M component raised a differential diagnosis problem. The slow decrease in Hb and PLT values and the increase in WBC count associated with the M component suggested that the pericardial mass was a plasmocytoma, but there were too few plasma cells in the mass. The hepatopathy and ascites were not related to viruses, and a correlation to TBC or MM was difficult to conceive. Amyloid liver deposition could be a good explanation. Moreover, deposits in the pericardium are frequently due to the presence of AL amyloidosis in the lymph nodes. In serous membranes, nontumor-related deposits are rare. However, a pericardial amyloid solitary mass has never been previously described.

We believe that the patient had a previous infection sustained by *Salmonella suinis* that triggered the normal immune response and inflammation. This could explain the fever. Perhaps, an amyloidogenic plasma cell (PC-AL) clone was already present at the time of infection, and its growth may have been stimulated by inflammatory cells. However, we do know how long an amyloid takes to have a production and deposition. The wrong immunoglobulin gene arrangement shifts the antibody production to a massive AL production that misfolds, producing amyloid. Moreover, bacteria inside the mass produce air due to their metabolism. These bubbles, that grow even bigger, participate in the heart compression and sudden heart tamponade. The presence of PCs inside the mass could be a good explanation of the FDG intake near the heart.

In conclusion, in AL amyloidosis, the diagnosis is commonly difficult. Many other diseases show a similar presentation. In our patient, TBC and MM could explain just a part of the symptoms. The fat-tissue biopsy result, related to the clinical data, ultimately suggested another possible yet still unknown presentation of amyloidosis. This case remains a paradigm of the clinical challenge that physicians have to face. In fact, many confounding factors are present together; so many different specialties need to be involved. In a nebulous clinical setting, a rare disease could be an explanation. After considering life-threatening conditions, related to the evidence-based approach, we quickly need to explore the possible differential diagnoses starting from the most frequent conditions. The unexpected finding of a monoclonal component drives a hematological approach in an apparently infective setting. This case should teach us never to exclude even the rarest conditions. In fact, due to the clinical presentation, amyloidosis was a really unexpected result, while the purulent pericarditis was a concomitant disease.

Conflicts of Interest

The authors declare that they have no conflicts of interest.

Authors' Contributions

All authors contributed equally to this work.

References

[1] G. Merlini and F. Dammacco, "Amiloidosi e manifestazioni cliniche correlate," *Internal and Emergency Medicine*, vol. 1, no. S1–3, pp. 83S–109S, 2006.

[2] G. Merlini, D. C. Seldin, and M. A. Gertz, "Amyloidosis: pathogenesis and new therapeutic options," *Journal of Clinical Oncology*, vol. 29, no. 4, pp. 1924–1933, 2011.

[3] A. D. Cohen and R. L. Comenzo, "Systemic light-chain amyloidosis: advances in diagnosis, prognosis, and therapy," *Hematology*, vol. 2010, no. 1, pp. 287–294, 2010.

[4] M. Rosenzweig and H. Landau, "Light chain (AL) amyloidosis: update on diagnosis and management," *Journal of Hematology and Oncology*, vol. 4, no. 1, p. 47, 2011.

[5] H. Agis, "News in AL amyloidosis ASH 2016: a rapidly evolving field of investigation," *Memo-Magazine of European Medical Oncology*, vol. 10, no. 2, pp. 66–71, 2017.

[6] M. A. Gertz, "Immunoglobulin light chain amyloidosis: 2011 update on diagnosis, risk-stratification, and management," *American Journal of Hematology*, vol. 86, no. 2, pp. 180–186, 2011.

[7] M. Grogan, A. Dispenzieri, and M. A. Gertz, "Light-chain cardiac amyloidosis: strategies to promote early diagnosis and cardiac response," *Heart*, vol. 103, no. 14, pp. 1065–1072, 2017.

[8] P. Westermark, "Localized AL amyloidosis: a suicidal neoplasm?," *Upsala Journal of Medical Sciences*, vol. 117, no. 2, pp. 244–250, 2012.

[9] T. Satani, T. Yokose, T. Kaburagi, Y. Asato, M. Itabashi, and R. Amemiya, "Amyloid deposition in primary pulmonary marginal zone B-cell lymphoma of mucosa-associated lymphoid tissue," *Pathology International*, vol. 57, no. 11, pp. 746–750, 2007.

[10] S. M. Said, C. Reynolds, R. E. Jimenez et al., "Amyloidosis of the breast: predominantly AL type and over half have concurrent breast hematologic disorders," *Modern Pathology*, vol. 26, no. 2, pp. 232–238, 2013.

[11] M. Hourseau, J. Virally, E. Habib, B. Juberthie, and L. Bienvenu, "Nodular amyloidoma associated with primary pulmonary Malt lymphoma," *Revue des Maladies Respiratoires*, vol. 25, no. 9, pp. 1123–1126, 2008.

[12] M. Kojima, S. Sugihara, M. Iijima, T. Ono, T. Yoshizumi, and N. Masawa, "Marginal zone B-cell lymphoma of minor salivary gland representing tumor-forming amyloidosis of the oral cavity. A case report," *Journal of Oral Pathology and Medicine*, vol. 35, no. 5, pp. 314–316, 2006.

[13] V. Sanchorawala, E. Blanchard, D. C. Seldin, C. O'Hara, M. Skinner, and D. G. Wright, "AL amyloidosis associated with B-cell lymphoproliferative disorders: frequency and treatment outcomes," *American Journal of Hematology*, vol. 81, no. 9, pp. 692–695, 2006.

[14] H. Y. Chiu, C. Y. Chu, and T. F. Tsai, "Localized AL amyloidosis in a patient with diffuse large B-cell lymphoma of the breast," *Acta Dermato Venereologica*, vol. 92, no. 3, pp. 284-285, 2012.

[15] R. J. H. Ryan, J. M. Sloan, A. B. Collins et al., "Extranodal marginal zone lymphoma of mucosa-associated lymphoid tissue with amyloid deposition: a clinicopathologic case series," *American Journal of Clinical Pathology*, vol. 137, no. 1, pp. 51–64, 2012.

[16] K. Suzuki, "Diagnosis and treatment of multiple myeloma and AL amyloidosis with focus on improvement of renal lesion," *Clinical and Experimental Nephrology*, vol. 16, no. 5, pp. 659–671, 2012.

[17] Y. M. Son, J. Y. Choi, C. H. Bak et al., "18F-FDG PET/CT in primary AL hepatic amyloidosis associated with multiple myeloma," *Korean Journal of Radiology*, vol. 12, no. 5, pp. 634–637, 2011.

[18] A. Mekinian, A. Jaccard, M. Soussan et al., "18F-FDG PET/CT in patients with amyloid light-chain amyloidosis: case-series and literature review," *Amyloid*, vol. 19, no. 2, pp. 94–98, 2012.

[19] A. Mekinian, E. Ghrenassia, G. Pop et al., "Visualization of amyloid arthropathy in light-chain systemic amyloidosis on F-18 FDG PET/CT scan," *Clinical Nuclear Medicine*, vol. 36, no. 1, pp. 52-53, 2011.

[20] B. Bogov, M. Lubomirova, and B. Kiperova, "Biopsy of subcutaneus fatty tissue for diagnosis of systemic amyloidosis," *Hippokratia*, vol. 12, no. 4, pp. 236–239, 2008.

[21] H. S. Yong, O. H. Woo, J. W. Lee, S. I. Suh, Y.-W. Oh, and E.-Y. Kang, "Primary localized amyloidosis manifested as supraclavicular and mediastinal lymphadenopathy," *British Journal of Radiology*, vol. 80, no. 955, pp. e131–e133, 2007.

[22] G. McKenzie, N. Raby, and D. Ritchie, "Non-neoplastic soft-tissue masses," *British Journal of Radiology*, vol. 82, no. 981, pp. 775–785, 2009.

[23] T. Prokaeva, B. Spencer, M. Kaut et al., "Soft tissue, joint, and bone manifestations of AL amyloidosis: clinical presentation, molecular features, and survival," *Arthritis and Rheumatism*, vol. 56, no. 11, pp. 3858–3868, 2007.

[24] S. Pasternak, B. A. Wright, and N. Walsh, "Soft tissue amyloidoma of the extremities: report of a case and review of the literature," *American Journal of Dermatopathology*, vol. 29, no. 2, pp. 152–155, 2007.

[25] T. Iguchi, M. Kizaki, A. Kurauchi, T. Yano, and Y. Ikeda, "Soft tissue *amyloidoma*," *Rinsho Ketsueki*, vol. 46, no. 7, pp. 507–512, 2005.

[26] M. L. Biewend, D. M. Menke, and K. T. Calamia, "The spectrum of localized amyloidosis: a case series of 20 patients and review of the literature," *Amyloid*, vol. 13, no. 3, pp. 135–142, 2006.

[27] J. Krishnan, W. S. Chu, J. P. Elrod, and G. Frizzera, "Tumoral presentation of amyloidosis (amyloidomas) in soft tissues. A report of 14 cases," *American Journal of Clinical Pathology*, vol. 100, no. 2, pp. 135–144, 1993.

[28] S. Takamori, H. Yano, A. Hayashi et al., "Amyloid tumor in the anterior mediastinum: report of a case," *Surgery Today*, vol. 34, no. 6, pp. 518–520, 2004.

[29] L. J. Costa, I. K. Brill, J. Omel, K. Godby, S. K. Kumar, and E. E. Brown, "Recent trends in multiple myeloma incidence and survival by age, race, and ethnicity in the United States," *Blood Advances*, vol. 1, no. 4, pp. 282–287, 2017.

[30] F. Cappelli, M. C. Porciani, F. Bergesio et al., "Right ventricular function in AL amyloidosis: characteristics and prognostic implication," *European Heart Journal-Cardiovascular Imaging*, vol. 13, no. 5, pp. 416–422, 2012.

[31] E. Kastritis, A. D. Wechalekar, M. A. Dimopoulos et al., "Bortezomib with or without dexamethasone in primary systemic (light chain) amyloidosis," *Journal of Clinical Oncology*, vol. 28, no. 6, pp. 1031–1037, 2010.

[32] M. Ntsekhe and M. Mayosi, "Tuberculous pericarditis with and without HIV," *Heart Failure Reviews*, vol. 18, no. 3, pp. 367–373, 2013.

[33] M. Imazio, F. Gaita, and M. LeWinter, "Evaluation and treatment of pericarditis: a systematic review," *JAMA*, vol. 314, no. 14, pp. 1498–1506, 2015.

32

Acute Lymphoblastic Leukemia following Lenalidomide Maintenance for Multiple Myeloma: Two Cases with Unexpected Presentation and Good Prognostic Features

Abdullah M. Khan, Jameel Muzaffar, Hermant Murthy, John R. Wingard, and Jan S. Moreb

Division of Hematology and Oncology, Department of Medicine, University of Florida, Gainesville, FL, USA

Correspondence should be addressed to Jan S. Moreb; morebjs@medicine.ufl.edu

Academic Editor: Marie-Christine Kyrtsonis

Lenalidomide maintenance following autologous stem cell transplant (ASCT) is considered the standard of care for eligible patients with multiple myeloma (MM). A recent meta-analysis has provided additional evidence that lenalidomide maintenance is associated with a higher incidence of second primary malignancies, including both hematologic and solid malignancies. Acute lymphoblastic leukemia (ALL) as a second primary malignancy is rarely described in the literature. Herein, we describe two patients with MM treated with induction therapy, ASCT, and lenalidomide maintenance that experienced cytopenias while on maintenance. ALL was unexpectedly diagnosed on bone marrow biopsy. One patient was diagnosed on routine biopsy performed as part of requirements of the clinical trial. Both patients had B-cell ALL, without known poor risk cytogenetics, and were managed with standard induction therapies resulting in complete remission. We also reviewed the literature for similar cases of secondary ALL (sALL) in MM patients exposed to immunomodulatory drugs (IMiDs). In conclusion, persistent cytopenias in responding MM patients receiving IMiDs maintenance should be an indication for bone marrow biopsy. Patients develop sALL after median of 32.5 months (range, 20–84) from being on lenalidomide or thalidomide maintenance, often presenting with cytopenias, display low tolerance to chemotherapy, but remission can often be achieved.

1. Introduction

Over 30,000 new cases of multiple myeloma (MM) are expected to be diagnosed in 2017 [1]. Arguably, the standard of care for eligible patients includes autologous stem cell transplant (ASCT) [2–4]. However, since MM is rarely cured with ASCT, there has been considerable interest in maintenance therapy with a goal to prolong progression free survival (PFS) and overall survival (OS). Three major trials have evaluated the role of lenalidomide maintenance in this regard [5–8]. In February 2017, on the basis of the Cancer and Leukemia Group B (CALGB) 100104 and Intergroup Francophone of Myeloma (IFM) 2005-02 studies, the Food and Drug Administration expanded its indications for lenalidomide to include maintenance therapy for patients with MM following ASCT. Furthermore, a meta-analysis of the three trials demonstrated OS benefit of lenalidomide maintenance, supporting the argument that it should be considered a standard of care after ASCT [9].

Further detailed in the meta-analysis was the association between second primary malignancies (SPM) and lenalidomide maintenance. The hazard ratio for a second primary hematologic malignancy was 2.03 ($P = 0.015$), and the hazard ratio for a second primary solid malignancy was 1.71 ($P = 0.032$) [9]. In the updated analyses of the two studies mentioned above, total of hematological SPMs reported was 34 and among those 8 cases of B-cell acute lymphoblastic leukemias (ALLs) [10]. It is not yet clear how lenalidomide contributes to ALL pathogenesis. Herein, we describe two cases of B-cell ALL, who received lenalidomide on the CALGB 100104 study, with unique presentation, generally with good prognostic features and with good response to standard chemotherapy. We also review the literature for similar ALL cases associated with immunomodulatory drugs (IMiDs) maintenance.

2. Case Presentation

We report here our two cases of secondary ALL (sALL) after exposure to lenalidomide maintenance. In addition, we reviewed the literature for any previously published similar cases in PubMed. We extracted pertinent information in regards to patient age, gender, prior IMiD exposure, length of exposure to IMiD therapy, phenotype of sALL, cytogenetics abnormalities, treatment given for the sALL and outcomes. Descriptive statistics were used.

2.1. Case 1. A 53-year-old female presented with back pain and was found to have a sacral mass in May 2009. After a thorough evaluation, she was diagnosed with a solitary plasmacytoma that was treated with radiation therapy. She had an IgG lambda monoclonal spike that was monitored for over a year before she showed progression to active MM according to her MM markers and new symptomatic bone lesions. Treatment was started with bortezomib and dexamethasone. She was enrolled to CALGB 100104 (supported by ECOG and BMT CTN) and underwent single autologous stem cell transplantation (ASCT). Her disease status after ASCT was very good partial response and, per trial protocol, she was started on lenalidomide maintenance therapy. Due to low absolute neutrophil counts (<1000), she initially required frequent lenalidomide dose interruptions and adjustments per the clinical trial. Six years into her maintenance therapy, her MM was in complete remission but developed low white blood cell and platelet counts prompting holding lenalidomide. Due to incomplete count recovery, a bone marrow biopsy was obtained. Morphology and flow cytometry revealed 50% blasts which expressed CD19, CD33, CD34, CD79a, HLA-DR, PAX5, and TdT but did not express CD117 or MPO. Of note, <5% plasma cells were detected and showed polyclonal kappa and lambda expression. Cytogenetics revealed trisomies of chromosomes 8, 10, and 21, monosomy chromosome 20. Fluorescent in situ hybridization (FISH) showed MYC and IGH gene locus copy number gain. The patient was treated using the CALGB study 8811 protocol [11]. The patient had severe hepatotoxicity with peg-asparaginase prompting long delays in her therapy; however, she had complete remission according to repeat bone marrow biopsy done one month after starting induction chemotherapy. Her subsequent therapy was interrupted due to significant myelosuppression that lead to the shortening of her intensification therapy. Currently, she is 12 months from diagnosis, in complete remission from her ALL, on maintenance with 6-mercaptopurine (Purinethol), vincristine (Oncovin), methotrexate, and prednisone (POMP). Her myeloma has remained in stable complete remission as well.

2.2. Case 2. A 69-year-old female transferred oncologic care to the University of Florida in February of 2013. She was diagnosed with IgG kappa multiple myeloma in February 2011 with Durie–Salmon stage 3B due to lytic bone lesions and elevated creatinine. She was initially treated with bortezomib and dexamethasone before adding lenalidomide due to inadequate treatment response. She was enrolled onto the CALGB 100104 clinical trial and underwent tandem autologous transplantation (conditioning regimen with melphalan 200 mg/m^2) followed by lenalidomide maintenance. At the time of evaluation in our institution, the patient had been on lenalidomide for 15 months. She had a hemoglobin content of 11.1 g/dL, platelets of 81,000/mm^3, and WBC of 2000/mm^3 with an absolute neutrophil count of 960. Chemistry revealed normal renal function and absence of hypercalcemia. Myeloma markers revealed hypogammaglobulinemia, an IgG kappa monoclonal spike of 0.5 g/dL, kappa 2.52 mg/dL, lambda 0.12 mg/dL, and a kappa/lambda ratio of 21. She had frequent lenalidomide dose adjustments or interruptions due to cytopenias. A required bone marrow biopsy, per the clinical trial, was obtained after cycle 23 of lenalidomide maintenance and revealed 1-2% of kappa restricted plasma cells. As part of the study requirements, a repeat bone marrow biopsy was obtained after three years of lenalidomide maintenance which revealed a hypocellular marrow with 25% abnormal B-lymphoblasts. Due to the unexpected results, a bone marrow biopsy was repeated with similar findings. The lymphoblasts expressed bright levels of CD34 and TdT, intermediate levels of CD19 and CD22, and diminished or absent expression of CD10, CD20, and CD45. Cytogenetics evaluation was normal but one cell had 46, XX, t(7;19). FISH testing was negative for BCR/ABL1, MLL, and RUNX1 gene loci fusion rearrangement as well as negative for chromosome 4 and chromosome 10 copy number changes. She was treated with hyper-CVAD [12] for 8 months followed by POMP maintenance. A postinduction bone marrow aspirate and biopsy showed a variably hypocellular marrow without overt morphologic evidence of B-cell ALL and ~6% abnormal plasma cells. She has not required further treatment for her myeloma and remained in a stable very good partial response. She is 36 months from her ALL diagnosis in continuous remission.

3. Discussion

The 5-year relative survival rate has improved from 24% for patients diagnosed with MM between 1975 and 1977 to 51% in patients diagnosed between 2007 and 2013 [13]. This increased life expectancy has raised concerns about the risks associated with prolonged exposure to antimyeloma therapy, including lenalidomide maintenance following ASCT [14]. Among the risks is the development of hematologic and solid SPM. Initial observations suggested a predilection for hematologic SPM of myeloid origin including myelodysplastic syndrome, acute myeloid leukemia, and chronic myeloid leukemia. However, updated clinical trial data and a number of case reports reveal an increased risk of lymphoid malignancies as well [9, 14].

The two cases we presented here describe unique asymptomatic presentation, the ones having been diagnosed on routine bone marrow biopsy. Both patients had pancytopenia that was thought to be related to lenalidomide effects. Thus, secondary acute leukemia should be suspected in

Table 1: Characteristics of patients with multiple myeloma who were exposed to IMiDs maintenance and developed acute lymphoblastic leukemia as a second primary malignancy.

Reference number	IMiD type	Time to Dx (mo)	Age (Y)/sex /presentation	Morphologic type	Cytogenetics/FISH	Treatment/outcome
[15]	Len[1]	20	62/F/pancytopenia	B cell (CD19, 20, 10, 22, 79a, TdT, IgMc+, and CD34−)	Normal	Death due to septicemia during induction
[16]	Len Thal	2 31	66/M/fatigue, low WBC	B cell (CD45, 19, 22, 34+, CD79±, TdT+)	Trisomy 4	Death 8 mo with no response to induction with CHOP
[17]	Len[1]	30	59/M/fatigue, pancytopenia	B cell (CD10, 19+, CD79a, Pax5, and TdT±)	Deletion 20q	Linker regimen, alive > 1 y after allo-SCT in CR
[17]	Len	36	34/M/pancytopenia and circulating blasts	B cell (CD10, 19, 22, 34, 79a, 38+)	Chr 14 rearrangement	CALGB 8811, death 1 month after induction due to CVS and septicemia
[17]	Len[1]	84	53/M/leukopenia	B cell (CD19, 34, 79a, PAX5, TdT+)	Small population of tetraploid cells by FISH	Linker regimen, >1 y after 2nd ASCT in CR
[18]	Thal[1,2]	29	61/F/pancytopenia	B cell (CD19, 38+)	NA	CALGB 9111
[19]	Len[1] Thal	4.5 32.5	65/F/dizziness	B cell (CD19, 22, 34, 79a+, HLA-DR+)	NA	No treatment, death after 14 mo
[19]	Thal	32	63/M/fatigue, cytopenias	B cell (CD10, 34+, HLA-DR, and CD33 dim)	NA	Lost to follow-up
[19]	Thal[1]	73	33/F/cough, fatigue and anemia	B cell (CD10, 34, 19, 22, 33, 79a+, HLA-DR+)	NA	No treatment, lost to follow-up
[20]	Thal	53	56/F/edema and dyspnea, pancytopenia	B cell (CD19, 20, 22, 10+, HLA-DR+)	Normal	Steroids only, DVT/PE, death within 10 days
[21]	Len	24–36	72/M/pancytopenia	B cell (CD10, 19, 20, 79a, and TdT+, CD34, 117, 38, 56−)	NA	Hyper-CVAD, POMP maintenance. CR for 26 mo, then relapse
Our case	Len[1]	23	69/F/none	B cell (CD34, 19, 22+)	t(7;19) in one metaphase	Hyper-CVAD, then POMP maintenance, in CR for 3 year
Our case	Len[1]	72	53/F/pancytopenia	B cell (CD19, 33, 34, 38, 79a+, PAX5+, TdT+)	+8, +10, +22, −20, and FISH showed MYC and IgH gene locus copy gain	Abbreviated CALGB 8811 due to intolerance, now on POMP maintenance, in CR for 1 year

[1]These patients had prior ASCT, while the others did not; [2]developed ALL 3 years after stopping Thal maintenance.

MM patients who develop unexplained persistent cytopenias. The other characteristics to note are that both of our patients did not display any of the known ALL bad prognostic features and were able to attain complete remission of their sALL with standard induction therapy. These two patients were most likely included in the recent updated analysis of the CALGB 100104 [8] which includes detailed description of all SPMs including the cases of B-cell ALL.

Eleven cases of ALL following IMiDs (lenalidomide and thalidomide) maintenance in the treatment of MM have been reported in the literature [15–21]. Only part of these reports made the connection to the IMiDs exposure. Table 1 shows the summary of the findings from our 2 patients and 11 patients described in the literature. We can summarize that B-cell ALL is the dominant morphological type and the usual presentation is cytopenias and fatigue while on IMiDs. Six patients had thalidomide as the main IMiD. The median time of exposure to the IMiDs before developing sALL was 32.5 months (range, 20–84). There were no unique chromosomal abnormalities associated with this diagnosis. When performed, FISH studies for the known bad prognostic ALL gene abnormalities were usually negative. Tolerance for intensive ALL chemotherapy could be challenging in these cases, and 2 patients died of septicemia, while few patients gave up and most likely died without treatment. However, the best treatment of these patients is not yet clear. In general, secondary leukemias have worse prognosis and require allo-SCT for curative purposes. Only one of these patients had that treatment with good outcome so far. Occasionally, MM patients may have autologous stem cell products frozen from their planned treatment for MM which can be used for second ASCT as a consolidation in the treatment of their sALL. Indeed, one patient was treated that way successfully. Our two patients seem to have done well with standard chemotherapy including CNS prophylaxis but required significant modification of drug doses due to severe myelosuppression.

Cases of sALL have been described in MM patients that were not exposed to IMiDs and was attributed to the melphalan, other chemotherapy used [22, 23], or possibly disease-related immune deficiency. At least some of these cases were associated with MLL gene rearrangement [23] which seems to be associated more frequently with sALL that develop after non-IMiD type of standard chemotherapy, discussed below.

In general, most secondary acute leukemias described in the literature have been secondary acute myeloid leukemia (AML), while sALL is much less common. It is believed to represent just 1–3% of all ALL and up to 10% of all secondary acute leukemia [24–27]. There are no large studies comparing sALL with de novo ALL, and most of the information has been derived from small case series reported in literature. Patients with sALL tend to be in elderly patients and have a worse outcome. Most of the sALL are of B-cell type and tend to have some high-risk cytogenetics and molecular features such as 11q23 rearrangement (especially after exposure to topoisomerase II inhibitors), as well as BCR-ABL and complex chromosomal abnormalities [25]. Treatments for breast cancer and lymphoma, both Hodgkin's and non-Hodgkin's, are the most common cancers associated with development of sALL [26]; however, in one series a sizable proportion of sALL patients were not treated with prior chemoradiotherapy [24]. The median latency period to development of sALL varied between 12 and 27 months, depending on the type of first malignancy and prior anticancer therapy, with a range between 0.8 and 9 years [25]. The largest retrospective studies have shown that type of first malignancy, previous treatment, interval to diagnosis, and cytogenetic abnormalities do not appear to affect the overall survival in sALL patients [24–27]. Median overall survival has been shown to be around 8 months as compared to 11 months for de novo ALL, and after adjusting for other variables, sALL itself appears to be an independent risk factor with dismal survival at 1, 3, and 5 years (35%, 16%, and 6.8%, resp., versus 47%, 31%, and 21% in de novo ALL for the same time periods). Age has been the only other factor affecting survival, with worse outcomes seen with increasing age [26]. Recent study published by Rosenberg et al. [28] extracts data on sALL from the Surveillance, Epidemiology, and End Results (SEER) cancer registry program between 1988 and 2012 and reports 3% of 14,470 patients with ALL were ALL with antecedent malignancy. According to this study, the most common prior malignancies were breast cancer (21%), hematologic malignancies (18%), and male genital system (15%).

Our findings show that the median latency period for sALL post-IMiDs seems to be longer (32 months) than that reported after other chemotherapy, and no cases were reported before 20 months from exposure to one of the IMiDs. On the other hand, sALL after other chemotherapy can present as early as few months after chemotherapy [24–28]. Also, in many but not all cases of sALL after non-IMiDs chemotherapy, MLL gene aberrations are reported [29], while none of the IMiDs-associated sALL cases, with known cytogenetics/FISH tests (Table 1), had such abnormality. These findings suggest different pathogenesis and mechanism for development of sALL after IMiDs. The exact mechanism is not known, but hints can be sought from published data on lenalidomide and thalidomide mechanism of actions and effects, especially on B lymphocytes. All IMiDs were reported to reactivate the Epstein–Barr virus lytic cycle in resting memory B cells, contributing to increased immunosuppression and possible mechanism for the development of secondary Hodgkin's lymphoma in post-ASCT/lenalidomide maintenance setting [30]. Another potential effect of lenalidomide on B cells could be through its known effect on the cereblon protein, changing the substrate specificity of the CRL4 (cereblon) E3 ubiquitin ligase complex, such that the proteins IKAROS (encoded by *IKZF1*) and AIOLOS (encoded by *IKZF3*) are selectively ubiquitinated and degraded in multiple myeloma cells [31, 32]. IKAROS and AIOLOS transcription factors are critical regulators of B-cell function in mice and humans [33]. IKAROS plays key roles in human B-cell development and malignancy, which is further studied by another recent publication [34]. Lenalidomide was also reported to expand the absolute lymphocytic counts in peripheral blood of patients treated for myelodysplastic syndrome, with expansion of the regulatory T cells (Treg) [35]. Treg could potentially promote immune tolerance towards any abnormal clonal expansion. On the other hand, the effect of IMiDs on Treg in myeloma patients is complex and seems controversial [36]. Whether any of these effects of lenalidomide play a role in the development of B-cell sALL in MM patients is worth further investigation.

In conclusion, persistent pancytopenia on IMiDs maintenance in MM patients should be investigated with bone marrow biopsy since it could be caused by secondary B-cell ALL. Our report shows that sALL can be seen not only after lenalidomide exposure but also after thalidomide, thus it could potentially be a class effect. Caution should be used in using intensive induction chemotherapy in these patients due to intolerance and risk of fatal infectious complications. However, in general, complete remission can be achieved in most patients and it can be durable, but long-term follow up (>5 years) is needed in order to determine curability and the subsequent behavior and outcome of the MM as well.

Conflicts of Interest

The authors declare that they have no conflicts of interest related to this publication.

References

[1] R. L. Siegel, K. D. Miller, and A. Jemal, "Cancer statistics, 2017," *CA: A Cancer Journal for Clinicians*, vol. 67, no. 1, pp. 7–30, 2017.

[2] P. Moreau and M. Attal, "All transplantation-eligible patients with myeloma should receive ASCT in first response," *Hematology*, vol. 2014, no. 1, pp. 250–254, 2014.

[3] M. Offidani, S. Gentili, F. Gay et al., "Stem cell transplantation in multiple myeloma," *Current Cancer Drug Targets*, 2016, in press.

[4] S. K. Kumar, V. Rajkumar, R. A. Kyle et al., "Multiple myeloma," *Nature Reviews Disease Primers*, vol. 3, p. 17046, 2017.

[5] P. L. McCarthy, K. Owzar, C. C. Hofmeister et al., "Lenalidomide after stem-cell transplantation for multiple myeloma," *New England Journal of Medicine*, vol. 366, no. 19, pp. 1770–1781, 2012.

[6] M. Attal, V. Lauwers-Cances, G. Marit et al., "Lenalidomide maintenance after stem-cell transplantation for multiple

myeloma," *New England Journal of Medicine*, vol. 366, no. 19, pp. 1782–1791, 2012.

[7] A. Palumbo, F. Cavallo, F. Gay et al., "Autologous transplantation and maintenance therapy in multiple myeloma," *New England Journal of Medicine*, vol. 371, no. 10, pp. 895–905, 2014.

[8] S. A. Holstein, S. H. Jung, P. G. Richardson et al., "Updated analysis of CALGB (Alliance) 100104 assessing lenalidomide versus placebo maintenance after single autologous stem-cell transplantation for multiple myeloma: a randomised, double-blind, phase 3 trial," *Lancet Haematology*, vol. 4, no. 9, pp. e431–e442, 2017.

[9] P. L. McCarthy, S. A. Holstein, M. T. Petrucci et al., "Lenalidomide maintenance after autologous stem-cell transplantation in newly diagnosed multiple myeloma: a meta-analysis," *Journal of Clinical Oncology*, vol. 35, no. 29, pp. 3279–3289, 2017.

[10] P. L. McCarthy and S. A. Holstein, "Role of stem cell transplant and maintenance therapy in plasma cell disorders," *Hematology*, vol. 2016, no. 1, pp. 504–511, 2016.

[11] R. A. Larson, R. K. Dodge, C. P. Burns et al., "A five-drug remission induction regimen with intensive consolidation for adults with acute lymphoblastic leukemia: cancer and leukemia group B study 8811," *Blood*, vol. 85, no. 8, pp. 2025–2037, 1995.

[12] J. Cortes, S. M. O'Brien, S. Pierce, M. J. Keating, E. J. Freireich, and H. M. Kantarjian, "The value of high-dose systemic chemotherapy and intrathecal therapy for central nervous system prophylaxis in different risk groups of adult acute lymphoblastic leukemia," *Blood*, vol. 86, no. 6, pp. 2091–2097, 1995.

[13] N. Howlader, A. M. Noone, M. Krapcho et al., *SEER Cancer Statistics Review, 1975–2014*, National Cancer Institute, Bethesda, MD, USA, 2017, https://seer.cancer.gov/csr/1975_2014/.

[14] P. Musto, K. C. Anderson, M. Attal et al., "Second primary malignancies in multiple myeloma: an overview and IMWG consensus," *Annals of Oncology*, vol. 28, no. 2, pp. 228–245, 2017.

[15] R. García-Muñoz, D. Robles-de-Castro, A. Muñoz-Rodríguez, and P. Rabasa, "Acute lymphoblastic leukemia developing during maintenance therapy with lenalidomide in a patient with multiple myeloma," *Leukemia & Lymphoma*, vol. 54, no. 12, pp. 2753–2755, 2013.

[16] J. Li, J. Zhan, F. Zhang, Z. Ye, and J. Ouyang, "Secondary lymphoblastic leukemia occurring 38 months after the primary diagnosis of multiple myeloma: a case report," *Oncology Letters*, vol. 12, no. 2, pp. 847–856, 2016.

[17] M. Tan, R. Fong, M. Lo, and R. Young, "Lenalidomide and secondary acute lymphoblastic leukemia: a case series," *Hematological Oncology*, vol. 35, no. 1, pp. 130–134, 2017.

[18] Y. Tsukada, Y. Hattori, H. Nakajima et al., "B-cell acute lymphoblastic leukemia developed 5 years after autologous stem cell transplantation for multiple myeloma," *Rinsho Ketsueki*, vol. 53, pp. 219–223, 2012, in Japanese.

[19] L. Junxun, L. Junru, C. Meilan et al., "Three patients with multiple myeloma developing secondary lymphoblastic leukemia: case reports and review of the literature," *Tumori Journal*, vol. 102, no. 2, pp. S131–S136, 2016.

[20] J. Piszcz, L. Bolkun, E. Cichocka, and J. Kloczko, "Secondary acute lymphoblastic leukaemia in a multiple myeloma patient," *Contemporary Oncology*, vol. 16, no. 6, pp. 593–595, 2012.

[21] M. M. Gonzalez, L. Kidd, J. Quesada, N. Nguyen, and L. Chen, "Acute myelofibrosis and acute lymphoblastic leukemia in an elderly patient with previously treated multiple myeloma," *Annals of Clinical and Laboratory Science*, vol. 43, no. 2, pp. 43176–43180, 2013.

[22] L. G. Lau, L. K. Tan, E. S. Koay, and T. C. Liu, "Acute lymphoblastic leukemia after tandem autologous stem cell transplantations for multiple myeloma," *Leukemia*, vol. 19, no. 2, pp. 299–301, 2004.

[23] K. Ueda, G. Yamamoto, A. Shinohara, A. Hangaishi, and M. Kurokawa, "Early onset of acute lymphoblastic leukemia with MLL rearrangement after autologous stem cell transplantation for multiple myeloma," *Annals of Hematology*, vol. 88, no. 8, pp. 813-814, 2009.

[24] L. Pagano, A. Pulsoni, M. E. Tosti et al., "Acute lymphoblastic leukaemia occurring as second malignancy: report of the GIMEMA archive of adult acute leukaemia," *British Journal of Haematology*, vol. 106, no. 4, pp. 1037–1040, 1999.

[25] R. Shivakumar, W. Tan, G. E. Wilding, E. S. Wang, and M. Wetzler, "Biologic features and treatment outcome of secondary acute lymphoblastic leukemia–a review of 101 cases," *Annals of Oncology*, vol. 19, no. 9, pp. 1634–1638, 2008.

[26] S. Giri, M. Chi, B. Johnson et al., "Secondary acute lymphoblastic leukemia is an independent predictor of poor prognosis," *Leukemia Research*, vol. 39, no. 12, pp. 1342–1346, 2015.

[27] C. Ganzel, S. Devlin, D. Douer, J. M. Rowe, E. M. Stein, and M. S. Tallman, "Secondary acute lymphoblastic leukaemia is constitutional and probably not related to prior therapy," *British Journal of Haematology*, vol. 170, no. 1, pp. 50–55, 2015.

[28] A. S. Rosenberg, A. Brunson, J. K. Paulus et al., "Secondary acute lymphoblastic leukemia is a distinct clinical entity with prognostic significance," *Blood Cancer Journal*, vol. 7, no. 9, p. e605, 2017.

[29] N. Douet-Guilbert, J. R. Eveillard, C. Meyer et al., "MLL partner genes in secondary acute lymphoblastic leukemia: report of a new partner PRRC1 and review of the literature," *Leukemia Research*, vol. 38, no. 11, pp. 1316–1319, 2014.

[30] R. J. Jones, T. Iempridee, X. Wang et al., "Lenalidomide, thalidomide, and pomalidomide reactivate the Epstein-Barr virus lytic cycle through phosphoinositide 3-kinase signaling and Ikaros expression," *Clinical Cancer Research*, vol. 22, no. 19, pp. 4901–4912, 2016.

[31] J. Kronke, N. D. Udeshi, A. Narla et al., "Lenalidomide causes selective degradation of IKZF1 and IKZF3 in multiple myeloma cells," *Science*, vol. 343, no. 6168, pp. 301–305, 2014.

[32] G. Lu, R. E. Middleton, H. Sun et al., "The myeloma drug lenalidomide promotes the cereblon-dependent destruction of Ikaros proteins," *Science*, vol. 343, pp. 305–309, 2014.

[33] T. A. Schwickert, H. Tagoh, S. Gultekin et al., "Stage-specific control of early B cell development by the transcription factor Ikaros," *Nature Immunology*, vol. 15, no. 3, pp. 283–293, 2014.

[34] L. A. Solomon, C. R. Batista, and R. P. DeKoter, "Lenalidomide modulates gene expression in human ABC-DLBCL cells by regulating IKAROS interaction with an intronic control region of SPI-B," *Experimental Hematology*, vol. 56, pp. 46. e1–57.e1, 2017.

[35] E. Balaian, C. Schuster, C. Schönefeldt et al., "Selective expansion of regulatory T cells during lenalidomide treatment of myelodysplastic syndrome with isolated deletion 5q," *Annals of Hematology*, vol. 95, no. 11, pp. 1805–1810, 2016.

[36] H. Quach, D. Ritchie, A. K. Stewart et al., "Mechanism of action of immunomodulatory drugs (IMiDS) in multiple myeloma," *Leukemia*, vol. 24, no. 1, pp. 22–32, 2010.

33

Primary Effusion Lymphoma without an Effusion: A Rare Case of Solid Extracavitary Variant of Primary Effusion Lymphoma in an HIV-Positive Patient

Hamza Hashmi,[1] Drew Murray,[1] Samer Al-Quran,[2] and William Tse[3]

[1]*Division of Hematology and Oncology, University of Louisville, Louisville, KY, USA*
[2]*Department of Pathology and Laboratory Medicine, University of Louisville, Louisville, KY, USA*
[3]*Division of Blood and Marrow Transplant, University of Louisville, Louisville, KY, USA*

Correspondence should be addressed to Hamza Hashmi; hamzahashmi87@hotmail.com

Academic Editor: Tatsuharu Ohno

Primary effusion lymphoma (PEL) is a unique form of non-Hodgkin lymphoma, usually seen in severely immunocompromised, HIV-positive patients. PEL is related to human herpesvirus-8 (HHV-8) infection, and it usually presents as a lymphomatous body cavity effusion in the absence of a solid tumor mass. There have been very few case reports of HIV-positive patients with HHV-8-positive solid tissue lymphomas not associated with an effusion (a solid variant of PEL). In the absence of effusion, establishing an accurate diagnosis can be challenging, and a careful review of morphology, immunophenotype, and presence of HHV-8 is necessary to differentiate from other subtypes of non-Hodgkin lymphoma. Treatment involves intensive chemotherapy, and prognosis is usually poor. We present a rare case of a PEL variant in an HIV-positive patient who presented with extensive lymphadenopathy without any associated effusions.

1. Introduction

Primary effusion (PEL) is an uncommon subtype of non-Hodgkin lymphoma seen in patients with human immunodeficiency virus (HIV). It is associated with human herpesvirus type 8 (HHV-8) also known as Kaposi sarcoma herpesvirus (KSHV). There is a rare solid extracavitary variant that can be mistaken morphologically for other types of aggressive diffuse large B-cell lymphoma (DLBCL).

2. Case Presentation

A 51-year-old Caucasian male, homosexual with a past medical history significant for controlled hypertension and ulcerative colitis treated with infliximab, presented with fatigue, intermittent night sweats, and significant weight loss of about 70 lbs over a period of 3 months. The patient reported productive cough and was nonbloody during this period of time accompanied by dry itchy skin with easy bruising.

CT scan of the chest, abdomen, and pelvis performed showed lymphadenopathy in the axillary area (Figures 1 and 2), lymphadenopathy in the abdominal cavity, and splenomegaly of 14.8 cm (Figure 3). Complete blood count revealed pancytopenia with white blood cell count of 9.8×10^3/microL, hemoglobin of 7.4 g/dl, and platelet count of $65{,}000 \times 10^3$/microL. INR was normal. Serum protein electrophoresis and immunofixation were normal. Serum HIV testing was positive with a high level of viral load, 5,900,000 copies/ml, CD4 count of 14 cells/mm^3, and CD8 count of 78 cells/mm^3. Serum Epstein–Barr virus testing was positive with a viral load of 14,000 copies/ml. Serum HHV-8 testing was positive with a viral load of 2,400,000 copies/ml. Whole-body PET scan revealed index lesions in the right axillary lymph node of 5.8×4.5 cm with a maximal SUV of 19.98 and a 6.6×5.5 cm left perisplenic mass with an SUV of 15.01. Left inguinal lymph node and right supraclavicular lymph node areas also showed mild PET avidity. Infectious disease service was consulted, and the patient was started on antiretroviral therapy with abacavir/lamivudine/dolutegravir. Given his

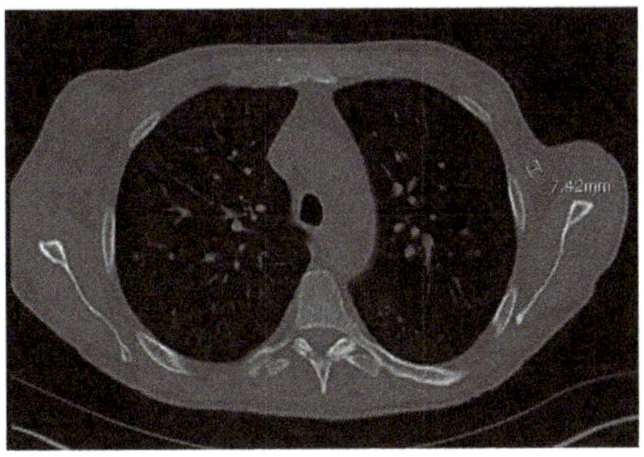

Figure 1: CT chest showing a 5.6 cm × 4.9 cm lymph node mass in the right axilla.

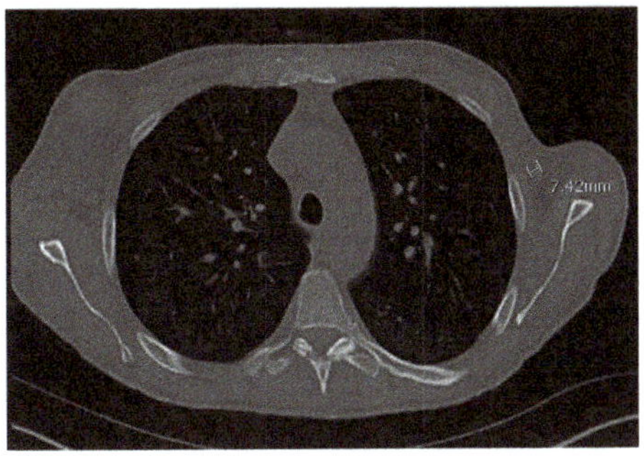

Figure 2: CT chest showing a 0.7 cm lymph node in the left axilla.

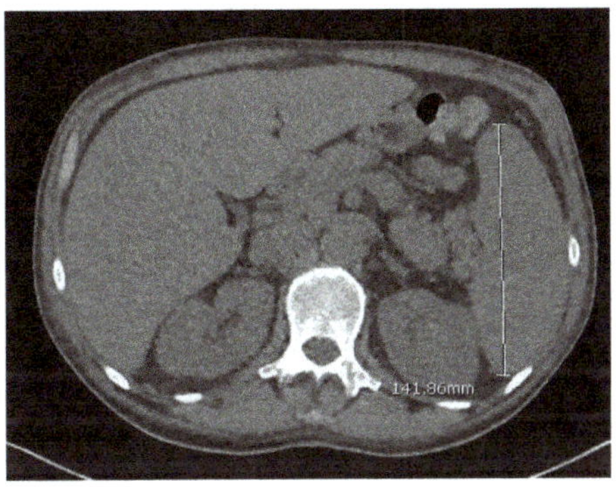

Figure 3: CT abdomen showing splenic enlargement of 14.8 cm.

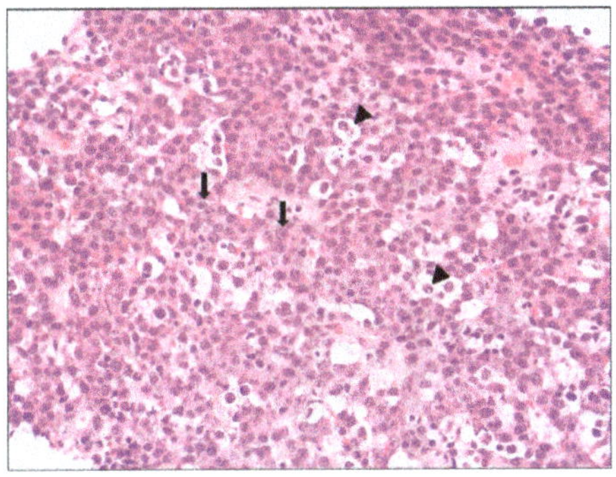

Figure 4: High-power photomicrograph of a hematoxylin and eosin- (H/E-) stained histologic section showing effacement of the lymph node architecture by the proliferation of immunoblastic cells (arrows) with abundant amphophilic cytoplasm, eccentric round large nuclei, and prominent single macronucleoli. Scattered apoptotic bodies and tangible body macrophages (arrowheads) were seen in background (original magnification: ×400).

extensive lymphadenopathy, the patient underwent a bone marrow biopsy as well as axillary lymph node biopsy.

A needle core of an axillary lymph node was performed. Microscopic examination of the histologic section showed diffuse effacement of the lymph node tissue architecture by the proliferation of immunoblastic cells with abundant amphophilic cytoplasm, eccentric round large nuclei, and prominent single macronucleoli (Figure 4). There was variable nuclear pleomorphism, with brisk mitotic activity and scattered apoptotic bodies and tangible body macrophages. Immunohistochemical studies (Figure 5) were performed with appropriate positive and negative controls according to established protocols. They demonstrated that the neoplastic cells were strongly CD30 (+), MUM1 (+), and diffusely HHV-8 (+) (using anti-LANA (latency-associated nuclear antigen) antibody), with high labeling of nuclei by Ki-67 (>95%), variable expression of CD138, and focal expression of CD45, CD79a, and p53. In situ hybridization study for EBV-encoded RNA (EBER) was diffusely positive. The neoplastic cells were negative for PAX5, CD117, CD56, ALK1, cyclin-D1, BCL2, BCL6, CD3, CD5, cytokeratin AE1/AE3, p63, CD20, S100 protein, CD15, and CD10. In situ hybridization studies for kappa and lambda light chain mRNA were negative. A portion of the fresh biopsy tissue was submitted for flow cytometric analysis which demonstrated the presence of large cells with bright expression of CD38. Cytogenetics performed revealed a normal male karyotype 46,XY.

The overall morphologic and immunophenotypic findings supported the diagnosis of an extracavitary (solid) variant of primary effusion lymphoma (PEL). The bone marrow biopsy did not reveal any evidence of lymphoma. There was no clinical, morphological, or radiographic evidence of other HIV-associated infectious or malignant complications including Kaposi sarcoma.

The patient was admitted to the hospital, and within 96 hours of starting his antiretroviral therapy, he received a first cycle of EPOCH (etoposide, prednisone, vincristine, cyclophosphamide, and doxorubicin). Two days after completing the first cycle, he developed neutropenic fever and acute hypoxic respiratory failure. He was started on broad-spectrum antibiotics and eventually required endotracheal intubation and mechanical ventilation. As CT scan of the chest revealed ground glass opacities, he was empirically started on Bactrim and prednisone. Bronchoscopy with bronchoalveolar lavage was performed which revealed PCR-positive pneumocystis. His clinical course was further complicated by septic shock by *Staphylococcus epidermidis* bacteremia, and the patient required vasopressor support along with broad-spectrum antibiotics. Antiretroviral therapy was continued throughout the course. Despite aggressive measures, his clinical condition continued to decline. As the patient experienced several episodes of generalized tonic-clonic seizures, CT head was done which showed right-sided intracranial bleed. Neurosurgery was consulted, and the patient was started on protamine drip for

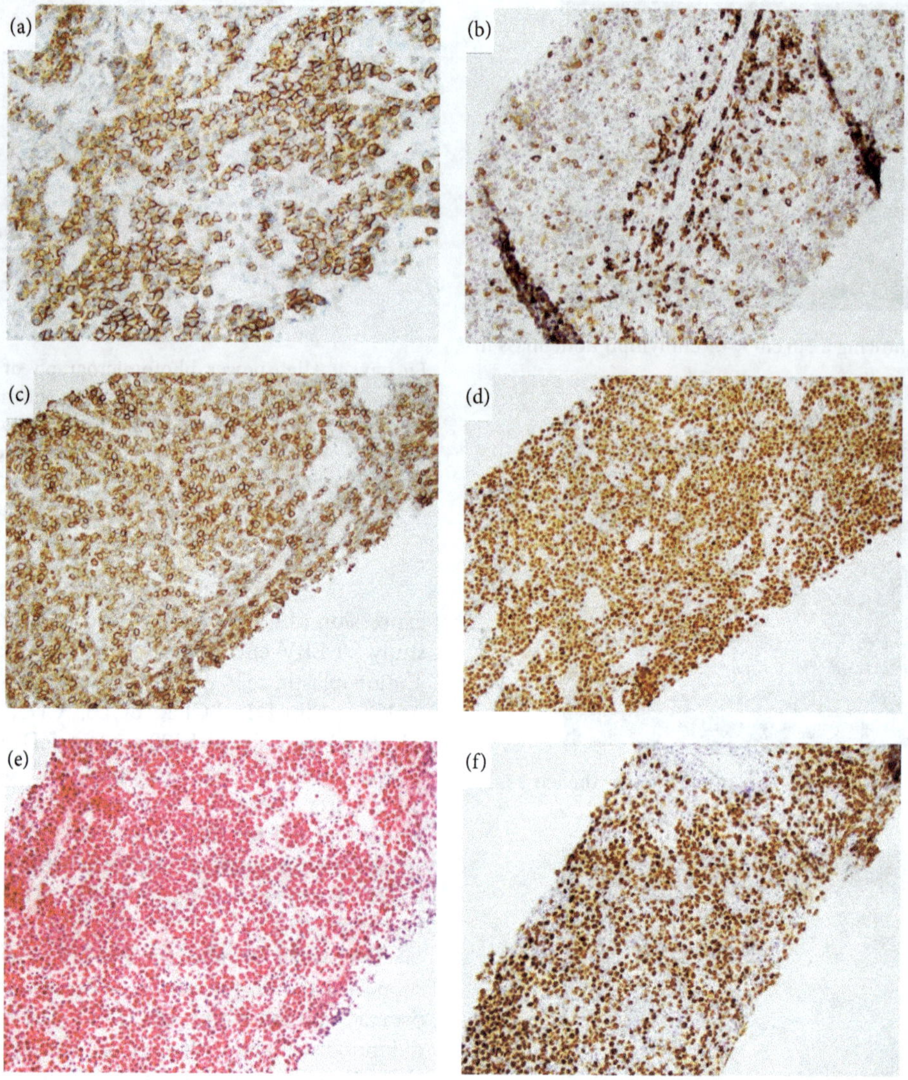

FIGURE 5: Composite photomicrograph of immunohistochemical and in situ hybridization studies showing that tumor cells are positive for (a) CD138 (variable), (b) CD79a (weak, variable), (c) CD30, (d) MUM1, (e) EBV (EBER), and (f) HHV-8.

reversal of the possible subcutaneous heparin effect. Given large hemorrhagic stroke, significant comorbidities including aggressive lymphoma, and overall poor prognosis, his family decided to pursue comfort care, and the patient passed away shortly after extubation. Although the patient was started on antiretroviral therapy within 96 hours and administered chemotherapy within one week from his HIV and primary effusion lymphoma (solid variant) diagnosis, his disease had an aggressive clinical course leading to death within 2 weeks after completing the first cycle of chemotherapy.

3. Case Discussion

3.1. Epidemiology. An estimated 5–20% of patients with human immunodeficiency virus (HIV)/acquired immunodeficiency syndrome (AIDS) will develop an NHL over their lifetime [1]. PEL, the more common serous form of KSHV large B-cell lymphoma, constitutes 1–4% of all HIV/AIDS-associated NHLs [2]. Due to its rarity and late discovery of KSHV in 1994, less than 100 cases of a solid variant of PEL have been reported to date. Although exceedingly uncommon PEL and its solid variant have been identified in patients without HIV/AIDS, these patients are typically HHV-8 negative and present with an existing immunocompromised state such as advanced age, malignancy, cirrhosis, hepatitis, immunosuppressant medications, and existing malignancies [3].

3.2. Presentation and Diagnostic Evaluation. Among HIV-associated NHLs, a solid variant of PEL primarily presents in extracavitary sites such as the lymph nodes, gastrointestinal tract, pharyngeal lymphoid tissue, bone marrow, liver, central nervous system, and spleen without the development of lymphomatous effusions seen in PEL [4]. A 2005 study noted that 100% of patients with a solid variant of PEL presented with generalized lymphadenopathy while only occurring in 20% of those with PEL [4]. Abnormal laboratory findings include for anemia, elevated LDH levels, and hypoalbuminemia due to development of nephrotic syndrome [4].

After initial evaluation of renal function, hepatic function, blood counts, electrolytes, and serum lactate dehydrogenase levels, diagnosis is helped by blood viral testing for HIV and HHV-8. Imaging with CT of the chest, abdomen, and pelvis or PET scan is used for evaluation of the extent of the disease. Biopsy of suspicious lesions is required for diagnosis, through morphologic examination and immunophenotyping by flow cytometry or immunohistochemistry. Pleural effusions should be analyzed for HHV-8 as positive pleural fluid is a characteristic of PEL.

Extracavitary (solid variant) PEL presents with solid masses exhibiting similar morphology, immunophenotype, and gene expression profiles to classic PEL, which arises predominantly as a lymphomatous effusion within body cavities, and is characteristically associated with HHV-8 infection. The major differential diagnosis includes plasmablastic lymphoma, a variant of large B-cell lymphoma with an unfavorable outcome that is commonly associated with HIV/immune suppression. These two entities have overlapping morphologic and immunophenotypic features; however, the presence of HHV-8 infection supports the diagnosis of extracavitary PEL.

4. Prognosis

It is not entirely clear whether the prognosis is better with a solid variant of PEL as compared to the classic PEL. One comparative study of 8 patients with extracavitary PEL and 29 with classic PEL suggested a better prognosis for extracavitary PEL (median survival rate, 11 months versus 3 months) [5]. Another study showed median overall survival of 10.2 months which was not different between groups but showed higher disease-free survival in the extracavitary group [6].

Another study looking at patients treated with similar anthracycline-based therapy reported higher CR rates in patients with classic PEL (66%) versus extracavitary variant (40%). However, patients with classic PEL had higher rates of relapse (40%) at median follow-up of 25 months [6].

Based on a retrospective series of 28 HIV-infected patients with PEL, two prognostic factors have been identified that are independently associated with shorter survival: [2] the poor performance status and [3] the absence of pre-existing HAART use [7].

5. Treatment

There is no standard of care established for the treatment of PEL, and prognosis remains dismal.

As in most patients with AIDS-associated lymphomas, the most common treatment used has been CHOP (cyclophosphamide, doxorubicin, vincristine, and prednisone) chemotherapy and concurrent HAART.

Initiation of HAART has been shown to be an essential component of successful therapeutic regimens in HIV+ patients with PEL. Retrospective case reports show prolonged survival and one case of complete remission in PEL treated with introduction of HAART [8, 9].

EPOCH (rituximab, etoposide, prednisone, vincristine, cyclophosphamide, and doxorubicin), with or without concomitant HAART, has also emerged as an alternative to CHOP and, in the context of HIV infection, might be associated with a slightly greater response rate [10].

Because PEL tumor cells rarely express CD20, rituximab has traditionally not been included in the treatment algorithms. If positive, rituximab can be employed as part of the treatment regimen.

The impact of combination antiretroviral therapy employed in patients with PEL has been documented [11]. However, awareness of the evolving knowledge of drug interactions with HAART, in particular protease inhibitors and chemotherapy, is important when creating a treatment plan [12].

Regardless of the treatment regimen, this immunocompromised population is at risk of opportunistic infections. Therefore, it is essential that they receive prophylactic antibiotics and, when the risk of febrile neutropenia exceeds 20%, adjuvant granulocyte colony-stimulating factor. Regardless of CD4 count, Bactrim should be used for PCP prophylaxis. In case of cytopenias related to chemotherapy or lymphoma, Bactrim can be substituted by pentamidine. Fluoroquinolone prophylaxis should be used in case of severe prolonged neutropenia [13, 14].

The potential efficacy of radiation therapy has been supported by a report of its successful use in a patient with chemotherapy-refractory PEL with solid pleural and chest masses who remained disease free at 12 months of follow-up. Hence, radiation therapy could be used in patients who are either refractory or relapsed to conventional chemotherapy [15].

More intensive regimens, such as high-dose chemotherapy followed by autologous hematopoietic cell transplantation (HCT) or allogeneic HCT, have had mixed results with two case reports showing success and another showing no response [16, 17]. The development of novel therapeutic agents for treatment of solid-variant PEL has not been reported in literature.

Conflicts of Interest

The authors declare that there are no conflicts of interest regarding the publication of this paper.

References

[1] R. F. Little, M. Gutierrez, and E. S. Jaffe, "HIV-associated non-Hodgkin lymphoma: incidence, presentation, and prognosis," *JAMA*, vol. 285, no. 14, pp. 1880–1885, 2001.

[2] Y. B. Chen, A. Rahemtullah, and E. Hochberg, "Primary effusion lymphoma," *The Oncologist*, vol. 12, no. 5, pp. 569–576, 2007.

[3] H.-B. Fan, D.-L. Yang, Y. Guo et al., "Human herpes virus 8-unrelated primary effusion lymphoma-like lymphoma in a patient with hepatitis B virus-related liver cirrhosis: a case report," *Journal of Research in Medical Sciences*, vol. 19, no. 2, pp. 190–192, 2014.

[4] A. Carbone, A. Gloghini, E. Vaccher et al., "Kaposi's sarcoma-associated herpesvirus/human herpesvirus type 8-positive

solid lymphomas: a tissue-based variant of primary effusion lymphoma," *Journal of Molecular Diagnostics (JMD)*, vol. 7, no. 1, pp. 17–27, 2005.

[5] A. Chadburn, E. Hyjek, S. Mathew, E. Cesarman, J. Said, and D. M. Knowles, "KSHV-positive solid lymphomas represent an extra-cavitary variant of primary effusion lymphoma," *American Journal of Surgical Pathology*, vol. 28, no. 11, pp. 1401-1416, 2004.

[6] S. Guillet, L. Gerard, V. Meignin et al., "Classic and extracavitary primary effusion lymphoma in 51 HIV-infected patients from a single institution," *American Journal of Hematology*, vol. 91, no. 2, pp. 233–237, 2016.

[7] E. Boulanger, L. Gerard, J. Gabarre et al., "Prognostic factors and outcome of human herpesvirus 8-associated primary effusion lymphoma in patients with AIDS," *Journal of Clinical Oncology*, vol. 23, no. 19, pp. 4372–4380, 2005.

[8] R. B. Berryman, "Primary effusion lymphoma complete remission with HAART (abstract 4741)," in *Presented at the 42nd Annual American Society of Hematology Meeting*, San Francisco, CA, USA, December 2000.

[9] E. Boulanger, F. Agbalika, O. Maarek et al., "A clinical, molecular and cytogenic study of 12 cases of human herpesvirus 8 associated primary effusion lymphoma (abstract 4683)," *Presented at the 42nd Annual American Society of Hematology Meeting*, San Francisco, CA, USA, December 2000.

[10] K. Dunleavy and W. H. Wilson, "How I treat HIV-associated lymphoma," *Blood*, vol. 119, no. 14, pp. 3245–3255, 2012.

[11] D. Ripamonti, B. Marini, A. Rambaldi, and F. Suter, "Treatment of primary effusion lymphoma with highly active antiviral therapy in the setting of HIV infection," *AIDS*, vol. 22, no. 10, pp. 1236-1237, 2008.

[12] H. A. Torres and V. Mulanovich, "Management of HIV infection in patients with cancer receiving chemotherapy," *Clinical Infectious Diseases*, vol. 59, no. 1, pp. 106–114, 2014.

[13] S. Okada, H. Goto, and M. Yotsumoto, "Current status of treatment for primary effusion lymphoma," *Intractable and Rare Diseases Research*, vol. 3, no. 3, pp. 65–74, 2014.

[14] A. G. Freifeld, E. J. Bow, K. A. Sepkowitz et al., "Clinical practice guideline for the use of antimicrobial agents in neutropenic patients with cancer: 2010 Update by the Infectious Diseases Society of America," *Clinical Infectious Diseases*, vol. 52, no. 4, pp. e56–e93, 2011.

[15] A. Cassoni, U. Ali, J. Cave et al., "Remission after radiotherapy for a patient with chemotherapy-refractory HIV-associated primary effusion lymphoma," *Journal of Clinical Oncology*, vol. 26, no. 32, pp. 5297–5299, 2008.

[16] T. W. Waddington and D. M. Aboulafia, "Failure to eradicate AIDS-associated primary effusion lymphoma with high-dose chemotherapy and autologous stem cell reinfusion: case report and literature review," *AIDS Patient Care and STDs*, vol. 18, no. 2, pp. 67–73, 2004.

[17] J. H. Won, S. H. Han, S. B. Bae et al., "Successful eradication of relapsed primary effusion lymphoma with high-dose chemotherapy and autologous stem cell transplantation in a patient seronegative for human immunodeficiency virus," *International Journal of Hematology*, vol. 83, no. 4, pp. 328–330, 2006.

34

Acquired Coagulopathy and Hemorrhage Secondary to Subcutaneous Heparin Prophylaxis

Maria Sunseri,[1] Tania Ahuja,[2] Tanya Wilcox,[1] and David Green[3]

[1]*Department of Medicine, New York University Langone Health, 550 First Avenue, New York, NY 10016, USA*
[2]*Department of Pharmacy, New York University Langone Health, 550 First Avenue, New York, NY, USA*
[3]*Department of Medicine, New York University Langone Health, Division of Hematology, 550 First Avenue, New York, NY, USA*

Correspondence should be addressed to Tania Ahuja; tania.ahuja@nyumc.org

Academic Editor: Simon Davidson

Unfractionated heparin and low-molecular-weight heparins are commonly used as thromboprophylaxis for hospitalized patients. Though generally considered safe at prophylactic doses, cases of catastrophic hemorrhage have been reported. The proposed mechanism involves bioaccumulation of heparin through saturation of the rapid-elimination pathway in its metabolism. We present an unusual case of an average-weight man with metastatic melanoma who suffered hemorrhage with syncope and end-organ damage while on prophylactic three times daily unfractionated heparin. Coagulation studies were consistent with heparin toxicity. Despite administration of protamine, the clearance of heparin was remarkably delayed, as demonstrated by serial coagulation studies. We review the suspected risk factors for heparin bioaccumulation and the emerging understanding of this unusual adverse event involving a nearly ubiquitous medication.

1. Background

Subcutaneous heparin is a common method of thromboprophylaxis used among heterogeneous populations of hospitalized patients for the prevention of venous thromboembolism (VTE) [1]. The benefit of VTE prophylaxis in medical and surgical inpatients has been widely demonstrated and is promoted by national guidelines [2], which use the available data to make graded recommendations for thromboprophylaxis based on an individual patient's risk of thrombosis or bleed. Further, organizations such as The Joint Commission have emphasized thromboprophylaxis as a key quality measure [2], such that many institutions are implementing computerized clinical decision support tools that prompt providers to order or withhold VTE prophylaxis for all patients at admission and at regular intervals throughout the hospitalization [2]. Patients with malignancy are known to suffer high rates of in-hospital morbidity and mortality from VTE [3, 4]. As such, available guidelines from sources such as the American Society for Clinical Oncology recommend routine thromboprophylaxis in cancer patients admitted for acute illness without apparent contraindication to anticoagulation [4]. Clinicians, in turn, are more likely to regularly order pharmacologic VTE prophylaxis in patients with known cancers.

Although there are tools available to assess thromboembolic risk, there is insufficient evidence to recommend which pharmacologic agent to use for VTE prophylaxis in hospitalized patients. Low-molecular-weight heparin may cause less bleeding complications compared to unfractionated heparin (UFH) and is easier to administer; however, its use is precluded by renal insufficiency and cost [5]. Heparin's widespread use as thromboprophylaxis is in part due to its relative safety profile at the doses effective in reducing risk of clinically significant VTE [1, 6–10]. However, clinically significant hemorrhage from heparin prophylaxis has been reported in the literature [11–14]. In fact, in hospitalized medical patients, prophylaxis with heparin is associated with an increase in all bleeding events (absolute increase, 9 events per 1000 persons treated) and a non-statistically significant increase in major bleeding events (absolute increase, 1 event per 1000 persons treated) [15].

Elimination of UFH is related to two mechanisms; initially, heparin is cleared through the reticuloendothelial system by a saturable, rapid, zero-order process [16]. At high doses, this system saturates, and further elimination occurs renally via a first-order process that is slower and nonsaturable [16]. It is suspected that prolonged use in a high-risk patient may lead to saturation of the rapid-elimination pathway and bioaccumulation of heparin, resulting in iatrogenic coagulopathy and increased risk of major hemorrhage. Furthermore, the dose of UFH for prophylaxis varies from 5000 units twice daily (BID) to three times daily (TID) without a head-to-head comparison. A meta-analysis provided a comparison between BID and TID UFH for prophylaxis in general medical inpatients and found that rates of minor bleeding were similar between the two dosing regimens; however, major bleeding occurred more frequently with TID than with BID dosing (0.73 versus 0.33 events per 100 patient-days; $P < 0.001$) [17]. Although not well studied, in a sub-analysis, data from the International Medical Prevention Registry on Venous Thromboembolism (IMPROVE) assessed in-hospital bleeding to identify risk factors on admission in acutely ill medical patients [18]. This analysis found independent factors associated with 14-day in-hospital bleeding to be active gastroduodenal ulcer, bleeding during the 3 months prior to admission, thrombocytopenia, advanced age, hepatic failure, renal failure, intensive care stay, presence of a central venous catheter, rheumatic disease, current cancer, and male sex [18]. In another study of elderly medical patients treated with prophylactic dosages of enoxaparin, the authors found renal impairment, defined as a creatinine clearance of <30 mL/min, and body weight < 50 kg to be associated with significantly higher antifactor Xa (anti-Xa) values [19]. There were no clinical conclusions drawn from this study regarding the safety of enoxaparin in elderly medical patients [19]. Given the paucity of data, clinicians must maintain a high index of suspicion for bleeding complications of pharmacologic thromboprophylaxis.

If heparin overdose is suspected clinically, the diagnosis can be supported by prolonged activated partial thromboplastin time (aPTT) or elevated anti-Xa assay. Prolonged thrombin time (TT) can help identify heparin effect, especially if a reptilase time (RT) is available. Reptilase time, like thrombin time, measures the conversion of fibrinogen to fibrin; however, it is not sensitive to the effects of heparin, and thus if normal can help localize the coagulopathy to a complication of heparin therapy [20].

Currently, there are no routine recommended monitoring parameters for low-dose heparin prophylaxis in hospitalized patients. In addition, without a head-to-head comparison, many clinicians consider dosing UFH TID for patients at highest risk for thromboembolism and BID for those at highest risk for bleeding [17]. Coagulation studies such as aPTT or anti-Xa may be useful for monitoring certain patients who are at increased risk of bioaccumulation and adverse outcome. We present a case of a patient on prolonged heparin thromboprophylaxis who experienced hemodynamically significant hemorrhage from probable bioaccumulation despite lacking the classic risk profile. Informed consent was obtained from the patient for publication of this case.

2. Case Presentation

A 68-year-old Colombian man who worked as an artist was diagnosed with stage IV metastatic melanoma two years prior to presentation after finding a lump in his groin. His past medical history was significant for well-controlled hypertension, hyperlipidemia, insulin-dependent type 2 diabetes, stage III chronic kidney disease, prostate cancer, and gout; he was also born with a single kidney. He experienced partial regression of his melanoma with pembrolizumab but developed acute interstitial nephritis; thus, therapy was suspended and the patient was treated with methylprednisolone followed by high-dose prednisone and furosemide. He then underwent gamma knife resection of a temporal lobe brain metastasis; his recovery was complicated by bilateral lower extremity deep vein thrombosis (DVT) treated with inferior vena cava filter; therapeutic anticoagulation was deferred in the setting of recent brain surgery. One week after discharge to an acute rehabilitation facility, he returned to the hospital complaining of urinary retention.

On presentation, the patient was found to have an enterococcal urinary tract infection and an acute kidney injury. He was started on ciprofloxacin for the infection; high-dose prednisone was resumed in light of his recent interstitial nephritis. His presentation was also notable for new acute occlusive DVTs in the bilateral lower extremities. Again, therapeutic anticoagulation was deferred given bleeding risk in the postoperative period. He was given prophylactically dosed enoxaparin, which was changed to heparin on hospital day 8 given worsening renal function. Heparin was administered subcutaneously and dosed TID as per institutional weight-based dosing protocols. Staging imaging revealed progression of his disease with diffuse lymphadenopathy and peritoneal carcinomatosis. Given worsening clinical status, it was decided to start vemurafenib, a B-type Raf (BRAF) inhibitor, and cobimetinib, a mitogen-activated protein kinase (MEK) inhibitor, at reduced doses.

On day 16 of hospitalization, the patient became unresponsive while sitting on the edge of his bed. On regaining consciousness, his blood pressure was 80/50 with heart rates ranging 120–130. He reported feeling dizzy and light headed. His vital signs quickly returned to baseline with symptomatic resolution. Physical exam was notable for right-sided supraclavicular fullness and tenderness to palpation, pain with passive range of motion of the right shoulder, and diffuse abdominal ecchymoses at sites of prior heparin injections. Immediate labs demonstrated elevated troponin and lactate. The following morning an acute drop in hemoglobin was noted, from 9.2 g/dL to 6.5 g/dL over 24 hours. Computed tomography (CT) of the chest revealed an expansive subcutaneous hematoma involving the posterior chest wall and right supraclavicular region (Figure 1). The hematoma appeared to be associated with sites of previously unknown metastatic lesions. Coagulation studies demonstrated markedly elevated aPTT (>200 s), thrombin time

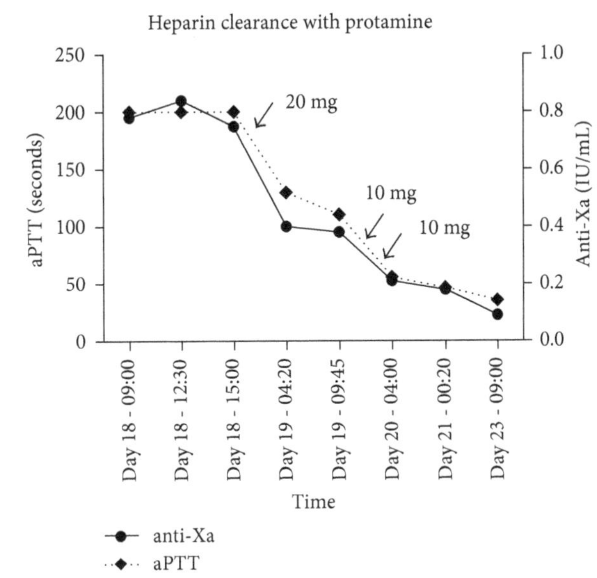

(a)

Day 1	Readmission for urinary retention; aPTT 24.6
Day 2	Acute occlusive venous thrombosis on lower extremity doppler
Day 3	Enoxaparin 30 mg by daily subcutaneous injection initiated
Day 4	Pre-existing post-surgical hemorrhage noted on brain imaging
Day 8	Enoxaparin transitioned to heparin 5000 units three times per day by subcutaneous injection
Day 9	Cobemetinib (MEK inhibitor) and vemurafenib (BRAF inhibitor) initiated
Day 14	BRAF/MEK inhibitors held due to mild liver injury
Day 16	Syncopal episode; hemoglobin 9.2 g/dL
Day 17	Hemoglobin drop identified; hemoglobin 6.5 g/dL
Day 18	0900: aPTT >200; anti-Xa 0.78; TT>200 1230: aPTT >200; anti-Xa 0.84 1500: aPTT >200; anti-Xa 0.75 1825: protamine sulfate 20 mg by intravenous injection
Day 19	0400: aPTT 129.7; anti-Xa 0.4 0945: aPTT 110.4 1500: protamine sulfate 10 mg by intravenous injection 1715: aPTT 68.9
Day 20	0100: protamine sulfate 10 mg by intravenous injection 0400: aPTT 55.9 1530: aPTT 45.3
Day 23	0600: aPTT 35.3

(b)

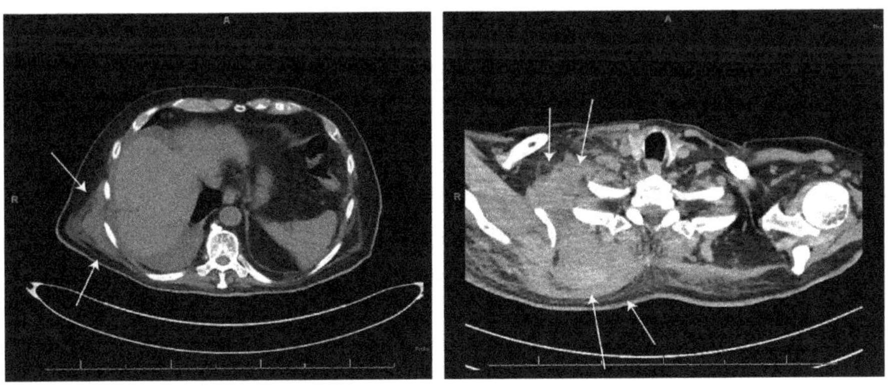

(c)

FIGURE 1: (a) Timeline of heparin clearance with protamine administration. Left y-axis: aPTT; right y-axis: anti-Xa. Arrows demarcate timing and dose of protamine administration. aPTT: activated partial thromboplastin time; reference range 27–38 seconds. Anti-Xa: antifactor Xa activity; reference 0 or <0.3 IU/mL for prophylactic dosing; reference range 0.3–0.7 for therapeutic anticoagulation. (b) Clinical timeline. Activated partial thromboplastin time and thrombin time measured in seconds. Anti-Xa measured in IU/mL. (c) Representative axial images from the patient's chest CT demonstrating multifocal soft tissue hematomas (arrows).

(>200 s), and anti-Xa (0.83 IU/mL). The constellation of lab findings indicated heparin toxicity.

The patient was supported with transfusions and reversed with several doses of intravenous (IV) protamine sulfate. The aPTT decreased after 20 mg of protamine from >200 s to 129.7 s and then 110.4 s. Two additional 10 mg doses were given with decrease to 68.9 s and 55.9 s, respectively. The aPTT normalized to 35.3 s the following day with no additional doses (Figure 1). Of note, despite the administration of protamine, the heparin clearance was remarkably delayed (Figure 1).

The patient recovered from his acute bleed, heparin was held indefinitely, and he did not have recurrence of his coagulopathy. Ultimately, however, his liver function worsened with the chemotherapy, requiring drug changes and further dose reductions. There was no reduction in his tumor burden despite trials of multiple agents, and his kidney function again declined. The patient was eventually transitioned to inpatient hospice.

3. Diagnostic Assessment

Measurement of aPTT, anti-Xa, and TT were made by standard specimen analysis in the clinical laboratory. Results may be spurious if the sample is drawn from a heparinized line or via traumatic venipuncture. In this case, each specimen was drawn from a peripheral indwelling central catheter; prior to collection, the line was appropriately flushed with normal saline, and the first 10 mL of collected blood was discarded.

4. Conclusions

This case describes an unusual adverse event involving a nearly ubiquitous medication. This patient's known malignancy and history of recurrent DVT made him a strong candidate for VTE prophylaxis. Although his recent brain surgery and metastatic melanoma precluded him from therapeutic anticoagulation due to risk of hemorrhage, he had no active bleeding and no history of significant bleed, suggesting minimal or no contraindication to low-dose TID heparin as thromboprophylaxis. The suggested risk factors for heparin bioaccumulation do not fit this patient, with exception of male sex and cancer. He was of average body weight, and his renal failure was acute with his creatinine clearance improving at the time of heparin administration. Despite this, he suffered hemodynamically significant hemorrhage with laboratory markers of end-organ damage that took several days to clear. The bleed appears to have originated from metastatic lesions visualized on his chest imaging. This case sheds further light on the emerging understanding of heparin bioaccumulation, suggesting that there may be as-yet unidentified factors placing certain patients at risk. Since heparin has been shown to be depolymerized by endothelial cell lysosomal enzymes [21], we hypothesize that the effects of this patient's malignancy or the BRAF or MEK inhibitors may have contributed to endothelial dysfunction and delayed heparin clearance. Reporting patients that suffer this outcome is important to elucidating the pathogenesis of bioaccumulation and eventually identifying parameters for patients that may require closer monitoring with targeted coagulation studies during prolonged use of heparin thromboprophylaxis.

Abbreviations

UFH: Unfractionated heparin
anti-Xa: Antifactor Xa activity
aPTT: Activated partial thromboplastin time
TT: Thrombin time
RT: Reptilase time
BID: Twice daily
TID: Three times daily
VTE: Venous thromboembolism
DVT: Deep vein thrombosis
BRAF: B-type Raf
MEK: Mitogen-activated protein kinase
CT: Computed tomography
IV: Intravenous.

Conflicts of Interest

The authors declare that there are no conflicts of interest.

Authors' Contributions

Maria Sunseri, Tania Ahuja, Tanya Wilcox, and David Green were all clinical providers for the patient and major contributors in writing the manuscript. All authors read and approved the final manuscript.

References

[1] S. R. Kahn, W. Lim, A. S. Dunn et al., "Prevention of VTE in nonsurgical patients: antithrombotic therapy and prevention of thrombosis, 9th ed: American College of Chest Physicians Evidence-Based Clinical Practice Guidelines," *Chest*, vol. 141, no. 2, pp. e195S–e226, 2012.

[2] K. C. Wilson and G. J. Merli, "Performance measures for improving the prevention of venous thromboembolism: achievement in clinical practice," *Journal of Thrombosis and Thrombolysis*, vol. 32, no. 3, pp. 293–302, 2011.

[3] K. Hogg and M. Carrier, "Prevention and treatment of venous thromboembolism in patients with cancer," *Therapeutic Advances in Hematology*, vol. 3, no. 1, pp. 45–58, 2012.

[4] N. M. Kuderer and G. H. Lyman, "Guidelines for treatment and prevention of venous thromboembolism among patients with cancer," *Thrombosis Research*, vol. 133, pp. S122–S127, 2014.

[5] D. Green, J. Hirsh, J. Heit, M. Prins, B. Davidson, and A. W. Lensing, "Low molecular weight heparin: a critical analysis of clinical trials," *Pharmacological Reviews*, vol. 46, no. 1, pp. 89–109, 1994.

[6] W. Alhazzani, W. Lim, R. Z. Jaeschke, M. H. Murad, J. Cade, and D. J. Cook, "Heparin thromboprophylaxis in medical-surgical critically ill patients: a systematic review and meta-analysis of randomized trials," *Critical Care Medicine*, vol. 41, no. 9, pp. 2088–2098, 2013.
[7] L. Wein, S. Wein, S. J. Haas, J. Shaw, and H. Krum, "Pharmacological venous thromboembolism prophylaxis in hospitalized medical patients: a meta-analysis of randomized controlled trials," *Archives of Internal Medicine*, vol. 167, no. 14, pp. 1476–1486, 2007.
[8] P. Mismetti, S. Laporte-Simitsidis, B. Tardy et al., "Prevention of venous thromboembolism in internal medicine with unfractionated or low-molecular-weight heparins: a meta-analysis of randomised clinical trials," *Thrombosis and Haemostasis*, vol. 83, no. 1, pp. 14–19, 2000.
[9] J. Park, J. M. Lee, J. S. Lee, and Y. J. Cho, "Pharmacological and mechanical thromboprophylaxis in critically ill patients: a network meta-analysis of 12 trials," *Journal of Korean Medical Science*, vol. 31, no. 11, pp. 1828–1837, 2016.
[10] A. O. Kanaan, M. A. Silva, J. L. Donovan, T. Roy, and A. S. Al-Homsi, "Meta-analysis of venous thromboembolism prophylaxis in medically ill patients," *Clinical Therapeutics*, vol. 29, no. 11, pp. 2395–2405, 2007.
[11] J. Hudcova and D. Talmor, "Life-threatening hemorrhage following subcutaneous heparin therapy," *Therapeutics and Clinical Risk Management*, vol. 5, no. 1, pp. 51–54, 2009.
[12] N. P. Tsapatsaris, "Low-dose heparin. A cause of hematoma of rectus abdominis," *Archives of Internal Medicine*, vol. 151, no. 3, pp. 597–599, 1991.
[13] D. M. Langguth, R. C. Wong, C. Archibald, and P. G. Hogan, "Haemorrhagic myositis associated with prophylactic heparin use in dermatomyositis," *Annals of the Rheumatic Diseases*, vol. 63, no. 4, pp. 464-465, 2004.
[14] S. T. String and P. J. Barcia, "Complications of small dose prophylactic heparinization," *American Journal of Surgery*, vol. 130, no. 5, pp. 570–574, 1975.
[15] A. Qaseem, R. Chou, L. L. Humphrey, M. Starkey, P. Shekelle, and Clinical Guidelines Committee of the American College of Physicians, "Venous thromboembolism prophylaxis in hospitalized patients: a clinical practice guideline from the American College of Physicians," *Annals of internal medicine*, vol. 155, no. 9, pp. 625–632, 2011.
[16] R. Tahir, "A review of unfractionated heparin and its monitoring," *U.S. Pharmacist*, vol. 32, no. 7, pp. HS-26–HS-36, 2007.
[17] C. S. King, A. B. Holley, J. L. Jackson, A. F. Shorr, and L. K. Moores, "Twice vs. three times daily heparin dosing for thromboembolism prophylaxis in the general medical population. A metaanalysis," *Chest*, vol. 131, no. 2, pp. 507–516, 2007.
[18] H. Decousus, V. F. Tapson, J. F. Bergmann et al., "IMPROVE investigators. Factors at admission associated with bleeding risk in medical patients," *Chest*, vol. 139, pp. 69–79, 2011.
[19] I. Mahe, I. Gouin-Thibault, L. Drouet et al., "Elderly medical patients treated with prophylactic dosages of enoxaparin: influence of renal function on anti-Xa activity level," *Drugs Aging*, vol. 24, no. 1, pp. 63–71, 2007.
[20] S. Niewiarowski, E. P. Kirby, and K. Stocker, "Throbocytin-a novel platelet activating enzyme from Bothrops atrox venom," *Thrombosis Research*, vol. 10, no. 6, pp. 863–869, 1977.
[21] T. Barzu, J. L. M. L. vanRijn, M. Petitou, G. Tobelem, and J. P. Caen, "Heparin degradation in the endothelial cells," *Thrombosis Research*, vol. 47, no. 5, pp. 601–609, 1987.

35

Coexistence of Antiphospholipid Syndrome and Heparin-Induced Thrombocytopenia in a Patient with Recurrent Venous Thromboembolism

Samuel Adediran and Nicole Agostino

Lehigh Valley Health Network, Departments of Hematology and Oncology and Medicine, Allentown, PA, USA

Correspondence should be addressed to Samuel Adediran; samuel.adediran@lvhn.org

Academic Editor: Kate Khair

Heparin-induced thrombocytopenia (HIT) is a prothrombotic adverse drug reaction in which heparin forms complexes with platelet factor 4 forming neoantigens that are recognized by autoantibodies. Antiphospholipid syndrome (APS) is similar to HIT in that it is mediated by autoantibodies that are also prothrombotic. We present a case of rare coexistence of antiphospholipid antibody syndrome and heparin-induced thrombocytopenia.

1. Introduction

Heparin-induced thrombocytopenia (HIT) is a prothrombotic adverse drug reaction in which heparin forms complexes with platelet factor 4 forming neoantigens that are recognized by autoantibodies (antiHPF4/HAPA). The Fc portions of the anti-HPF4 bind Fc receptors on platelets causing platelets activation, aggregation, release of α and dense granules, and formation of procoagulants [1]. The hallmark of this is thrombocytopenia and thrombosis. HIT occurs in about 2% of all patients who receive heparin of whom about 35% develop thrombosis [2]. Antiphospholipid syndrome (APS) is similar to HIT in that it is mediated by autoantibodies that are also prothrombotic. Autoantibodies are generated to phospholipids or to phospholipid-binding proteins which are recognized risk-factors for thrombosis and pregnancy morbidity. Diagnosis of APS requires the elevation of at least one of the phospholipid autoantibodies and a clinical manifestation (Procedure 1). In this report we present a patient with recurrent venous thromboembolism despite being on full anticoagulation who was found to have concurrent HIT and APS.

2. Case Report

A 37-year-old Caucasian female with history of obesity and iron-deficiency anemia presented with painful left lower extremity swelling. A physical examination revealed an edematous, tender, and mildly erythematous left lower extremity. Mild tachycardia was noted. A lower extremity venous duplex ultrasound showed an extensive, occlusive deep venous thrombosis (DVT) from the left common femoral vein to the calf veins. Also, there was occlusive DVT within the left common and external iliac veins. A computer tomographic (CT) imaging of the chest with contrast revealed pulmonary emboli within the subsegmental pulmonary artery branches in the right lower lobe. Heparin was administered intravenously. Catheter-directed venous thrombolysis was done, and complete clearing of the left iliofemoral DVT was achieved. Intravenous heparin was switched to rivaroxaban, and the patient was discharged home. A week later, the patient presented with right-sided pleuritic chest pain. A CT of the chest with contrast revealed new acute pulmonary emboli within the distal left lower lobar artery and the basilar segmental pulmonary arteries of the left lower lobe. A venous

Diagnosis of APS
At least one clinical criterion and one laboratory criterion
(1) Clinical criteria
(a) ≥1 episodes of venous, arterial or small-vessel thrombosis confirmed and documented.
(b) Pregnancy-related morbidity:
≥1 unexplained deaths of a normal fetus at or beyond the 10th week of gestation.
≥1 premature births of a normal neonate before the 34th week of gestation
≥3 unexplained consecutive spontaneous abortions before the 10th week of gestation
(2) Laboratory criteria
(a) IgG and/IgM anticardiolipin antibodies present in medium or high titer on two or more occasions, at least 12 weeks apart.
(b) Lupus anticoagulant on two or more occasions at least 12 weeks apart
(c) IgG and IgM $\beta 2$ glycoprotein antibodies present in medium or high titer on two or more occasions, at least 12 weeks apart.

PROCEDURE 1: The Sydney classification criteria for antiphospholipid syndrome.

TABLE 1: Antiphospholipid profile at the time of presentation and at twelve-week follow-up.

Tests	At presentation (normal)	Three months after (normal)
Anticardiolipin IgG	140 (<15 GPL units)	135
Anticardiolipin IgM	30.4 (<12.5 MPL units)	60.6
Anti-$\beta 2$ glycoprotein 1 IgG	>150 (<20 SGU)	>150
Anti-$\beta 2$ glycoprotein 1 IgM	38 (<20 SMU)	42
PTT, lupus sensitive	82.5 (32–45 s)	
DRVVT screen	69.1 (31.4–45 s)	
DRVVT confirmation	1.6 (<1.3 s)	
Hexagonal phase phospholipid	39.7 (0–8 s)	

duplex ultrasound showed extensive left lower extremity DVT from the left common femoral vein to the calf veins and occlusive thrombus within the left external iliac vein and the left common iliac vein. Intravenous heparin drip was initiated. Inferior vena cava filter was placed. Catheter-directed venous thrombolysis was performed, and complete thrombolysis of the left lower extremity DVT was noted within 24 hours. Three days later, heparin was stopped, and a low molecular weight heparin, lovenox, was started. Within 24 hours of starting lovenox, the patient noticed increased left leg tightness and worsening pain. A venous duplex ultrasound was performed and again revealed extensive, occlusive DVT from the left common femoral vein to the left popliteal vein and a nonocclusive DVT in a small left external iliac vein. By this time, platelet count had decreased from 448 × 109/L at the time of admission to 147 × 109/L (normal, 150–400 × 109/L). Enzyme-linked immunosorbent assays (ELISA) were performed in order to evaluate for the presence of heparin associated platelet antibodies (HAPA) and antiphospholipid antibodies (APLA). Lovenox was stopped, and argatroban was started. TPA thrombolysis with aspiration thrombectomy was performed, and a follow-up venography demonstrated complete removal of thrombus from the popliteal, femoral, and common femoral veins. Three days later, while the patient was on argatroban, a venous duplex ultrasound again demonstrated extensive, occlusive DVT in the distal veins (posterior tibial, peroneal, and gastrocnemius) extending to the popliteal, femoral, deep femoral, and common femoral veins. Argatroban was stopped; arixtra, 10 mg daily, was started, and monitoring with serial venous duplex ultrasound was continued. Three days after starting arixtra, partial recanalization of DVT within the left external iliac vein and the left femoral popliteal system was demonstrated. Platelet count nadir at 134 × 109/L. HAPA was strongly positive 1.412 (normal, <0.4 OD). Serotonin release assay was positive with 82% (normal, ≥20%) serotonin release with low-dose heparin (0.1 U/mL) and 0% (normal, =20%) serotonin release with high-dose heparin (100 U/mL). Antiphospholipid antibody profile demonstrated elevated anti-$\beta 2$ glycoprotein 1, anticardiolipin, and positive lupus anticoagulant (Table 1). Once platelet count stabilized and DVT recanalization was achieved, Coumadin was started. Coumadin was overlapped with arixtra for 5 days after INR reached therapeutic level. Three months after the initial hospital encounter, antiphospholipid antibodies levels were still elevated, confirming the diagnosis of antiphospholipid syndrome. We recommended against pregnancy giving her significant thrombotic risk, and the risk of fetal toxicity with Coumadin.

3. Discussion

The coexistence of antiphospholipid antibody syndrome and clinical heparin-induced thrombocytopenia is not often seen. This case demonstrates the simultaneous occurrence of both entities in an otherwise healthy patient. A similar case was reported by Tun et al. wherein a 42-year-old female found to have pulmonary embolism, superior mesenteric artery thrombus, and multiple infarctions had thrombocytopenia and positive HAPA. However, serotonin release assay was not reported [3]. While HAPA as measured by ELISA is very sensitive, serotonin release assay, a functional assay that determines the ability of heparin-dependent IgG to activate platelet to secrete serotonin, is more specific. Correlation between APS and HAPA/anti-HPF4 has been suggested. Lasne et al. reported twenty patients with APS three of whom tested positive for HAPA. One of the patients had positive serotonin release 26% (normal, ≥20%). None of these patients reported history of HIT or received heparin in at least thirty months. They suggested that APS may increase predisposition to HIT [4]. In a study in which sixty-nine patients had positive APLA with or without APS, ten patients (14.5%) were reported positive for HAPA, three of whom had prior heparin exposure. No HIT was reported [5]. Another small retrospective study reported that out of thirty-three patients with APLA, twenty of whom had primary APS, seven developed HAPA. Two of the seven patients had positive aggregation tests concerning for HIT. Two had no prior exposure to heparin [6]. It has been proposed that the distortion of vascular endothelium seen in APS causes the exposure of glycosaminoglycans such as heparin sulfate that may then complex with platelet factor 4. This may cause molecular modification that produces neoantigens and HAPA [7].

On the other hand, Martin-Toutain et al. found poor correlation between two different ELISA tests for HAPA on the same blood sample. This prompted them to suggest that the presence of HAPA may be related to cross-reactivity between APLA and antibodies used in various ELISA and not necessarily a pathogenic antibody responsible for development of clinical HIT [8]. Martinuzzo et al. found no cross-reactivity between HAPA and IgG anticardiolipin or IgG anti-β2-glycoprotein 1 [6]. Other studies have shown partial cross-reactivity [9]. Therefore, it is still not clear whether or not the presence of APLA predisposes a patient to developing HAPA. To further complicate matters, there are at least two reported cases of heparin-related thrombocytopenia in patient with APS who developed thrombosis but had negative HAPA. It was suggested that the presence of antiphospholipid antibodies possibly interferes with HIT diagnostic tests causing a lack of antigen recognition by the antibodies used in the tests [10, 11]. Our patient clearly had elevated antiphospholipid antibodies, markedly positive HAPA, and high positive serotonin release. Thus, it represents a true case of concurrent antiphospholipid syndrome and clinical heparin-induced thrombocytopenia in an otherwise healthy patient.

The mainstay of treatment for venous thromboembolism (VTE) secondary to APS is heparin in the acute setting and vitamin K antagonist (VKA) in the long term. Warfarin has numerous dietary and drug interactions and there is need for frequent monitoring of INR making its use somewhat challenging. Also, variable responsiveness of reagents used in INR test to lupus anticoagulant can complicate monitoring. As a result, the use of new oral anticoagulants (NOACS) like dabigatran, apixaban, and rivaroxaban has been advocated. However, there are no good data to recommend the use of NOACs in APS [12]. A few case reports have shown VTE recurrences in patients with APS who were treated with rivaroxaban and dabigatran, indicating that NOACS may not be as effective as VKAs in APS [13]. After our patient's first episode of pulmonary embolism and DVT, she was discharged home on rivaroxaban. She presented a week after with extension of DVT and PE. In retrospect, this was likely a failure of rivaroxaban in APS. Positive serotonin release confirmed HIT, indicating that two process were probably happening concurrently. Despite no good supporting data, some have suggested that it is reasonable to consider NOACs in patients who do not tolerate VKAs [12]. In a retrospective review of thirty-five patients with APS who were switched to rivaroxaban after VKA intolerance, no recurrent VTE was observed after a median follow-up of ten months [14]. The ongoing prospective randomized control trial "rivaroxaban in antiphospholipid syndrome" will shed more light on the use of rivaroxaban as compared to VKAs in the secondary prevention of VTE in antiphospholipid syndrome.

Heparin-induced thrombocytopenia is treated by stopping heparin and administering non-heparin anticoagulants. Argatroban is the only FDA-approved anticoagulant for this indication. However, other non-heparin anticoagulants, namely, bivalirudin, fondaparinux, and danaparoid, have been used successfully. Warkentin et al. reviewed sixteen patients with HIT who were treated with fondaparinux. None of the patients developed new, recurrent, or progressive thrombosis. A few other reports have described successful treatment of HIT with fondaparinux [15].

In a patient with both HIT and APS, the 14th international congress on APL task force suggests anticoagulation with argatroban or danaparoid. The use of danaparoid has been discontinued in the United States. Our patient received argatroban, but her clot burden worsened necessitating a change to fondaparinux. We found four other case reports in the literature, detailing the successful use of fondaparinux in patients with concurrent APS and HIT [16–18]. Two of these cases were pediatric. Our case further adds to the point that fondaparinux can be successfully used to treat VTE in patient with HIT and APS at least in the acute setting.

For a child-bearing female with history of HIT and APS who requires indefinite anticoagulation, the choice of anticoagulant to use during pregnancy is complicated. The only anticoagulant recommended during pregnancy for a patient with APS is low molecular weight heparin (LMWH). However, LMWH is better avoided in HIT. Warfarin is contraindicated in pregnancy due to high risk of fetal malformations especially in the first trimester [19]. No good data exist on the potential risks of the NOACs in pregnancy. Animal studies have shown reproductive toxicity, embryo-fetal toxicity, and increase incidence of common malformations with the NOACs. Because the potential risk of NOAC in human is unknown, they should be avoided during pregnancy and breastfeeding [20]. Other treatment considerations in pregnancy are fondaparinux and danaparoid. There is no good quality data to support their use in pregnancy. However there are a few case reports and case series about the safety of fondaparinux in pregnancy. A retrospective study reviewed 13 women with 15 pregnancies who were treated with fondaparinux because of hypersensitivity to LMWH. For six of the pregnancies, fondaparinux was started in the first trimester, in the second trimester for eight, and in the third trimester for one. Five pregnancy complications were observed: two miscarriages, one voluntary termination due to congenital malformation, one cerebral palsy due to delay in delivery, and one recurrent DVT due to drug underdosing [21]. A prospective study of twelve pregnancies showed no adverse effect from fondaparinux [22]. It is also worth noting that while Coumadin has been successfully used in some pregnant women with mechanical heart valves, its use is associated with significant complications such has embryopathy, subchorionic hemorrhage, and fetal bleeding [23]. Given the high thrombotic risk of APS, the fetal toxicity of Coumadin, and the uncertainty of fondaparinux in pregnancy, our patient chose not to become pregnant.

Conflicts of Interest

The above named authors certify that they have no affiliations with or involvement in any organization or entity with any financial interest or nonfinancial interest in the subject matter or materials discussed in this manuscript.

References

[1] T. E. Warkentin, D. M. Arnold, I. Nazi, and J. G. Kelton, "The platelet serotonin-release assay," *American Journal of Hematology*, vol. 90, no. 6, pp. 564–572, 2015.

[2] Y. Levy and M. Berla, "The complexities of anticoagulation in the antiphospholipid syndrome," *The Israel Medical Association journal*, vol. 16, no. 1, pp. 54–56, 2014.

[3] N. T. Tun, M. Krishnamurthy, and R. Snyder, "Catastrophic anti-phospholipid syndrome and heparin-induced thrombocytopenia-related diseases or chance association?" *Blood Coagulation and Fibrinolysis*, vol. 26, no. 2, pp. 214–219, 2015.

[4] D. Lasne, R. Saffroy, C. Bachelot et al., "Tests for heparin-induced thrombocytopenia in primary antiphospholipid syndrome," *British Journal of Haematology*, vol. 97, no. 4, p. 939, 1997.

[5] G. De Larrañaga, M. Martinuzzo, A. Bocassi, M. M. Fressart, and R. Forastiero, "Heparin-platelet factor 4 induced antibodies in patients with either autoimmune or alloimmune antiphospholipid antibodies," *Thrombosis and Haemostasis*, vol. 88, no. 2, pp. 371–373, 2002.

[6] M. E. Martinuzzo, R. R. Forastiero, Y. Adamczuk, G. Pombo, and L. O. Carreras, "Antiplatelet factor 4—heparin antibodies in patients with antiphospholipid antibodies," *Thrombosis Research*, vol. 95, no. 6, pp. 271–279, 1999.

[7] D. A. Hoppensteadt and J. M. Walenga, "The Relationship Between the Antiphospholipid Syndrome and Heparin-Induced Thrombocytopenia," *Hematology/Oncology Clinics of North America*, vol. 22, no. 1, pp. 1–18, 2008.

[8] I. Martin-Toutain, J. C. Piette, M. C. Diemert, C. Faucher, L. Jobic, and A. Ankri, "High prevalence of antibodies to platelet factor 4 heparin in patients with antiphospholipid antibodies in absence of heparin-induced thrombocytopenia," *Lupus*, vol. 16, no. 2, pp. 79–83, 2007.

[9] D. Alpert, L. A. Mandl, D. Erkan, W. Yin, E. I. Peerschke, and J. E. Salmon, "Anti-heparin platelet factor 4 antibodies in systemic lupus erythaematosus are associated with IgM antiphospholipid antibodies and the antiphospholipid syndrome," *Annals of the Rheumatic Diseases*, vol. 67, no. 3, pp. 395–401, 2008.

[10] J. Perunicic, N. M. Antonijevic, P. Miljic et al., "Clinical challenge: heparin-induced thrombocytopenia type II (HIT II) or pseudo-HIT in a patient with antiphospholipid syndrome," *Journal of Thrombosis and Thrombolysis*, vol. 26, no. 2, pp. 142–146, 2008.

[11] L. Zeller, Y. Almog, A. Tomer, S. Sukenik, and M. Abu-Shakra, "Catastrophic thromboses and severe thrombocytopenia during heparin therapy in a patient with anti-phospholipid syndrome," *Clinical Rheumatology*, vol. 25, no. 3, pp. 426–429, 2006.

[12] D. Erkan, C. L. Aguiar, D. Andrade et al., "14th International Congress on Antiphospholipid Antibodies: task force report on antiphospholipid syndrome treatment trends," *Autoimmunity Reviews*, vol. 13, no. 6, pp. 685–696, 2014.

[13] K. Win and G. M. Rodgers, "New oral anticoagulants may not be effective to prevent venous thromboembolism in patients with antiphospholipid syndrome," *American Journal of Hematology*, vol. 89, no. 10, p. 1017, 2014.

[14] S. Savino, K. Breen, and B. J. Hunt, "Rivaroxaban use in patients with antiphospholipid syndrome and previous venous thromboembolism," *Blood Coagulation and Fibrinolysis*, vol. 26, no. 4, pp. 476–477, 2015.

[15] T. E. Warkentin, M. Pai, J. I. Sheppard, S. Schulman, A. C. Spyropoulos, and J. W. Eikelboom, "Fondaparinux treatment of acute heparin-induced thrombocytopenia confirmed by the serotonin-release assay: a 30-month, 16-patient case series," *Journal of Thrombosis and Haemostasis*, vol. 9, no. 12, pp. 2389–2396, 2011.

[16] S. G. Holtan, S. K. Knox, and A. Tefferi, "Use of fondaparinux in a patient with antiphospholipid antibody syndrome and heparin-associated thrombocytopenia," *Journal of Thrombosis and Haemostasis*, vol. 4, no. 7, pp. 1632–1634, 2006.

[17] H. Tokgoz, U. Caliskan, and M. Demir, "Successful use of fondaparinux in a child with heparin-induced thrombocytopenia," *Blood Coagulation and Fibrinolysis*, vol. 23, no. 8, pp. 769–771, 2012.

[18] M. J. Manco-Johnson, M. Wang, N. A. Goldenberg et al., "Treatment, survival, and thromboembolic outcomes of thrombotic storm in children," *Journal of Pediatrics*, vol. 161, no. 4, pp. 682.el–688.el, 2012.

[19] C. B. Chighizola, M. Moia, and P. L. Meroni, "New oral anticoagulants in thrombotic antiphospholipid syndrome," *Lupus*, vol. 23, no. 12, pp. 1279–1282, 2014.

[20] D. J. Arachchillage and H. Cohen, "Use of new oral anticoagulants in antiphospholipid syndrome," *Current Rheumatology Reports*, vol. 15, no. 6, p. 331, 2013.

[21] E. Elsaigh, J. Thachil, M. J. Nash et al., "The use of fondaparinux in pregnancy," *British Journal of Haematology*, vol. 168, no. 5, pp. 762–764, 2015.

[22] H. M. Knol, L. Schultinge, J. J. H. M. Erwich, and K. Meijer, "Fondaparinux as an alternative anticoagulant therapy during pregnancy," *Journal of Thrombosis and Haemostasis*, vol. 8, no. 8, pp. 1876–1879, 2010.

[23] W. S. Chan, S. Anand, and J. S. Ginsberg, "Anticoagulation of pregnant women with mechanical heart valves: A systematic review of the literature," *Archives of Internal Medicine*, vol. 160, no. 2, pp. 191–196, 2000.

36

A Rare Case of Systemic AL Amyloidosis with Muscle Involvement: A Misleading Diagnosis

Fabrizio Accardi,[1] Valentina Papa,[2] Anna Rita Capozzi,[3] Gian Luca Capello,[4] Laura Verga,[4] Cristina Mancini,[5] Eugenia Martella,[5] Roberta Costa,[2] Laura Notarfranchi,[1] Benedetta Dalla Palma,[1] Franco Aversa,[1] Vladimiro Pietrini,[3] Giovanna Cenacchi,[2] and Nicola Giuliani[1]

[1]*UO di Ematologia e CTMO, Azienda Ospedaliero-Universitaria di Parma and Department of Medicine and Surgery, University of Parma, Parma, Italy*

[2]*Department of Biomedical and Neuromotor Sciences, Alma Mater University of Bologna, Bologna, Italy*

[3]*Muscle and Nerve Histopathology Laboratory, Neurology Unit, Azienda Ospedaliero-Universitaria di Parma, University of Parma, Parma, Italy*

[4]*Department of Diagnostic Medicine, Electron Microscopy Laboratory, IRCCS Fondazione Policlinico San Matteo and University of Pavia, Pavia, Italy*

[5]*Pathology Unit, Azienda Ospedaliero-Universitaria di Parma, Parma, Italy*

Correspondence should be addressed to Nicola Giuliani; nicola.giuliani@unipr.it

Academic Editor: Uma Dasgupta

Muscle involvement in AL amyloidosis is a rare condition, and the diagnosis of amyloid myopathy is often delayed and underdiagnosed. Amyloid myopathy may be the initial manifestation and may precede the diagnosis of systemic AL amyloidosis. Here, we report the case of a 73-year-old man who was referred to our center for a monoclonal gammopathy of undetermined significance (MGUS) diagnosed since 1999. He reported a progressive weakness of proximal muscles of the legs with onset six months previously. Muscle biopsy showed mild histopathology featuring alterations of nonspecific type with a mixed myopathic and neurogenic involvement, and the diagnostic turning point was the demonstration of characteristic green birefringence under cross-polarized light following Congo red staining of perimysial vessels. Transmission electron microscopy (TEM) confirmed amyloid fibrils around perimysial vessels associated with collagen fibrils. A stepwise approach to diagnosis and staging of this disorder is critical and involves confirmation of amyloid deposition, identification of the fibril type, assessment of underlying amyloidogenic disorder, and evaluation of the extent and severity of amyloidotic organ involvement.

1. Introduction

Immunoglobulin light chain (AL) amyloidosis is the more frequent type of acquired amyloidosis.

The disease originates from a monoclonal misfolded light chain, produced by a plasma cell or B-cell clone, with a tendency to aggregation and tissue deposition leading to organ dysfunction. Mostly, it is a systemic disease, with a potentially generalized organ injury, but localized deposits are described [1]. Muscle involvement in AL amyloidosis is a rare condition, and the diagnosis of amyloid myopathy is often delayed and underdiagnosed. Amyloid myopathy may be the initial manifestation and may precede the diagnosis of systemic AL amyloidosis.

2. Case Presentation

Here, we report the case of a 73-year-old man who was referred to our center in November 2014 for a monoclonal gammopathy of undetermined significance (MGUS) diagnosed since 1999. He reported a progressive weakness of proximal muscles of the legs with onset six months previously. He did not present bone or muscle pain nor experienced limitations in instrumental activities of daily living. Laboratory data showed that blood count, electrolytes, including calcium, and renal and liver function were within normal range. A monoclonal component on γ-region on serum protein electrophoresis was described, equal to 2 gr/dl. Serum immunofixation was positive for IgG-κ, Bence Jones proteinuria was 244 mg in 24 hours, κ free light chains were 338 mg/L, and λ free light chains were 10.8 mg/L with an abnormal ratio equal to 31.3. A complete bone marrow examination and several imaging studies were performed. A bone marrow aspirate showed 30% of plasma cells restricted to κ chain by immunohistochemistry. Fluorescence in situ hybridization (FISH) analysis was negative for the presence of del(13q), del (17p), and chromosome 14 rearrangements. Conventional skeletal radiography excluded lytic lesions.

^{18}FDG-PET did not display areas of increased uptake. A spine gadolinium-enhanced MRI detected normal bone marrow signals and two herniated discs at the lumbar and sacral levels (L4-L5 and L5-S1). The bone densitometry study revealed osteoporosis, and the patient was treated with vitamin D supplementation and bisphosphonates. Considering the absence of an event defining the disease as active, the plasma cell dyscrasia was classified as smoldering multiple myeloma (SMM).

During the follow-up period, the patient reported the appearance of pain and stiffness at the shoulders and hips and jaw claudication. Antinuclear antibodies (ANA) were negative, TSH was in normal range, creatinine phosphokinase (CPK) was 116 UI/L (normal value: 5–174), and B12 level was 162 pg/ml (192–1037). The mild B12 deficiency was corrected. Suspecting polymyalgia oral predinisone was started but without any clinical benefit therapy was interrupted. An electromyography revealed normal motor unit potentials.

Because of the persistent symptoms, a clarifying left quadriceps muscle biopsy was taken on June 2016. It showed mild histopathology featuring alterations of nonspecific type with a mixed myopathic and neurogenic involvement (Figures 1(a)–1(d)). Considering the diagnosis of SMM, a light chain deposition could be suspected; the diagnostic turning point was the demonstration of characteristic green birefringence under cross-polarized light following Congo red staining of perimysial vessels (Figures 1(e) and 1(f)). In addition to the standard stainings, a differential diagnosis with other myopathies was performed by including histoenzymatic reactions. Moreover, the metabolic component was analyzed with the appropriate reactions, and any inflammatory aspects were explained by immunohistochemistry (data not shown). For further confirmation of the presence of amyloid in the wall of some muscle vessels, we also stained with Thioflavin S which showed the localization of amyloid in the same zones dyed with Congo red but in greater quantity (Figure 1(g)).

Transmission electron microscopy (TEM) confirmed amyloid fibrils around perimysial vessels associated with collagen fibrils (Figure 2(a)); endomysial capillaries only showed a thickened wall (Figure 2(b)). On muscle biopsy, immunoelectron microscopy showed a strong staining by polyclonal anti-kappa light chain antibody, thus identifying the fibril type (Figure 2(c)). The abdominal fat pad was negative for the presence of amyloid deposition; on the contrary, the obtained salivary gland biopsies were positive for Congo red staining (Figures 3(a) and 3(b)) as confirmed by immunoelectron microscopy (Figure 3(c)).

A biochemical reevaluation of the patient showed the lack of increase of cardiac serum biomarkers (BNP: 55 pg/ml, normal value: 0–100, and troponin I: <0.01 ng/ml, normal value: 0.01–0.06). Urinary albumin was negative, and a mild CPK increase was noticed. Echocardiography revealed normal left ventricular volume and thickness and a sigmoid-shaped ventricular septum. The systolic function was preserved. A diagnosis of AL amyloidosis with muscle involvement was made, and a treatment with cyclic oral melphalan and dexamethasone was started. The patient is currently under treatment.

3. Discussion

The identification of the muscle as the unique site of amyloid accumulation is a very rare event. In a recent report on 3434 patients diagnosed with AL amyloidosis, 51 (1.5%) had a muscle biopsy positive for amyloid deposition. Among these, amyloid muscle involvement was isolated in 11 patients (22%). Common presenting symptoms of patients with amyloid myopathy are muscle weakness, myalgia, skeletal pseudohypertrophy, dysphagia, macroglossia, jaw claudication, and hoarseness [2]. Our patient showed progressive muscle weakness of lower limbs with subsequent appearance of pain and stiffness at the shoulders and hips and jaw claudication without marked biochemical signs of muscle involvement.

The conclusive diagnosis was systemic AL amyloidosis with myopathic involvement as amyloid deposits were also detected in the salivary gland. However, the myopathy was the only clinical manifestation of the disease because any other symptoms and signs of systemic AL amyloidosis involvement, like cardiac dysfunction or renal proteinuria, were not present. In a recent study, Liewluck and Milone reported that, in nearly 70% of patients with AL amyloidosis muscle involvement, myopathy was the only sign at the clinical presentation [3]. AL systemic amyloidosis-associated myopathy differs from pure isolated amyloid myopathy caused by other amyloidogenic protein subtypes for some clinical characteristics such as older age at onset and less frequent CPK elevation [3].

In this case, the time from the first muscular symptom onset and amyloidosis diagnosis was 25 months. Diagnostic delay of amyloidosis is often reported, as recently described in a patient experience survey where 37.1% of interviewed patients received the correct diagnostic formulation after more than one year from the initial symptoms [4].

In Mayo Clinic case series of biopsy-confirmed muscle AL amyloidosis, the median time from the first disease manifestations and diagnosis was 23 months [2]. Unlike other amyloid proteins, in AL amyloidosis, any organ can be affected by amyloid deposition, and well-defined criteria of

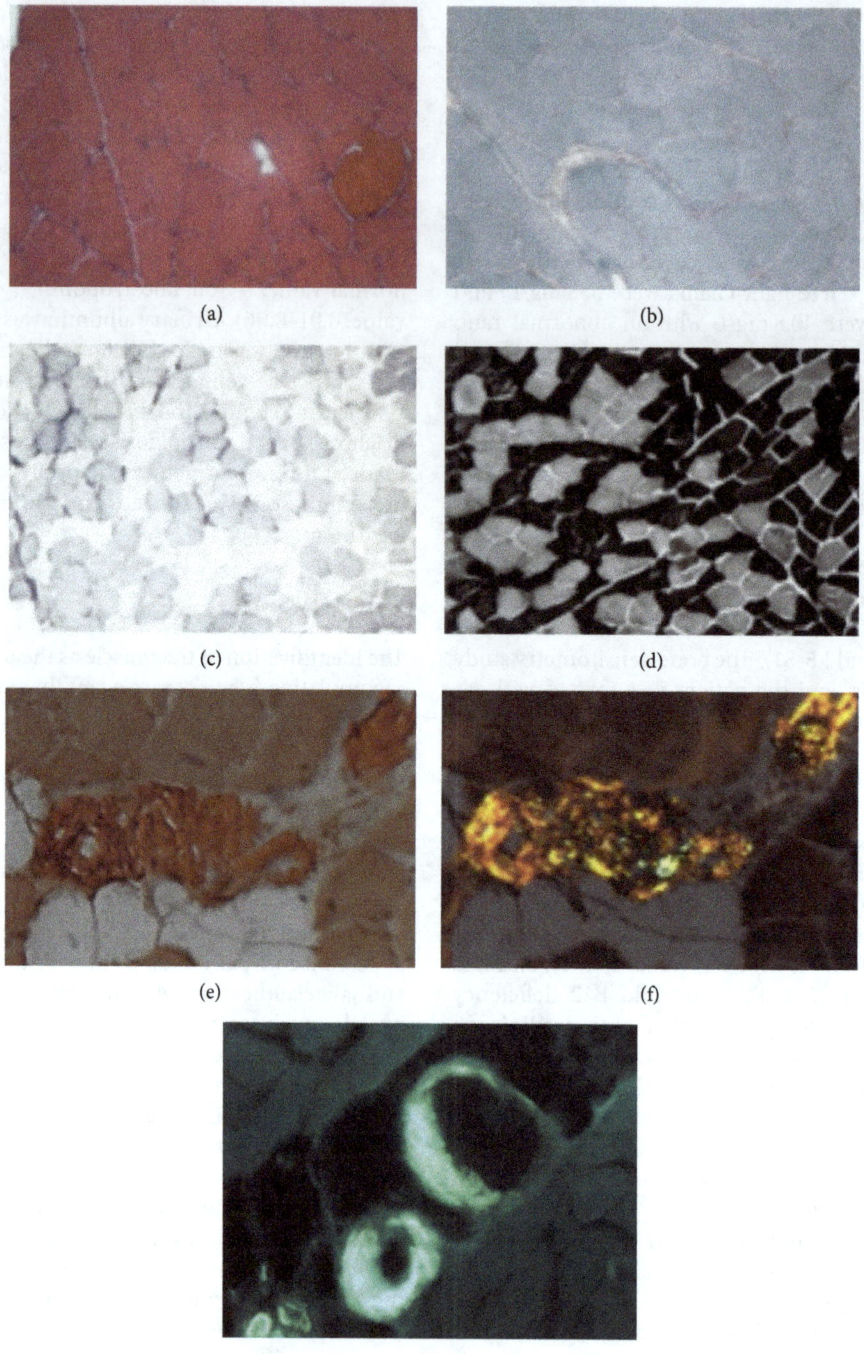

FIGURE 1: Muscle biopsy general features and the presence of amyloid substance. (a) Hematoxylin and eosin staining: the muscle cells show regular morphological characteristics with the exception of one hypercontracted cell; (b) Gomori staining: normal histological picture; (c) succinate dehydrogenase staining (SDH): the staining shows mild changes in myofibrillar texture; (d) ATPase pH 9.4: normal muscle fiber typing and distribution. Congo red staining without (e) or with polarized light (f): presence of amyloid around/inside the wall of perimysial vessels (×20); (g) Thioflavin S staining with fluorescence microscope: amyloid substance appears bright green in dark field. It completely includes the vessel wall of some perimysial arterioles (×20).

organ involvement were described [5, 6]. The diagnostic pitfall may be of particular relevance when the amyloid deposition and the resulting organ damage involve, solely, a less common site such as the striated muscle.

In 19 of 79 cases reviewed by Chapin et al., the initial muscle biopsy was unable to identify the presence of amyloid deposition [7]. This was due to different reasons such as the lack of involvement of that specific muscle district by a "random" biopsy or the absence of Congo staining [8]. In agreement with this observation, Muchtar et al. reported that a different muscle disease was diagnosed in about 40% of the patients before the histological revision [2]. The delay in

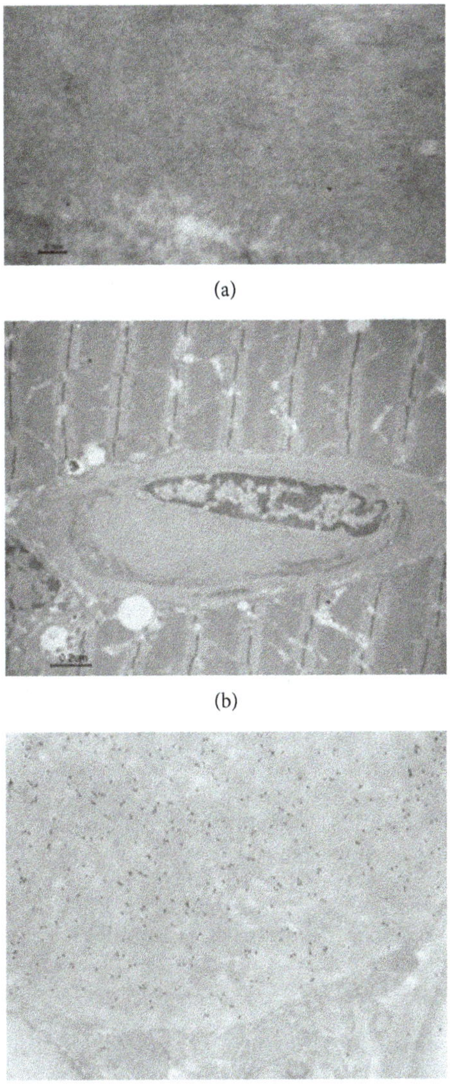

(a)

(b)

(c)

Figure 2: Presence of amyloid fibrils confirmed by electron microscopy. Muscle biopsy was routinely fixed in 2.5% glutaraldehyde in cacodylate buffer, postfixed in osmium tetroxide, and dehydrated and embedded in Araldite; thin sections were studied under Philips CM100 TEM fibrillary structures likely resembling amyloid fibrils in the perimysial pericapillary area (a) (bar = 0.1 μm); an endomysial capillary lumen with a lightly thicker wall without amyloid fibrils (b) (bar = 0.2 μm). Postembedding immunostaining with a polyclonal anti-kappa light chain antibody (Dako, 1 : 100) thin section was studied under a Jeol JEM-1400 Plus electron microscope (c).

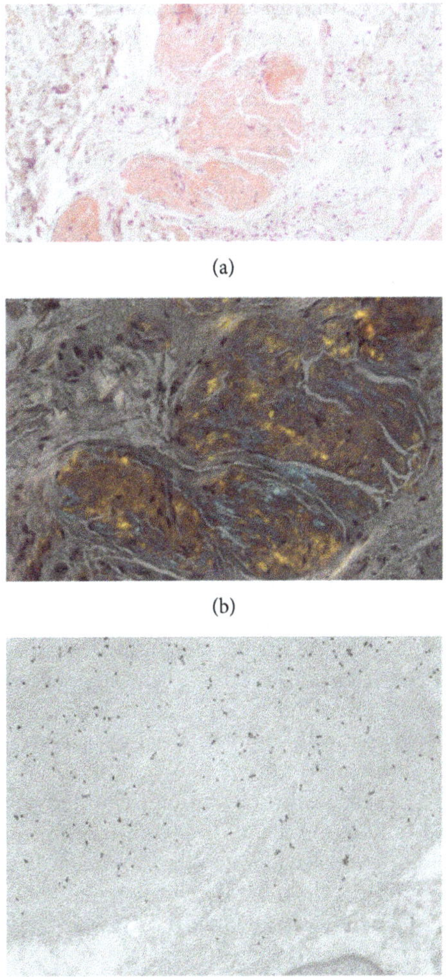

(a)

(b)

(c)

Figure 3: Presence of amyloid in the salivary gland. (a) Hematoxylin and eosin staining: some more dark areas between the muscle fibers are observed (×10). Olympus Bx51 optical microscope. (b) Congo red staining with polarized light: apple green birefringence. (c) Postembedding immunostaining: amyloid fibrils are intensely and specifically immunostained with anti-kappa light chain antibody (Dako, 1 : 100). Jeol JEM-1400 Plus electron microscope.

diagnosis is an important issue and increases the risk of disease aggravation, particularly with cardiac involvement, that determines the disease stage and prognosis [9, 10].

Interestingly, three main clinical presentation patterns of amyloid myopathy are described in literature case series and case reports [2, 7, 11]. The first group reveals the distinctive feature of skeletal pseudohypertrophy with palpable nodules in muscles and "wood-like" atypical consistency often associated with macroglossia. The second group includes patients affected by muscle weakness, predominantly proximal, possibly accompanied by atrophy without other signs of amyloid tissue deposition. The "atrophic form" represents a clinical challenge because the diagnosis is difficult and should take into account all possible differential diagnoses of myopathy [12]. The third group is a mixed clinical phenotype.

The pathophysiological mechanism of muscle fiber injury is poorly clarified. In muscle amyloidosis, the fibril deposition is universally observed on endomysial and perimysial vessels, as in our case, suggesting as a possible mechanism the chronic ischemia derived from endothelial damage [13]. Less frequently described are denervation atrophy and necrotic fibers with regeneration signs [2, 7]. An increase in protein synthesis and cell fusion of human myoblasts in culture was reported by Delaporte et al. after the exposure to a purified kappa chain serum of a patient affected by muscle pseudohypertrophy [14]. A striking characteristic of AL amyloidosis is the enormous inter-patient variability in the protein structure and tissue tropism that was also observed in amyloid proteins derived from the same variable light chain gene. A little change in the amino acid sequence acquired during hypersomatic mutation of immunoglobulin genes may greatly influence the specificity and type of organ damage [15].

In the present case, chemotherapy was promptly started after diagnosis as the therapeutic goals in AL systemic amyloidosis should be the eradication of the underlining clone, the suppression of the production of the dangerous light chain, and the prevention of further organ damage [1].

The accurate characterization of muscle biopsy was essential for the correct diagnosis.

The adoption of Congo red staining, in histopathological examination of an undetermined myopathy, represents an important teaching point in order to avoid a failure in diagnosis. An unexplained muscle disorder in patients with monoclonal gammopathies, by including MGUS, should evoke, among other possible diagnoses, the suspicion of amyloid deposition, and the analysis of biomarkers of early amyloid organ involvement, like albuminuria and cardiac markers, together with abdominal fat or salivary gland biopsies should be performed.

This report suggests that a multidisciplinary approach is the cornerstone of the diagnostic work-up to recognize the rare amyloid myopathy. A stepwise approach to diagnosis and staging of this disorder is critical and involves muscle biopsy, confirmation of amyloid deposition, identification of the fibril type, assessment of underlying amyloidogenic disorder, and evaluation of the extent and severity of amyloidotic organ involvement.

Conflicts of Interest

The authors declare that there are no conflicts of interest.

Acknowledgments

Funding was provided by Associazione Italiana per la Ricerca sul Cancro. The authors thank Giorgio Giaccone from Neuropatologia-Istituto Neurologico C. Besta, Milan, for the support in Figure 1(g).

References

[1] G. Merlini, A. D. Wechalekar, and G. Palladini, "Systemic light chain amyloidosis: an update for treating physicians," *Blood*, vol. 121, no. 26, pp. 5124–5130, 2013.

[2] E. Muchtar, D. Derudas, M. Mauermann et al., "Systemic immunoglobulin light chain amyloidosis–associated myopathy: presentation, diagnostic pitfalls, and outcome," *Mayo Clinic Proceedings*, vol. 91, no. 10, pp. 1354–1361, 2016.

[3] T. Liewluck and M. Milone, "Characterization of isolated amyloid myopathy," *European Journal of Neurology*, vol. 24, no. 12, pp. 1437–1445, 2017.

[4] I. Lousada, R. L. Comenzo, H. Landau, S. Guthrie, and G. Merlini, "Light chain amyloidosis: patient experience survey from the Amyloidosis Research Consortium," *Advances in Therapy*, vol. 32, no. 10, pp. 920–928, 2015.

[5] G. Merlini and V. Bellotti, "Molecular mechanisms of amyloidosis," *New England Journal of Medicine*, vol. 349, no. 6, pp. 583–596, 2003.

[6] M. A. Gertz, R. Comenzo, R. H. Falk et al., "Definition of organ involvement and treatment response in immunoglobulin light chain amyloidosis (AL): a consensus opinion from the 10th International Symposium on Amyloid and Amyloidosis," *American Journal of Hematology*, vol. 79, no. 4, pp. 319–328, 2005.

[7] J. E. Chapin, M. Kornfeld, and A. Harris, "Amyloid myopathy: characteristic features of a still underdiagnosed disease," *Muscle & Nerve*, vol. 31, no. 2, pp. 266–272, 2005.

[8] L. W. Ostrow, A. M. Corse, B. M. Morrison et al., "Expanding the spectrum of monoclonal light chain deposition disease in muscle," *Muscle & Nerve*, vol. 45, no. 5, pp. 755–761, 2012.

[9] A. Dispenzieri, M. A. Gertz, R. A. Kyle et al., "Serum cardiac troponins and N-terminal pro-brain natriuretic peptide: a staging system for primary systemic amyloidosis," *Journal of Clinical Oncology*, vol. 22, no. 18, pp. 3751–3757, 2004.

[10] A. D. Wechalekar, S. O. Schonland, E. Kastritis et al., "A European collaborative study of treatment outcomes in 346 patients with cardiac stage III AL amyloidosis," *Blood*, vol. 121, no. 17, pp. 3420–3427, 2013.

[11] M. A. Gertz and R. A. Kyle, "Myopathy in primary systemic amyloidosis," *Journal of Neurology, Neurosurgery & Psychiatry*, vol. 60, no. 6, pp. 655–660, 1996.

[12] R. J. Walters, "Muscle diseases: mimics and chameleons," *Practical Neurology*, vol. 14, no. 5, pp. 288–298, 2014.

[13] S. Spuler, A. Emslie-Smith, and A. G. Engel, "Amyloid myopathy: an underdiagnosed entity," *Annals of Neurology*, vol. 43, no. 6, pp. 719–728, 1998.

[14] C. Delaporte, B. Varet, M. Fardeau, D. Nochy, and A. Ract, "In vitro myotrophic effect of serum kappa chain immunoglobulins from a patient with kappa light chain myeloma and muscular hypertrophy," *Journal of Clinical Investigation*, vol. 78, no. 4, pp. 922–927, 1986.

[15] S. Enqvist, K. Sletten, F. J. Stevens, U. Hellman, and P. Westermark, "Germ line origin and somatic mutations determine the target tissues in systemic AL-amyloidosis," *PLoS One*, vol. 2, no. 10, article e981, 2007.

Acquired Elliptocytosis as a Manifestation of Myelodysplastic Syndrome with Ring Sideroblasts and Multilineage Dysplasia

Jacob D. Kjelland,[1] Denis M. Dwyre,[2] and Brian A. Jonas[3,4]

[1]*Department of Internal Medicine, University of California Davis Medical Center, Sacramento, CA 98517, USA*
[2]*Department of Pathology, University of California Davis Medical Center, Sacramento, CA 98517, USA*
[3]*Department of Internal Medicine, Division of Hematology and Oncology, University of California Davis Medical Center, Sacramento, CA 98517, USA*
[4]*VA Northern California Health Care System, Mather, CA 95655, USA*

Correspondence should be addressed to Brian A. Jonas; bajonas@ucdavis.edu

Academic Editor: Sudhir Tauro

Acquired elliptocytosis is a known but rarely described abnormality in the myelodysplastic syndromes (MDS). Here we report the case of an elderly male who was admitted to the hospital with chest pain, dyspnea, and fatigue and was found to be anemic with an elliptocytosis that had only recently been noted on peripheral smears of his blood. After bone marrow biopsy he was diagnosed with MDS with ring sideroblasts and multilineage dysplasia and acquired elliptocytosis. Here we report a rare case of acquired elliptocytosis cooccurring with MDS with ring sideroblasts and multilineage dysplasia.

1. Introduction

The myelodysplastic syndromes (MDS) are a heterogeneous group of clonal myeloid hemopathies that result in ineffective development of one or more hematopoietic lineages. The genetic alterations and other pathologic processes in the bone marrow causing dysfunctional hematopoiesis lead to a wide range of disease phenotypes which can range from mild single lineage cytopenia to severe pancytopenia or transformation to acute leukemia. Similarly diverse are the microscopic characteristics of the dysplastic cells in the bone marrow and peripheral blood.

In this report, we present the case of an elderly male who was diagnosed with MDS after being admitted to our hospital for symptomatic anemia. Review of his bone marrow biopsy showed two morphological findings of particular note. The first finding was ring sideroblasts, which are present in about 25% of cases of MDS [1]. Ring sideroblasts are erythroid precursor cells in which iron is unable to be exported from the mitochondria due to one of a variety of defects. This leads to an excess of iron within the mitochondria, which stains with Prussian blue, revealing the so-called ring sideroblast. As with most findings in MDS, ring sideroblasts are not specific to MDS but are found in numerous congenital and acquired conditions encompassing many genetic and acquired defects. Recently, mutations in a gene coding for a portion of the U2 snRNP have been linked to the development of ring sideroblasts in MDS. In one study, *SF3B1*, located on chromosome 2 (http://genome.ucsc.edu) was found to be mutated in 20% of all MDS cases and 65% of those with ring sideroblasts [2]. In another recent study, 81% of MDS subtypes with ring sideroblasts had *SF3B1* mutations [3]. It has been speculated that the mutated protein may cause generalized downregulation of several core pathways within the mitochondria, potentially accounting for the higher frequency of ring sideroblasts observed in patients with mutated *SF3B1* [2]. The second finding in our case was elliptocytosis, a finding which can be hereditary or can be acquired. Hereditary elliptocytosis is caused by mutations in in structural components of the erythrocyte cell membrane. Mutations in genes coding for protein 4.1, alpha spectrin, beta spectrin, band 3, and Glycophorin C have all been implicated in hereditary elliptocytosis [4, 5]. Of note, other hereditary conditions, such as sickle cell anemia, thalassemias, and pyruvate kinase deficiency can have elliptocytosis as a feature [4]. Acquired elliptocytosis is sometimes seen in myeloid malignancies (including MDS) as well as in iron deficiency anemia, megaloblastic anemias, polycythemia, and myelofibrosis [5].

2. Case

A 70-year-old Caucasian male immigrant from Eastern Europe with a 6-year history of anemia and an 8-year history of thrombocytopenia was admitted to our hospital for chest pain and dyspnea. At the time of his admission, his exam was notable for mild scleral icterus and a palpable spleen 2 cm below the costal margin.

He had undergone prior workup for his cytopenias without a clear diagnosis. There was no family history of anemia. He did not use alcohol. His medications included amiodarone and ranolazine (medications associated with bone marrow suppression), but no other medications known to affect hematopoiesis. Records obtained documenting the outpatient workup included studies showing normal vitamin B12 and folate levels, decreased haptoglobin with a negative Coombs test, and a bone marrow biopsy performed 2 years earlier which showed a hypercellular marrow, moderate erythroid hyperplasia, a deletion of chromosome 20q by cytogenetics, 3-4% ring sideroblasts, and normal flow cytometry studies. Based on these findings, there was concern for a pre-MDS state, such as clonal cytopenia of undetermined significance (CCUS). One month prior to admission, a peripheral smear showed elliptocytosis. Physician's notes from the outpatient workup indicate that a peripheral smear was reviewed 2 years earlier and there was no mention of elliptocytosis or spherocytosis at that time.

At time of admission, the patient's hemoglobin was 7.6 g/dL with an MCV of 91.1 μm^3, a platelet count of 28,000/mm^3, white blood cell count of 5,200/mm^3, and absolute neutrophil count of 4,600/mm^3. He had 6.7% reticulocytes with an absolute reticulocyte count of 190,000/mm^3. His total bilirubin was elevated at 4.5 mg/dL with direct bilirubin of 2.4 mg/dL. Transaminases were normal. LDH was elevated at 349 U/L, but haptoglobin levels were normal and a direct Coombs test was negative. Methylmalonic acid level was slightly elevated at 0.48 μmol/L (normal up to 0.40 μmol/L). Thyroid studies and vitamin B12 levels were normal. Folate was not checked. Ferritin was 540 ng/mL, with normal serum iron and transferrin levels. No paroxysmal nocturnal hemoglobinuria clone was detected by peripheral blood flow cytometry. Osmotic fragility was tested and found to be normal. HIV screen was negative. Hematology was consulted for diagnostic assistance. Review of the peripheral smear showed marked elliptocytosis (Figure 1). A bone marrow biopsy was performed which showed a hypercellular marrow with erythroid hyperplasia, dyserythropoiesis and dysmegakaryopoiesis, and adequate stainable iron with >15% ring sideroblasts and 3% blasts (Figure 2). Cytogenetic analysis showed 46,XY,del(20)(q11.2q13.3)/47,idem,+del(20)[6].

Based on these findings, the patient was diagnosed with MDS with ring sideroblasts and multilineage dysplasia (MDS-RS-MLD). His IPSS-R score was 5.5, stratifying him to the high risk IPSS-R group, with an estimated median overall survival of 1.6 years [7]. During his hospital stay he received a total of 2 units of packed red blood cells and 1 unit of platelets, with resolution of his chest pain and dyspnea. Prior to this time, he had not required transfusion for his marrow disorder and had only received blood product transfusions in the postoperative setting (distant open heart surgery and others). He was discharged on hospital day 6 with a follow-up appointment in hematology clinic scheduled. He rescheduled the appointment for unknown reasons and, unfortunately, passed away at home approximately three weeks after discharge. No autopsy was performed.

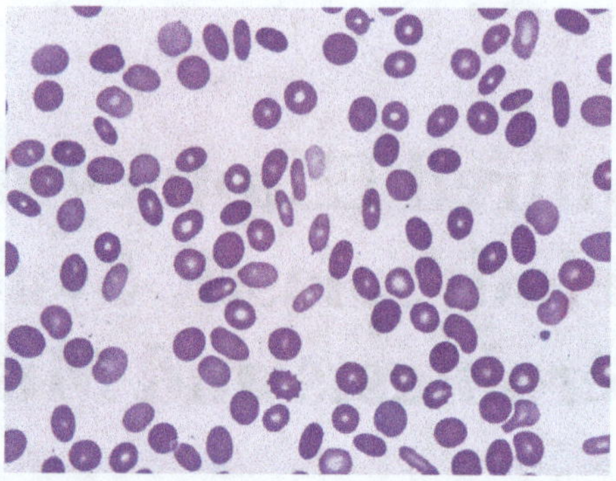

FIGURE 1: Peripheral blood smear (Wright-Giemsa stained, 100x): peripheral smear showing anemia, with numerous elliptocytes and thrombocytopenia.

3. Discussion

Over the last 4 decades, understanding of the pathophysiology of MDS has advanced considerably. As a result, there have been revisions in classification and risk scoring of MDS leading to improvements in the ability of clinicians to offer a more accurate prognosis for affected patients. Still, with the considerable heterogeneity and incomplete understanding of MDS, additional investigations into the mechanisms underlying the development of MDS will likely yield new information and insight into disease progression and refinements to MDS classification.

This case report describes a unique case of acquired elliptocytosis presumably related to MDS, with a high percentage of ring sideroblasts. MDS with ring sideroblasts is a relatively common subtype of MDS, found in approximately 25% of all MDS cases [1]. Acquired elliptocytosis in MDS, however, is rare. Only 14 such cases are available in the literature to date (Table 1). According to the 2016 WHO guidelines, a majority of previously reported cases of acquired elliptocytosis in MDS would be classified as either MDS with single lineage dysplasia or multilineage dysplasia (10 of 14 cases) [8]. The case reported in this paper is classified as MDS with ring sideroblasts and multilineage dysplasia (MDS-RS-MLD) and is now the 15th documented case of acquired elliptocytosis in MDS. Of the 15 cases of MDS with an acquired elliptocytosis,

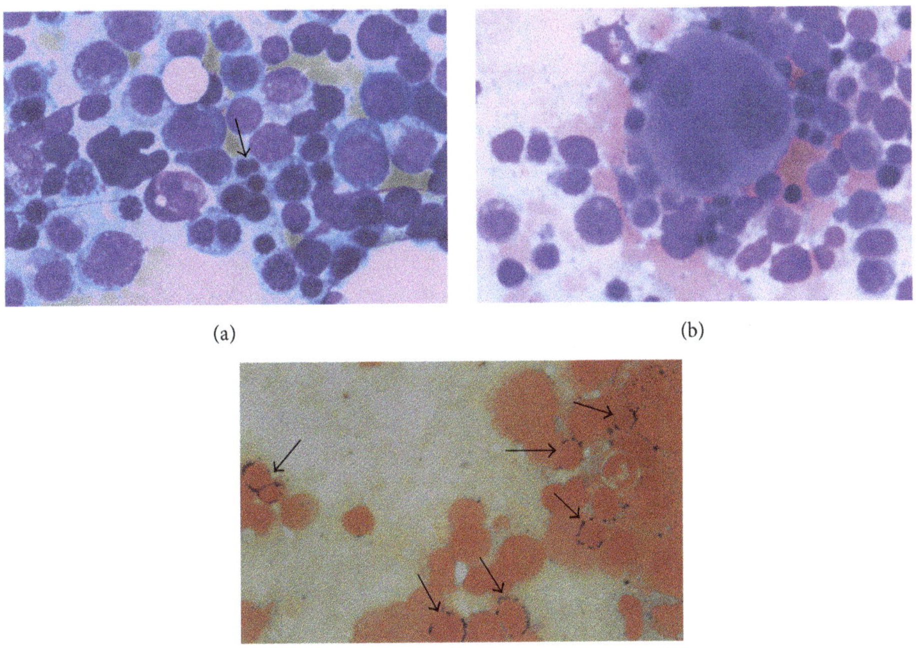

(a) (b) (c)

FIGURE 2: (a) Bone marrow aspirate (Wright-Giemsa stain, 100x). High magnification of the bone marrow aspirate shows a marrow with erythroid hyperplasia, megaloblastic maturation, and a dysplastic erythroid cell (arrow). (b) Bone marrow aspirate (Wright-Giemsa stained, 100x). High magnification of the bone marrow aspirate shows a dysplastic megakaryocyte with separate lobes. (c) Bone marrow aspirate (Iron stain, 100x). The iron stained aspirate shows multiple ring sideroblasts (>15%) (arrows).

14 reported cytogenetics, and, of those 14 patients, 11 had deletions of chromosome 20q.

While the causal factor(s) leading to acquisition of elliptocytosis in cases of MDS have not been definitively identified, several cases have noted decreased levels of human erythroid protein 4.1 in association with del(20q) [9–11]. This protein is a major cytoskeleton component in erythrocytes and reductions in its levels are implicated in a small percentage of cases of hereditary elliptocytosis [4, 5]. Interestingly, the *EPB41* gene, which codes for human erythroid protein 4.1 is found on chromosome 1 (http://genome.ucsc.edu) [9]. Since the common location of lost genetic material in most of the cases of MDS with acquired elliptocytosis is on chromosome 20, it has been hypothesized that the association between del(20q) and reduced levels of human erythroid protein 4.1 is a consequence of loss of factors affecting transcription or splicing of the *EPB41* gene's mRNA [9]. Of note, among the 14 known patients with MDS and acquired elliptocytosis who have cytogenetic data available, only one had a chromosome 1 abnormality and this patient also had a deletion on chromosome 20 [12]. We can speculate that there may be a role for cooperating mutations, possibly involving splice factors such as the one coded for by *SF3B1* and downregulation of *EPB41* or another gene coding for an erythrocyte membrane protein, leading to peripheral elliptocytosis in MDS. Such a mechanism would provide an explanation for the development of elliptocytosis in MDS and at the same time link the seemingly unrelated observations of decreased levels of human erythroid protein 4.1 and deletion of chromosome 20q in MDS with acquired elliptocytosis [9–11]. To evaluate this idea, future cases of MDS with acquired elliptocytosis should be studied using techniques such as next-generation sequencing based myeloid mutation profiling, RNA-sequencing to evaluate mRNA expression, and gene expression profiling.

A correlation between deletions on the long arm of chromosome 20 and acquisition of elliptocytosis in MDS has emerged since the first patient with acquired elliptocytosis in what we now call MDS was reported by Hartz et al. in 1984 (then called preleukemic syndrome) and the first such case where cytogenetic studies were performed by Rummens et al. in 1986 [13, 14]. The focus of this report is on a rare and interesting finding, but it should be noted that chromosome 20 deletions are not uncommon in MDS. Chromosome 20 deletions were found in 7% of MDS cases in one large case series and are common enough to be included as a variable in the IPSS-R for MDS [7, 15]. While del(20q) has been shown to confer good cytogenetic risk, the impact of acquired elliptocytosis on prognosis is unknown and may benefit from further study [16]. The observation that acquired elliptocytosis seems to be related to del(20q) in MDS leads one to question why acquired elliptocytosis is so rare, given that 20q deletions are relatively common in MDS. To our knowledge, this question has yet to be addressed. Future research aimed at resolving this paradox may help to further refine the categorization or risk stratification for patients with MDS if a causative link between del(20q) and acquired elliptocytosis can be established.

Table 1: Characteristics of the current and previously published cases of myelodysplastic syndrome with acquired elliptocytosis.*

Age and gender	FAB classification	2016 WHO classification	Cytogenetics	IPSS-R score	Reported outcome	Reference number
81, male	RA	MDS-like CMML	46,XY,i(14)(q10)[5]/46,XY[35]	3-4 (blasts <5% but may be >2%)	NR	[6]
67, female†	RA-EB	MDS-EB-2	del(20)(q11q13)[20]	5	NR	[17]
72, male	RA	MDS-MLD	NR	0–5 (cytogenetics NR, blasts <5% but may be >2%)	Death, 8 years after diagnosis	[13]
75, male	RA	MDS-MLD	Del(20q)(q11.2)	2-3 (blasts <5% but may be >2%)	NR	[18]
59, male	RA	MDS-MLD	44, XY; -3, -5, 12p+, -15, 17p and 45, XY; -5, 12p+, -15,17p	7	NR	[14]
60, male	RA-EB	MDS-EB-1	Del(20q)	4	Progressed to AML within 1 year of MDS diagnosis, death 1 year later	[14]
82, male	RA	MDS-SLD or MLD	46 XY, del(20q)(q11.2)	1.5–3 (blasts <5% but may be >2%, ANC NR)	NR	[19]
79, male	RA	MDS-SLD or MLD	46 XY, del(20q)(q11.2)	1.5–2.5 (blasts <5% but may be >2%)	NR	[19]
78, male	RA	MDS-SLD or MLD	Del(20)(q11.2)	1-2 (blasts <5% but may be >2%)	NR	[9]
74, female	RA	MDS-SLD or MLD	t(14)	3-4 (blasts <5% but may be >2%)	NR	[9]
77, male	RA	MDS-SLD or MLD	Del(20q)	1-2 (blasts <5% but may be >2%)	NR	[9]
66, male	RA	MDS-U or CCUS	46,XY,del(20)(q11.2)[20]	2.5–3 (ANC NR)	Progressed to RA-EB, achieved remission with therapy	[10]
59, male	RA	MDS-MLD	Del(20q)	2.5–4.5 (platelets NR, blasts <5% but may be >2%)	NR	[11]
72, male	RA	MDS-SLD	+1,der(1;5)(q10;p10),t(1;5)(p10;q10),del(20)(q11)	5	Reported to have remained well for 18 months at publication	[12]
70, male	*RARS*	*MDS –RS-MLD*	*46,XY,del(20)(q11.2q13.3)/47,idem,+del(20)*	*5.5*	*Death, 1 month after diagnosis*	*Currently reported case*

FAB and 2016 WHO classifications were determined using data from published cases. Where data are not sufficient to determine classification, the possible classifications based on available information are shown. IPSS-R score calculated using data from published cases. Where insufficient data is available, the range of possible scores is presented with missing information noted in parentheses. *General abbreviations*: ANC: absolute neutrophil count, MPN: myeloproliferative neoplasm, NA: not applicable, NR: not reported, *FAB abbreviations*: RA: refractory anemia, RA-EB: refractory anemia with excess blasts, RARS: refractory anemia with ring sideroblasts. *WHO 2016 abbreviations*: MDS-SLD: MDS with single lineage dysplasia, MDS-MLD: MDS with multilineage dysplasia, MDS-MLD-RS: MDS with multilineage dysplasia and ring sideroblasts, MDS-EB-1/2: MDS with excess blasts 1 or 2, MDS-U: MDS unclassifiable, AML: acute myeloid leukemia, CMML: chronic myelomonocytic leukemia, CCUS: clonal cytopenia of unclear significance.

*One case not included in this report was classified as MDS/MPN when published in 2008 but would now be classified as AML based on 25% blasts on bone marrow biopsy. †Molecular data available for this case; reported findings included no mutation in *JAK2*, *CALR*, or *MPL*.

Disclosure

The content is solely the responsibility of the authors and does not necessarily represent the official views of the National Institutes of Health.

Conflicts of Interest

The authors declare that there are no conflicts of interest regarding the publication of this article.

Authors' Contributions

Jacob D. Kjelland and Brian A. Jonas designed the study. Denis M. Dwyre contributed the images. Jacob D. Kjelland, Denis M. Dwyre, and Brian A. Jonas wrote and edited the manuscript. All authors agree on the final manuscript.

Acknowledgments

Brian A. Jonas is supported by the National Cancer Institute of the National Institutes of Health under Award no. K12CA138464.

References

[1] I. Navarro, M. A. Ruiz, A. Cabello et al., "Classification and scoring systems in myelodysplastic syndromes: a retrospective analysis of 311 patients," *Leukemia Research*, vol. 30, no. 8, pp. 971–977, 2006.

[2] E. Papaemmanuil, M. Cazzola, J. Boultwood et al., "Somatic SF3B1 Mutation in Myelodysplasia with Ring Sideroblasts," *The New England Journal of Medicine*, vol. 365, no. 15, pp. 1384–1395, 2011.

[3] L. Malcovati, M. Karimi, E. Papaemmanuil et al., "SF3B1 mutation identifies a distinct subset of myelodysplastic syndrome with ring sideroblasts," *Blood*, vol. 126, no. 2, pp. 233–241, 2015.

[4] P. G. Gallagher, "Hereditary elliptocytosis: spectrin and protein 4.1R," *Seminars in Hematology*, vol. 41, no. 2, pp. 142–164, 2004.

[5] W. T. Tse and S. E. Lux, "Red blood cell membrane disorders," *British Journal of Haematology*, vol. 104, no. 1, pp. 2–13, 1999.

[6] M. G. Boavida, P. Ambrósio, D. Dhermy, C. Silva, and M. E. Correia Jr., "Isochromosome 14q in refractory anemia," *Cancer Genetics and Cytogenetics*, vol. 97, no. 2, pp. 155-156, 1997.

[7] P. L. Greenberg, H. Tuechler, J. Schanz et al., "Revised international prognostic scoring system for myelodysplastic syndromes," *Blood*, vol. 120, no. 12, pp. 2454–2465, 2012.

[8] D. A. Arber, A. Orazi, R. Hasserjian et al., "The 2016 revision to the World Health Organization classification of myeloid neoplasms and acute leukemia," *Blood*, vol. 127, no. 20, pp. 2391–2405, 2016.

[9] C. Alanio-Bréchot, P.-O. Schischmanoff, M. Fénéant-Thibault et al., "Association between myeloid malignancies and acquired deficit in protein 4.1R: a retrospective analysis of six patients," *American Journal of Hematology*, vol. 83, no. 4, pp. 275–278, 2008.

[10] M. Hur, K. M. Lee, H. C. Cho et al., "Protein 4.1 deficiency and deletion of chromosome 20q are associated with acquired elliptocytosis in myelodysplastic syndrome," *Clinical and Laboratory Haematology*, vol. 26, no. 1, pp. 69–72, 2004.

[11] H. Ideguchi, Y. Yamada, S. Kondo, K. Tamura, S. Makino, and N. Hamasaki, "Abnormal erythrocyte band 4.1 protein in myelodysplastic syndrome with elliptocytosis," *British Journal of Haematology*, vol. 85, no. 2, pp. 387–392, 1993.

[12] F. Ishida, S. Shimodaira, H. Kobayashi et al., "Elliptocytosis in myelodysplastic syndrome associated with translocation (1;5)(p10;q10) and deletion of 20q," *Cancer Genetics and Cytogenetics*, vol. 108, no. 2, pp. 162–165, 1999.

[13] J. W. Hartz, D. H. Buss, D. R. White, M. G. Bond, and M. Scharyj, "Marked elliptocytosis and schistocytosis in hematopoietic dysplasia," *American Journal of Clinical Pathology*, vol. 82, no. 3, pp. 354–359, 1984.

[14] J. L. Rummens, C. Verfaillie, A. Criel et al., "Elliptocytosis and schistocytosis in myelodysplasia: report of two cases," *Acta Haematologica*, vol. 75, no. 3, pp. 174–177, 1986.

[15] D. Haase, U. Germing, J. Schanz et al., "New insights into the prognostic impact of the karyotype in MDS and correlation with subtypes: evidence from a core dataset of 2124 patients," *Blood*, vol. 110, no. 13, pp. 4385–4395, 2007.

[16] J. Schanz, H. Tüchler, F. Solé et al., "New comprehensive cytogenetic scoring system for primary myelodysplastic syndromes (MDS) and oligoblastic acute myeloid leukemia after MDS derived from an international database merge," *Journal of Clinical Oncology*, vol. 30, no. 8, pp. 820–829, 2012.

[17] R. Boutault and M. Eveillard, "Acquired elliptocytosis in the setting of a refractory anemia with excess blasts and del(20q)," *Blood*, vol. 127, no. 21, p. 2646, 2016.

[18] J. Knight and D. R. Czuchlewski, "Acquired elliptocytosis of myelodysplastic syndrome," *Blood*, vol. 121, no. 4, p. 572, 2013.

[19] M. Baweja, A. Moreno-Aspitia, D. Menke et al., "Marked elliptocytosis in myelodysplastic syndromes (MDS) is associated to deletion of chromosome 20q," *Blood*, vol. 106, article 4927, 2005.

38

Venetoclax in Combination with Decitabine for Relapsed T-Cell Acute Lymphoblastic Leukemia after Allogeneic Hematopoietic Cell Transplant

Leena T. Rahmat ,[1] Anna Nguyen,[2] Haifaa Abdulhaq,[3] Sonam Prakash,[2] Aaron C. Logan,[1] and Gabriel N. Mannis[1]

[1]*Department of Hematologic Malignancies and Blood and Marrow Transplant, University of California, San Francisco, CA, USA*
[2]*Department of Pathology, University of California, San Francisco, CA, USA*
[3]*Department of Hematology and Oncology, University of California, San Francisco, CA, USA*

Correspondence should be addressed to Leena T. Rahmat; leenarahmatmd@gmail.com

Academic Editor: Salah Aref

Long-term disease-free survival in adults with T-cell acute lymphoblastic leukemia (T-ALL) remains poor, particularly after relapse, with few available salvage options. Preclinical data suggest that inhibition of the antiapoptotic protein BCL-2 (B-cell lymphoma 2) either alone or in combination with other agents, may be a unique therapeutic approach for the treatment of T-ALL. We present a case of a young male with T-ALL, relapsed after allogeneic hematopoietic stem cell transplant, who achieved a second complete remission following salvage therapy with combined venetoclax and decitabine. Assessment of measurable residual disease by next generation sequencing showed no evidence of residual disease of a sensitivity of 1×10^{-6}. While the combination of venetoclax and hypomethylating agents has shown promise in the treatment of relapsed/refractory AML, and to our knowledge, this is the first report of this combination demonstrating clinical activity in relapsed/refractory T-ALL.

1. Introduction

T-cell acute lymphoblastic leukemia (T-ALL) is an aggressive hematologic malignancy that accounts for approximately 25% of all adult ALL cases [1]. Despite an improved cure rate in the pediatric ALL population, long-term disease-free survival in adults remains poor [2]. Outcomes for patients with relapsed or refractory T-ALL are particularly dismal, with few available therapeutic options. Recent preclinical studies have demonstrated that inhibition of the antiapoptotic protein BCL-2 (B-cell lymphoma 2) may be a novel therapeutic strategy for the treatment of T-ALL, either alone or in combination with other agents [3, 4]. Venetoclax (ABT-199) is a highly specific BCL-2 inhibitor, currently approved for the treatment of chronic lymphocytic leukemia. Genetic studies in T-ALL have also recognized recurrent somatic alterations involved in DNA methylation and posttranslational histone modifications, suggesting a potential rationale for the combination of venetoclax and hypomethylating agents [5].

2. Case Presentation

A 20-year-old male with no past medical history presented with acute hypoxic respiratory failure requiring intubation. CT scans revealed a 9.1×7.3 cm mediastinal mass encasing the aortic arch with extension into the lower neck resulting in tracheal deviation. Laboratory evaluation demonstrated a white blood cell count of 2.5×10^9/L with 78% blasts on differential, hemoglobin 7.1 g/dL, and platelets 51×10^9/L. Bone marrow evaluation revealed a hypercellular marrow with 98% blasts by morphology. By flow cytometry, blasts expressed CD34, CD117, CD33, CD38, CD56, and CD7 and lacked expression of myeloperoxidase (MPO) and monocytic markers. A subset of blasts expressed low levels of cytoplasmic CD3 although subsequent assessment by immunohistochemistry for CD3 was negative. The blasts were negative for CD2, CD4, CD5, CD8, CD19, and cCD79a. Cytogenetic analysis revealed 10 metaphases with a complex karyotype including rearrangement of chromosome 4, loss of chromosomes 12 and 13, and a rearrangement between chromosome 13 and 1-2 unidentified markers. Molecular testing was positive for a FLT3-ITD mutation. A fine needle aspiration of the mediastinal mass demonstrated acute leukemia with an immunophenotype similar to that of the bone. T-cell gene rearrangement analysis by PCR on the mediastinal biopsy showed no evidence of clonal T-cell gene rearrangement. While it was difficult to assign a definite lineage for this acute leukemia, diagnostic considerations included acute myeloid leukemia (AML), T-ALL, and mixed phenotype acute leukemia T/myeloid (MPAL). To meet criteria for MPAL T/myeloid, blasts must express lineage-defining markers for both T and myeloid lineages [6]. This acute leukemia lacked MPO as well as monocytic markers and therefore did not meet criteria for the myeloid component of MPAL T/myeloid. While flow cytometry demonstrated weak cytoplasmic CD3 on the blasts suggestive of T-lineage differentiation, this could not be confirmed by immunohistochemical stains. Additionally, the blasts lacked expression of CD2, CD4, CD5, CD8, and CD1a. Therefore, a diagnosis of AML, NOS was initially favored.

The patient was induced with daunorubicin in combination with high-dose cytarabine and achieved complete remission (CR). He was consolidated with 2 cycles of high-dose cytarabine and in light of the FLT3-ITD mutation, sorafenib was added. Because his leukemia was considered "poor-risk" given the extramedullary disease at presentation, complex karyotype, and FLT3-ITD mutation, he underwent a 7/10 haploidentical allogeneic hematopoietic cell transplant (alloHCT) from his father in first remission. Conditioning included fludarabine, cyclophosphamide, and low-dose total body irradiation as per the standard Hopkins regimen [7]. Prior to alloHCT, multiparameter flow cytometry from the University of Washington showed no evidence of measurable residual disease (MRD). Post transplant immunosuppression consisted of cyclophosphamide, tacrolimus, and mycophenolate mofetil. A bone marrow biopsy and restaging PET CT at approximately day +60 confirmed an ongoing CR and 100% donor chimerism in the CD3, CD14/15, and CD19 compartments. For posttransplant maintenance, he received 6 cycles azacitidine (given daily for 5 days at 32 mg/m^2 in 28-day cycles)—initiated at approximately day +100—followed by maintenance sorafenib 200 mg twice daily. His tacrolimus was discontinued at approximately 6 months posttransplant with no evidence at any point of either acute or chronic graft-versus-host disease (GVHD).

At 13 months posttransplant, he developed progressive neutropenia. Bone marrow evaluation revealed relapsed leukemia with 42% blasts expressing a slightly different immunophenotype than that of his original disease (CD117-negative and CD5-positive). Immunohistochemical stains on the core biopsy demonstrated that blasts were positive for CD34, TdT, CD5, and CD7, with a small subset that was weakly positive for CD3. Cytogenetic studies demonstrated a complex karyotype similar to that of his original leukemia. FLT3-ITD PCR was negative but extended mutational testing—not previously performed—revealed mutations in FBXW7, NOTCH1, and EZH2, all of which are recurrently mutated in T-ALL [8]. Additionally, bone marrow chimerism studies showed for the first time a decline in CD3 donor chimerism from 100% to 91%.

Based on emerging data to support the use of venetoclax in T-ALL, he began salvage therapy with venetoclax (given daily, initially at 800 mg then dose reduced to 400 mg due to the interaction with his azole for fungal prophylaxis) in combination with decitabine (given daily for 5 days at 20 mg/m^2 in 28-day cycles). After 2 cycles, his peripheral blood counts had normalized, formal CR criteria were met, and a restaging bone marrow evaluation demonstrated no morphologic evidence of residual leukemia. MRD assessment—again performed via multiparameter flow cytometry at the University of Washington—also showed no evidence of persistent disease. CD3 chimerism in the bone marrow was restored to 100% donor.

In light of the lymphoid origin of his relapsed leukemia, next generation sequencing (NGS) was performed (ClonoSEQ, Adaptive Biosciences) on his relapse specimen, identifying a dominant T-cell receptor (TCR) clone comprising 8.249% of total nucleated cells. We retrospectively also assessed his original diagnostic bone marrow specimen and found that the same TCR clone was present in 11% of total nucleated cells. MRD assessment from a bone marrow specimen after 2 cycles of venetoclax and decitabine—also via ClonoSEQ—showed no detectable residual leukemia at a sensitivity of 1 leukemic cell per 10^6 cells. He received a total of 5 cycles of decitabine and venetoclax, with intermittent dose interruptions of venetoclax due to neutropenia. He remained MRD negative via multiparameter flow cytometry and ClonoSEQ and subsequently underwent a second haploidentical alloHCT with fludarabine, cyclophosphamide, and low-dose TBI conditioning. Decitabine and venetoclax were discontinued shortly prior to the second haploidentical alloHCT. He achieved full donor chimerism at day +18 posttransplant and continues in follow-up.

3. Discussion

We present the case of a young male—initially diagnosed with AML, NOS but which, in retrospect, was T-ALL—who achieved a first complete remission following induction chemotherapy and subsequently underwent haploidentical alloHCT. He relapsed 13 months later with disease that was immunophenotypically and genetically consistent with T-ALL. He achieved a second complete remission following 2 cycles of the BCL-2 inhibitor venetoclax in combination with the hypomethylating agent (HMA) decitabine, with no evidence of MRD by either multiparameter flow cytometry or NGS. He remained in remission following completion of 5 cycles of decitabine and venetoclax and subsequently underwent a second haploidentical alloHCT. At the time of this writing, he remains in remission and continues in routine posttransplant follow-up.

While the combination of venetoclax and HMAs have shown significant promise in the treatment of relapsed/refractory AML, to our knowledge, this is the first report of the combination showing clinical activity in relapsed/refractory T-ALL [9]. *In vitro* studies demonstrate that some T-ALL cell lines are highly sensitive to BCL-2 inhibition [4]. One subgroup of T-ALL, early T-cell progenitor (ETP) T-ALL, has historically been characterized by treatment-resistance and high risk for relapse. Preclinical data show that ETP T-ALL is highly BCL-2 dependent and is sensitive to both *in vitro* and *in vivo* treatment with venetoclax [10]. Early T-cell precursors have high expression of BCL-2 but this gradually decreases during normal T-cell differentiation. Variations in venetoclax sensitivity could therefore be mediated in part by varying stages of differentiation arrest between different subtypes of T-ALL [4].

Studies by both Bogenberger et al. [11] and Tsao et al. [12] initially showed that the combination of azacitidine and BCL-2 inhibition synergistically induced apoptosis in AML cells. As monotherapy, HMAs have limited data to support their use in ALL, although several *in vitro* studies suggest that epigenetic regulation may be important in the pathogenesis of ALL [5, 13]. Preclinical studies have shown that promoter regions of several genes associated with biological and prognostic significance in ALL—including the tumor suppressor gene, FHIT (fragile histidine triad), and ERG isoforms—are methylated in ALL and can be demethylated with exposure to hypomethylating agents [14, 15]. The limited clinical data supporting the use of HMAs in ALL include a case report of an adult patient with concurrent MDS and B-ALL who achieved a morphologic remission of both ALL and MDS with azacitidine monotherapy, as well as an older study evaluating the efficacy of single agent azacitidine in a variety of acute leukemias [16]. This study found that only 2 of 23 patients with ALL achieved a CR.

In light of this patient's prior posttransplant exposure to HMAs, it seems unlikely that an HMA alone would have been sufficient to induce an MRD-negative second remission. Although impossible to know if the disease may have responded to venetoclax monotherapy, we hypothesize that—similar to what has been described in the AML setting—venetoclax and HMAs are likely to work synergistically to eradicate relapsed T-ALL [17]. If proven to be effective in larger, prospective studies, the combination of venetoclax and HMAs would be particularly attractive in the posttransplant relapse setting given its relatively nontoxic profile.

4. Conclusion

The prognosis of relapsed/refractory T-ALL is poor, with few available therapeutic options. Preclinical studies have shown both that BCL-2 inhibitors may be effective in T-ALL and that epigenetic regulation plays a role in ALL pathogenesis. In addition to the emerging data suggesting mechanistic synergy between BCL-2 inhibition and HMA therapy in AML, this case provides rationale for further study of venetoclax and HMAs in relapsed T-ALL, particularly in the posttransplant setting.

Conflicts of Interest

The authors declare that there are no conflicts of interest to disclose.

References

[1] C.-H. Pui, M. V. Relling, and J. R. Downing, "Acute lymphoblastic leukemia," *New England Journal of Medicine*, vol. 350, no. 15, pp. 1535–1548, 2004.

[2] S. Faderl, S. O'Brien, C.-H. Pui et al., "Adult acute lymphoblastic leukemia: concepts and strategies," *Cancer*, vol. 116, no. 5, pp. 1165–1176, 2010.

[3] S. Peirs, V. Frismantas, F. Matthijssens et al., "Targeting BET proteins improves the therapeutic efficacy of BCL-2 inhibition in T-cell acute lymphoblastic leukemia," *Leukemia*, vol. 31, no. 10, pp. 2037–2047, 2017.

[4] S. Peirs, F. Matthijssens, S. Goossens et al., "ABT-199 mediated inhibition of BCL-2 as a novel therapeutic strategy in T-cell acute lymphoblastic leukemia," *Blood*, vol. 124, no. 25, pp. 3738–3747, 2014.

[5] S. Peirs, J. Van der Meulen, I. Van de Walle et al., "Epigenetics in T-cell acute lymphoblastic leukemia," *Immunological Reviews*, vol. 263, no. 1, pp. 50–67, 2015.

[6] M. J. Borowitz, M. C. Bene, N. L. Harris et al., "Acute leukemias of ambiguous lineage," in *WHO Classification of Tumours of Haematopoietic and Lymphoid Tissues. Revised Fourth Edition*, S. H. Swerdlow, E. Campo, N. L. Harris et al., Eds., p. 181, IARC Press, Lyon, France, 2017.

[7] P. V. O'Donnell, L. Luznik, R. J. Jones et al., "Nonmyeloablative bone marrow transplantation from partially HLA-mismatched related donors using posttransplantation cyclophosphamide," *Biology of Blood and Marrow Transplantation*, vol. 8, pp. 377–386, 2002.

[8] J. Feng, Y. Li, Y. Jia et al., "Spectrum of somatic mutations detected by targeted next-generation sequencing and their prognostic significance in adult patients with acute lymphoblastic leukemia," *Journal of Hematology & Oncology*, vol. 10, no. 1, p. 61, 2017.

[9] C. D. DiNardo, K. W. Pratz, A. Letai et al., "Safety and preliminary efficacy of venetoclax with decitabine or azacitidine in elderly patients with previously untreated acute myeloid leukemia: a non-randomised, open-label, phase 1b study," *The Lancet Oncology*, vol. 19, no. 2, pp. 216–228, 2018.

[10] T. N. Chonghaile, J. E. Roderick, C. Glenfield et al., "Maturation stage of T-cell acute lymphoblastic leukemia determines BCL-2 versus BCL-XL dependence and sensitivity to ABT-199," *Cancer Discovery*, vol. 4, no. 9, pp. 1074–1087, 2014.

[11] J. M. Bogenberger, S. M. Kornblau, W. E. Pierceall et al., "BCL-2 family proteins as 5-azacitidine-sensitizing targets and determinants of response in myeloid malignancies," *Leukemia*, vol. 28, no. 8, pp. 1657–1665, 2014.

[12] T. Tsao, Y. Shi, S. Kornblau et al., "Concomitant inhibition of DNA methyltransferase and BCL-2 protein function synergistically induce mitochondrial apoptosis in acute myelogenous leukemia cells," *Annals of Hematology*, vol. 91, no. 12, pp. 1861–1870, 2012.

[13] G. Garcia-Manero, S. Jeha, J. Daniel et al., "Aberrant DNA methylation in pediatric patients with acute lymphocytic leukemia," *Cancer*, vol. 97, no. 3, pp. 695–702, 2003.

[14] R. W. Stam, M. L. den Boer, and M. M. Passier, "Silencing of the tumor suppressor gene FHIT is highly characteristic for MLL gene rearranged infant acute lymphoblastic leukemia," *Leukemia*, vol. 20, no. 2, pp. 264–271, 2006.

[15] A. Bohne, C. Schlee, and M. Mossner, "Epigenetic control of differential expression of specific ERG isoforms in acute T-lymphoblastic leukemia," *Leukemia Research*, vol. 33, no. 6, pp. 817–822, 2009.

[16] K. Paulson, R. Kumar, A. Ahsanuddin et al., "Azacitidine as a novel agent in the treatment of acute lymphoblastic leukemia," *Leukemia & Lymphoma*, vol. 52, no. 1, pp. 136–138, 2011.

[17] J. M. Bogenberger, D. Delman, N. Hansen et al., "Ex vivo activity of BCL-2 family inhibitors ABT-199 and ABT-737 combined with 5-azacytidine in myeloid malignancies," *Leukemia & Lymphoma*, vol. 56, no. 1, pp. 226–229, 2015.

Solitary Lytic Bone Metastasis: A Rare Presentation of Small Lymphocytic Leukemia

Heather Katz,[1] Steven Sagun,[2] Doreen Griswold,[3] and Mohamed Alsharedi[1]

[1]*Department of Hematology/Oncology, Joan C. Edwards School of Medicine Marshall University, 1600 Medical Center Dr, Huntington, WV 25701, USA*
[2]*Joan C. Edwards School of Medicine Marshall University, 1600 Medical Center Dr, Huntington, WV 25701, USA*
[3]*Department of Pathology, Joan C. Edwards School of Medicine Marshall University, 1600 Medical Center Dr, Huntington, WV 25701, USA*

Correspondence should be addressed to Heather Katz; katzh@marshall.edu

Academic Editor: Massimo Breccia

Chronic lymphocytic leukemia (CLL)/small lymphocytic lymphoma (SLL) is a hematologic malignancy characterized by an over accumulation of incompetent neoplastic lymphocytes. Bone metastasis in CLL/SLL is very rare. We report a case of a 76-year-old Caucasian female presented with an unresolving pulmonary infiltrate with mediastinal lymphadenopathy concerning for malignancy. Positron emission tomography (PET)/computed tomography (CT) showed an infiltrative mass in the mediastinum with diffuse uptake and a hypermetabolic mass within the left iliac bone. Transbronchial biopsy revealed morphology and features of SLL. However, with concern for another primary cancer, a CT-guided biopsy of the PET avid left iliac bone was performed and revealed bone and marrow with involvement of CLL/SLL similar to the chest lymphadenopathy. To our knowledge and after extensive review of medical literature, this is first reported case of SLL with solitary bone metastasis to the hip.

1. Introduction

Chronic lymphocytic leukemia (CLL)/small lymphocytic lymphoma (SLL) is an insidious malignancy in which the bone marrow produces too many lymphocytes thus accruing neoplastic lymphocytes within the lymph nodes, blood, or bone marrow [1, 2]. CLL/SLL is currently the most common leukemia in the USA and will account for approximately one-third of all adult leukemia incidences in 2018 [1–3]. Identification of ≥5000 lymphocytes per μL with proper immunophenotype is diagnostic CLL while SLL requires lymphadenopathy and/or splenomegaly with <5000 lymphocytes per μL in the peripheral blood [2, 4, 5]. Bone metastasis in CLL/SLL is very rare, generally osteolytic, and affects less than 5% of CLL patients [6–9]. We report a very rare case of a 76-year-old female who was incidentally found to have diffuse lymphadenopathy on imaging, subsequently diagnosed with CLL/SLL and found to have a solitary left iliac bone lesion consistent with CLL/SLL.

2. Case Report

A 76-year-old Caucasian female with a past medical history of chronic obstructive pulmonary disease (COPD), hypertension, and osteoarthritis had developed a COPD exacerbation requiring steroids and antibiotics. Her primary care physician ordered a chest X-ray (CXR) due to persistent cough and abnormal breath sounds on physical exam. The CXR revealed a moderate-sized infiltrate in the inferior portion of lingular segment which likely represented a pneumonic infiltrate. She was treated with a 10-day course of antibiotics. Repeat chest X-ray revealed minimal clearing of parenchymal infiltrate from the lingular segment. A subsequent computed tomography (CT) scan of the chest showed evidence of residual infiltrative changes involving the right middle lobe as well as the lingular division of the left upper lobe. There was also evidence of diffuse low-attenuation density involving the mediastinum highly suggestive of diffuse adenopathy which was concerning for lymphoma.

At initial consultation by oncology, her vital signs were stable, and she denied B symptoms including fevers, night sweats, and weight loss. She denied any hemoptysis or worsening shortness of breath. Physical exam was unremarkable with no palpable cervical, axillary, or inguinal adenopathy or hepatosplenomegaly, and respiratory exam was clear to auscultation bilaterally. CBC with differential showed a white blood cell count of $4.4 \times 10\,mm^3$ with an absolute lymphocyte count of $0.66 \times 10\,mm^3$, hemoglobin of 13.7 gm/dL, and platelet count of $178 \times 10\,mm^3$. She had an unremarkable complete metabolic panel (CMP) and mildly elevated lactate dehydrogenase (LDH) at 235. Due to concern for lymphoma and findings on CT of the chest, a PET/CT was ordered which showed an infiltrative mass in the mediastinum with diffuse uptake (maximum standardized uptake value (SUV) 5.94 (Figure 1).

There were small lymph nodes in the left axilla showing low level uptake with maximum SUV 1.73 and 1.52, respectively. Finally, there was a hypermetabolic mass within the left iliac bone with a maximum SUV 11.71 (Figure 2).

She underwent an endobronchial ultrasound and transbronchial biopsy of station 7 lymph node which revealed lymphoid tissue composed of small, mitotically inactive cells with round to slightly irregular nuclear contours and scant cytoplasm (Figure 3).

Flow cytometric analysis demonstrated an abnormal CD5+ B cell population. Immunohistochemical stains showed that the cells were positive for CD20 (Figure 4) and CD5 (Figure 5) and negative for Cyclin D1 (Figure 6).

Scattered CD3 positive T cells were also present. The morphology and phenotype supported the diagnosis of small lymphocytic leukemia (SLL). Since SLL does not typically present with bone lesions and there was concern for another primary cancer, a CT-guided biopsy was performed of the PET avid left iliac bone. Pathology from that biopsy showed both bone and marrow with involvement of CLL/SLL (Figure 7).

Flow cytometry from the left iliac bone biopsy revealed monoclonal kappa light chain restricted B-cell population phenotypically consistent with CLL/SLL (Figure 8).

No specific abnormalities were detected by CLL fluorescence in situ hybridization (FISH) including centromere 12, 13q14 (DLEU1), ATM/11q, TP53/17p13, and CCNDQ/IGH–t(11; 14).

Currently, she does not have cytopenias, B symptoms, or bulky disease; however, there was concern that the mediastinal adenopathy may be contributing to her pulmonary symptoms and that the left hip lesion was causing discomfort. Consequently, systemic therapy was offered as was radiation to the hip; however, the patient declined and opted for observation and close surveillance. She will return for further evaluation of symptoms and laboratory data in 2 months.

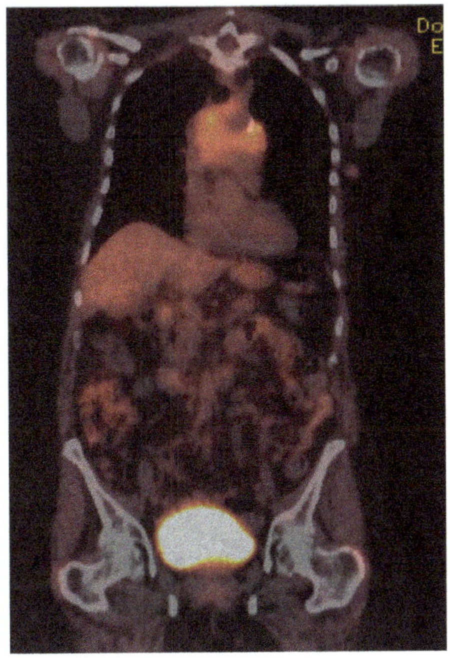

Figure 1: PET/CT with an infiltrative mass in the mediastinum with diffuse uptake.

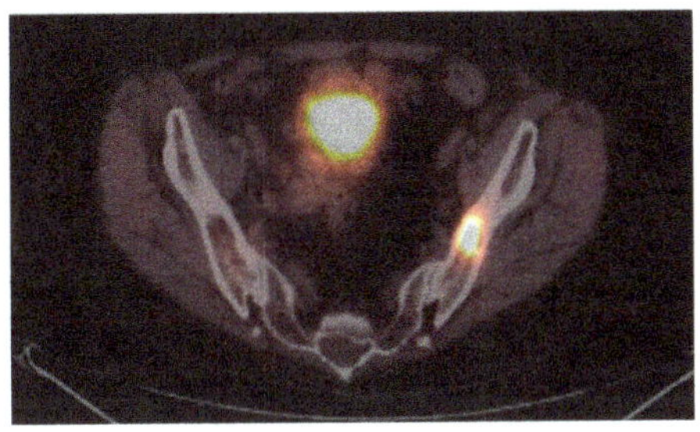

Figure 2: PET CT with hypermetabolic mass within the left iliac bone.

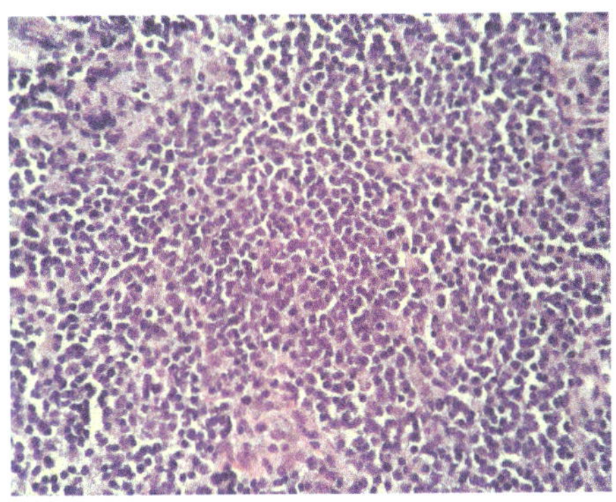

Figure 3: Hematoxylin and eosin stain: lymphoid tissue composed of small, mitotically inactive cells with round to slightly irregular nuclear contours and scant cytoplasm.

3. Discussion

CLL/SLL is a chronic disease characterized by an over accumulation of small dysfunctional neoplastic lymphocytes. Hypothesized pathogenesis of the dysfunctional lymphocytes includes environmental factors, chromosomal deletions, genetic or epigenetic modifications, and altered miRNA expression [1, 2]. The resulting lymphoproliferation causes harm to the patient due to suboptimally functioning B-cells

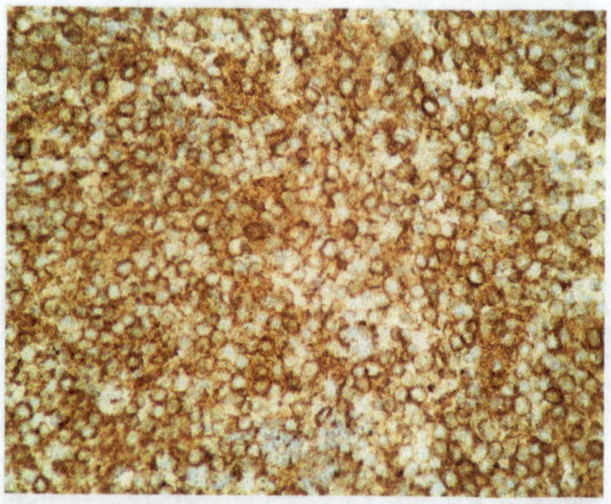

Figure 4: Immunohistochemistry positive for CD20.

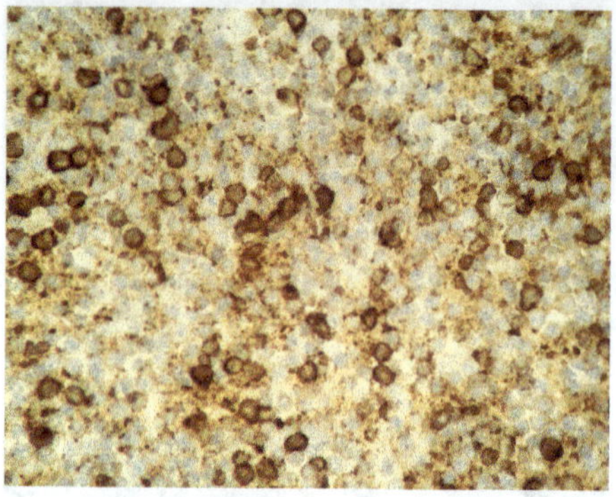

Figure 5: Immunohistochemistry positive for CD5.

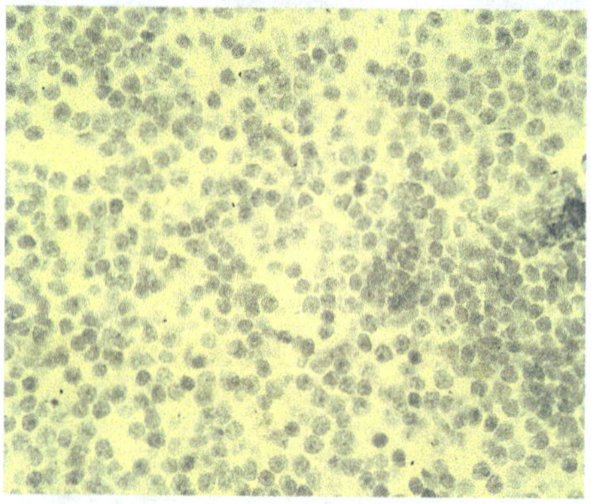

Figure 6: Immunohistochemistry negative for Cyclin D1.

and overcrowding of the blood, bone marrow, lymph nodes [2].

CLL/SLL is currently the most common leukemia in the USA and will account for approximately one-third of all adult leukemia incidence in 2018 [1–3]. The median age at diagnosis is 70 years, and there is a 1.7 : 1 male: female ratio [1, 4]. The symptoms and signs of CLL/SLL are variable. Although many patients are asymptomatic at time of diagnosis, late-stage CLL/SLL can present with B symptoms (fever, night sweats, and weight loss), lymphadenopathy, hepatosplenomegaly, or skin lesions. The most common laboratory abnormalities are lymphocytosis, anemia, and thrombocytopenia, or hypogammaglobulinemia [2, 10].

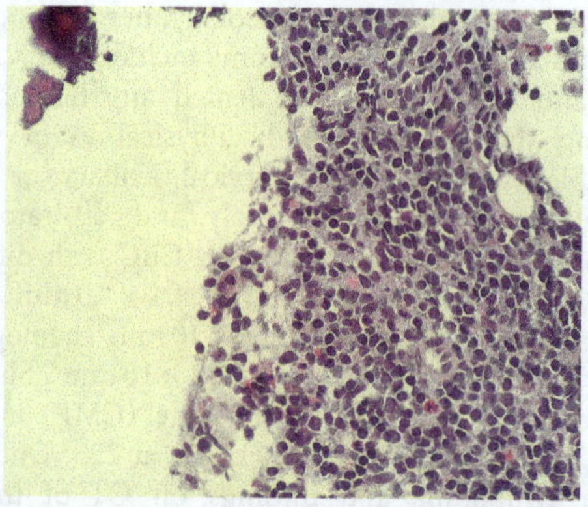

Figure 7: Hematoxylin and eosin stain: a malignant infiltrate of small, mitotically inactive lymphocytes replacing the marrow space in the biopsy from left iliac bone.

The workup for CLL/SLL includes a complete blood count (CBC) with differential, peripheral smear evaluation, and flow cytometry of the atypical lymphocytes. Identification of ≥5000 B-cells per μL with proper immunophenotype is diagnostic of CLL while SLL requires lymphadenopathy and/or splenomegaly with <5000 B-cells per μL in the peripheral blood with proper immunophenotype [2, 4, 5]. The typical immunophenotype of CLL is CD5 positive, CD23 positive, CD10 negative, CD19 positive, CD20 dim, surface immunoglobulin dim positive, and cyclin D1 negative [2, 4, 5].

While CLL is the most common leukemia, CLL associated solitary lytic bone lesions are very uncommon and affects less than 5% of CLL patients [6–9]. Secondary nonlymphoid malignancies should also be considered, and large retrospective cohort studies have shown increased relative risk and prevalence of lung cancer in CLL patients [11].

Bone lesions associated with CLL are generally osteolytic, and the pathogenesis of bone osteolysis is thought to be caused by localized osteoclast stimulating factors and cytokines released by the abnormal lymphocytes [1, 6, 9, 12, 13]. Narayan et al. suggests that CLL bone lesions are most common in the axial skeleton and proximal long bones [6]. A review of 14 case reports supports this hypothesis as 87% of the reviewed cases were CLL bone lesions involving the axial skeleton or proximal long bones [6–9, 12–16]. The most common site of metastasis was to the femur and vertebral column [6–9, 12–16]. In 70% of the reports, patients had multiple bone lesion sites [6–9, 12–16]. After extensive review of the literature, solitary lytic bone lesions of the hip from SLL/CLL were not reported.

4. Conclusion

Solitary bone lesions due to chronic lymphocytic leukemia are extremely rare, and this is the first case presenting as a solitary hip lesion. This case highlights the importance of a multidisciplinary and comprehensive workup in patients who present with mediastinal lymphadenopathy and solitary bone lesions. We sought to highlight this case for its rarity

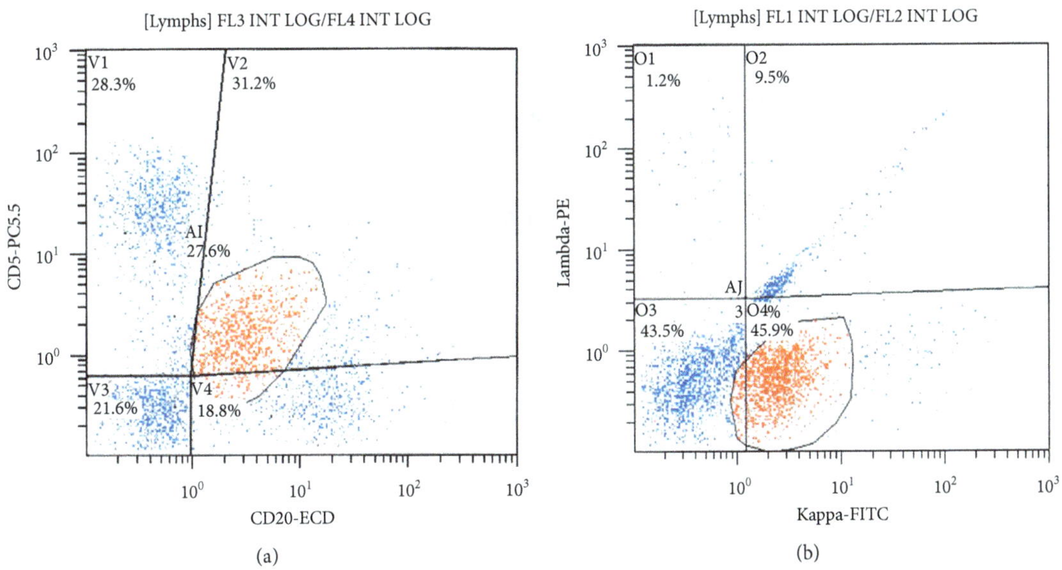

FIGURE 8: Flow cytometry from the left iliac bone biopsy revealed monoclonal kappa light chain restricted B-cell population phenotypically consistent with CLL/SLL.

and unusual presentation and to add further information in the literature about atypical metastatic involvement in SLL/CLL.

Conflicts of Interest

The authors declare that they have no conflicts of interest.

References

[1] C. S. Boddy and M. Shuo, "Frontline therapy of CLL: evolving treatment paradigm," *Current Hematologic Malignancy Reports*, vol. 13, no. 2, pp. 69–77, 2018.

[2] T. J. Kipps, F. Stevenson, C. J. Wu et al., "Chronic lymphocytic leukaemia," *Nature Reviews Disease Primers*, vol. 3, p. 16096, 2016.

[3] R. L. Siegel, K. D. Miller, and A. Jemal, "Cancer statistics," *CA: A Cancer Journal for Clinicians*, vol. 68, no. 1, pp. 7–30, 2018.

[4] M. Hallek, "Chronic lymphocytic leukemia: 2015 update on diagnosis, risk stratification, and treatment. Annual Clinical updates in hematological malignancies," *American Journal of Hematology*, vol. 90, no. 5, pp. 447–460, 2015.

[5] National Comprehensive Cancer Network, "Chronic lymphocytic leukemia/small lymphocytic lymphoma," *NCCN Guidelines Version*, vol. 5, 2018.

[6] H. Narayan, D. Bandyopadhyay, K. Schmidt et al., "Successful treatment of a patient with chronic lymphocytic leukaemia (CLL) presenting with bony metastases with aggressive antibody and chemotherapy," *Clinical and Laboratory Haematology*, vol. 27, no. 6, pp. 405–408, 2005.

[7] G. Hatouma, C. Meshkinb, S. Alkhunaizib, R. Levenec, and J. Formoso-Onofrioc, "The risk of misdiagnosing the primary site responsible for bone metastases in patients with chronic lymphocytic leukemia and a second primary carcinoma," *World Journal of Oncology*, vol. 6, no. 2, pp. 332–334, 2015.

[8] C. H. Dunphy, Y. V. Oza, and M. E. Skelly, "Previously undescribed form of B-cell chronic lymphoid leukemia with IgA expression/secretion and lytic bone lesions," *American Journal of Hematology*, vol. 55, no. 4, pp. 208–211, 1997.

[9] P. McMillen and G. Mundy, "Hypercalcaemia and osteolytic bone lesions in chronic lymphocytic leukaemia," *BMJ*, vol. 281, no. 6248, p. 1107, 1980.

[10] K. R. Rai, A. Sawitsky, E. P. Cronkite, A. D. Chanana, R. N. Levy, and B. S. Pasternack, "Clinical staging of chronic lymphocytic leukemia," *Blood*, vol. 46, no. 2, pp. 219–234, 1975.

[11] C. A. Dasanu and D. T. Alexandrescu, "Risk for second nonlymphoid neoplasms in chronic lymphocytic leukemia," *Medscape General Medicine*, vol. 9, no. 4, p. 35, 2007.

[12] G. Alanoglu, S. Dagdas, Z. Aki, F. Yagmurlu, and G. Ozet, "Hypercalcemia and multiple pathological fractures in chronic lymphocytic leukaemia: a case report," *Turkish Journal of Haematology*, vol. 20, no. 3, pp. 167–170, 2003.

[13] P. Soni, N. Aggarwal, A. Rai et al., "Chronic lymphocytic leukemia: a rare cause of pathological fracture of the femur," *Journal of Investigative Medicine High Impact Case Reports*, vol. 5, no. 4, article 2324709617735135, 2017.

[14] J. Redmond, D. P. Stites, J. H. Beckstead, C. B. George, C. H. Casavant, and D. R. Gandara, "Chronic lymphocytic leukemia with osteolytic bone lesions, hypercalcemia, and monoclonal protein," *American Journal of Clinical Pathology*, vol. 79, no. 5, pp. 616–620, 1983.

[15] T. Jiya, R. B. Van, S. Sugihara, D. P. Van, R. Manoliu, and P. Wuisman, "Lumbar intervertebral disc involvement in chronic lymphocytic leukemia. A case report," *Spine*, vol. 23, no. 17, pp. 1895–1899, 1998.

[16] V. Yau, M. Christakis, N. Ismiil, E. Chow, S. Sedhev, and A. Cuthbert, "Chronic lymphocytic leukemia resembling metastatic bone disease-- an unusual manifestation," *Journal of Pain and Symptom Management*, vol. 26, no. 6, pp. 1074–1076, 2003.

Incorporating Cystatin C to Predict Methotrexate Elimination in Patients with CNS Lymphoma and Suspicious Renal Function

Jason N. Barreto[1] **Allison L. McClanahan,**[2] **Andrew D. Rule,**[3,4] **Carrie A. Thompson,**[2] **and Erin Frazee**[1,5]

[1]*Department of Pharmacy, Mayo Clinic, Rochester, MN, USA*
[2]*Division of Hematology, Department of Internal Medicine, Mayo Clinic, Rochester, MN, USA*
[3]*Division of Nephrology and Hypertension, Department of Internal Medicine, Mayo Clinic, Rochester, MN, USA*
[4]*Division of Epidemiology, Department of Health Sciences Research, Mayo Clinic, Rochester, MN, USA*
[5]*Robert D. and Patricia E. Kern Center for the Science of Health Care Delivery, Mayo Clinic, Rochester, MN, USA*

Correspondence should be addressed to Jason N. Barreto; barreto.jason@mayo.edu

Academic Editor: Akimichi Ohsaka

High-dose methotrexate (MTX; ≥1 g/m^2) is a renally eliminated and nephrotoxic first-line therapy for central nervous system (CNS) lymphoma. Creatinine-based estimation of renal function is the recommended approach to dosing MTX in these cases, but nonrenal determinants of creatinine production and elimination in cancer patients such as malnutrition and cachexia lead to overestimation of glomerular filtration rate (GFR) by this method and a heightened risk for drug toxicity. Serum cystatin C is one of the first readily available, relatively inexpensive, endogenous biomarkers to emerge as a practical adjunct to creatinine for estimation of renal function for drug dosing. In this report, we describe two cases where cystatin C was used in conjunction with creatinine to inform MTX dosing for CNS lymphoma. In both cases, the estimated GFR was nearly 40% lower with the combination of the two biomarkers compared to creatinine-only estimates. Empiric MTX dose reductions as a product of these results likely spared the patients sustained exposure to toxic drug concentrations and facilitated earlier administration of supportive care interventions. Further prospective investigations with validated dosing regimens including cystatin C are warranted for high-dose MTX.

1. Introduction

High-dose methotrexate (MTX) is currently the treatment of choice for central nervous system (CNS) lymphoma [1]. Although the dose for MTX has ranged in previous studies from 3.5–12 g/m^2, doses in excess of 1 g/m^2 have been shown to achieve sufficient CNS penetration for prophylaxis and treatment of lymphoma [2]. MTX is a renally eliminated, nephrotoxic antineoplastic agent that requires an accurate assessment of preexisting kidney function as determined by glomerular filtration rate (GFR) for optimal dosing [3]. Use of high-dose MTX in patients with unrecognized renal dysfunction could lead to acute kidney injury (AKI), increased risk of systemic toxicity from prolonged drug exposure, and an extended hospitalization due to prolonged MTX clearance [4]. Exposure to exceedingly high concentrations of MTX for a protracted period of time is known to cause dermatitis, hepatitis, debilitating mucositis, and life-threatening myelosuppression [4, 5].

A serum creatinine-based estimation of GFR calculated using the Cockcroft-Gault (CG) formula is the recommended equation to estimate renal function when determining the MTX dose for a patient with CNS lymphoma [6, 7]. Measured creatinine clearance with a timed urine collection may also be used, but it is cumbersome, time consuming, and may be inaccurate in patients without an indwelling urinary catheter. Creatinine production is often reduced in patients with malignancies due to reduced skeletal muscle mass (the source

TABLE 1: Laboratory values for patients longitudinally followed with serum creatinine and cystatin C during methotrexate administration for treatment of CNS lymphoma.

Day	SCr (mg/dL)	CysC (mg/L)	UOP (mL/kg/hr)[a]	eGFR-CG (mL/min)	eGFR CKD EPI_{cysC} mL/min/1.73 m^2	eGFR CKD EPI_{cysC} mL/min	eGFR CKD $EPI_{cr\text{-}cysC}$ mL/min/1.73 m^2	eGFR CKD $EPI_{cr\text{-}cysC}$ mL/min	MTX (μmol/L)
Case 1 (51-year-old male, 172 cm, 72.7 kg, BSA 1.88 m^2)									
−1	0.4	1.81	5.46	>120	37	40	69	75	—
0	<0.4	—	4.48	>120	—	—	—	—	—
1	<0.4	—	5.36	>120	—	—	—	—	—
2	0.4	1.86	5.41	>120	35	38	68	74	0.44
3	<0.4	1.94	4.79	>120	33	36	66	72	0.18
4	<0.4	1.46	4.30	>120	49	53	81	88	0.16
5	<0.4	1.64	4.81	>120	42	46	75	82	0.13
6	<0.4	—	2.08	>120	—	—	—	—	0.12
7	0.2	1.63	2.15	>120	42	46	86	93	0.07
Case 2 (38-year-old male, 177 cm, 78.6 kg, BSA 1.97 m^2)									
−1	1.3	1.99	—	87	34	39	47	54	—
0	1.1	1.76	2.99	101	40	46	56	64	—
1	1.6	1.85	2.23	70	38	43	44	50	—
2	1.2	1.92	2.65	93	36	41	50	57	1.7
3	1.1	1.85	4.00	101	38	43	54	61	0.21
4	1.1	1.88	2.99	101	37	42	54	61	0.16
5	—	—	3.26	—	—	—	—	—	0.10

CKD EPI = Chronic Kidney Disease Epidemiology Collaborative; eGFR-CG = estimated GFR calculated from the Cockcroft-Gault equation; CysC = cystatin C; eGFR = estimated glomerular filtration rate; MTX = methotrexate; SCr = serum creatinine; [a]the daily fluid balance for Case 1 ranged from −5.1 L to +2.1 L and for Case 2 from −1.6 L to +2.4 L.

of creatinine generation), and acute or chronic deconditioning, which can lead to overestimation of GFR with serum creatinine [8]. Cystatin C is one of the first endogenous GFR markers to emerge as a practical alternative to creatinine in the last several decades. It is much less influenced by muscle mass than creatinine, though it does have different nonrenal confounders. Its use has been widely validated across the continuum of care, and evidence indicates that the combined use of serum creatinine and cystatin C to estimate GFR more accurately predicts true renal function than use of either marker alone [9].

It is unclear whether use of cystatin C combined with serum creatinine to estimate GFR at the time of MTX dosing could more accurately predict MTX concentrations than a standard creatinine-only approach. More complete characterization of a patient's renal profile surrounding MTX administration could be the first step to identifying methods to optimize both efficacy and safety of this drug for CNS lymphoma and other malignancies. Herein, we present two cases with CNS lymphoma where the Chronic Kidney Disease Epidemiology Collaborative equation with both serum creatinine and cystatin C (CKD $EPI_{Cr\text{-}CysC}$) was used for GFR estimation at the time of MTX dosing and throughout the therapy.

2. Case Presentation

2.1. Case 1. A 51-year-old (172 cm, 72.7 kg) man with a history of diffuse large B-cell lymphoma (DLBCL) presented with acute neurologic decline including a witnessed generalized tonic-clonic seizure prompting hospital admission. The patient underwent an extensive workup encompassing 28 days of persistent functional decline and progressive paralysis. The investigation concluded with a sural nerve biopsy that revealed neurolymphomatosis (DLBCL) with secondary nerve microvasculitis.

The decision was made to treat with 8 grams/m^2 and administer 15 grams of MTX based on a CG estimated creatinine clearance of >120 mL/min calculated using a serum creatinine of <0.4 mg/dL (comparable to available creatinine values in 1 month prior to admission) and body surface area (BSA) of 1.88 m^2. Unfortunately, dysautonomia associated with the neurologic syndrome precipitated a hypotensive event requiring vasopressor support and a delay of chemotherapy. This acute decompensation prompted increased scrutiny of the patient's renal function beyond standard serum creatinine measurements. A cystatin C measurement returned at 1.81 mg/L, which indicated a CKD $EPI_{Cr\text{-}CysC}$ eGFR of 69 mL/min/1.73 m^2 (70 mL/min). The MTX dose was subsequently decreased by 20% to 12 grams in accordance with the impaired renal function. MTX was administered followed by leucovorin rescue according to protocol [7]. Routine monitoring included daily serum creatinine and cystatin C concentrations, urine output, and serum MTX concentrations 48 hours after the infusion initiation and every 24 hours thereafter. On day +2 of MTX therapy, serum creatinine remained 0.4 mg/dL, cystatin C was 1.86 mg/L (CKD $EPI_{Cr\text{-}CysC}$ eGFR of 68 mL/min/1.73 m^2, 74 mL/min), and the corresponding serum MTX level was 0.44 μmol/L (desired level < 0.1 μmol/L). Daily serum MTX concentrations are shown in Table 1. During this timeframe, the patient experienced mild hypokalemia, grade 1 elevation in aspartate aminotransferase without clinically evident symptoms. MTX concentrations were measured until a level of <0.1 μmol/L was achieved at day +6 at which point supportive care measures (leucovorin, intravenous fluids, sodium bicarbonate, and furosemide) were discontinued. Continued observation over the next 7 days demonstrated no change in the patient's neurologic status, and rituximab (375 mg/m^2) in combination with 5 days of high-dose methylprednisolone (1 gram) were administered. Unfortunately, the patient still showed no improvement over the next several days. The decision was made to pursue comfort measures, and the patient expired soon after.

2.2. Case 2. A 38-year-old (177 cm, 78.6 kg) man with a history of relapsed Burkitt's lymphoma with neurolymphomatosis, positive CSF cytology, and likely parenchymal disease based on imaging was admitted for high-dose MTX 8 grams/m^2 as part of combination chemotherapy. During the previous admission for cycle-1 day 1, 15.8 grams of MTX was administered based on a CG estimated creatinine clearance of >90 mL/min calculated using a serum creatinine of 1.2 mg/dL and BSA of 1.97 m^2. The 48-hour MTX concentration from this first dose in the cycle was elevated at 5.1 μmol/L, which resulted in a prolonged hospital length of stay until day +8 when the level had fallen to less than 0.1 μmol/L. With the exception of severe nausea and vomiting, the patient experienced no clinical or laboratory abnormalities. By day +8, his nausea and vomiting had resolved, and the patient was discharged.

Evaluation prior to dose 2 (cycle 1, day 15) revealed no appreciable changes to body habitus or serum creatinine concentration. The recommended dose would have again been 15.8 grams of MTX, but given the previous elevations in serum MTX concentrations, an empiric 20% dose decrease was planned and a cystatin C was checked. The serum cystatin C measurement prior to dose 2 was 1.99 mg/L corresponding to a CKD EPI$_{Cr\text{-}CysC}$ estimated GFR of 47 mL/min/1.73 m^2 (54 mL/min). Based on this information, the MTX dose was reduced an additional 30% to 9 grams and leucovorin rescue was preemptively increased from the standard 25 mg to 100 mg every 6 hours and ordered to start 24 hours after the MTX infusion as per protocol.

As with Case 1, routine monitoring included daily serum creatinine and cystatin C concentrations, urine output, a serum MTX concentration at day +2 and as clinically indicated thereafter. On day +2 of MTX therapy (cycle 1 day 17), serum creatinine increased to 1.6 mg/dL from 1.1 mg/dL while cystatin C remained steady at 1.85 mg/L and the serum MTX level returned at 1.7 μmol/L. Throughout treatment with dose 2, the patient never experienced any adverse clinical effects. By day +5, the MTX concentration declined to the goal level of less than 0.1 μmol/L, and the patient was discharged without signs and symptoms of any toxicity. Unfortunately, shortly after this discharge, the patient returned to an outpatient visit with debilitating leg pain and a white blood cell count of 52,400 cells/mm^3 and was confirmed to have disease progression. Systemic combination chemotherapy was changed to rituximab, gemcitabine, vinorelbine, and prednisone.

3. Discussion

These two cases highlight the potential utility of cystatin C to assist with drug dosing in patients with lymphoma receiving MTX. In both of these circumstances, the serum creatinine and corresponding estimated CG creatinine clearance overestimated the patients' GFR. In the second case, an overestimated creatinine-based GFR led to a larger MTX dose than what was appropriate, resulting in a prolonged hospital stay. In both cases, cystatin C incorporated into the GFR estimation predicted more acceptable serum concentrations of MTX.

An accurate assessment of renal function is critical at the time of MTX initiation to ensure that the selected dose optimizes tumor kill without subjecting the host to unnecessary toxicity [10]. Although direct GFR measurement with an exogenous agent such as iothalamate would be ideal, application of this method to all patients receiving nephrotoxic pharmacotherapies is time intensive, resource demanding, and impractical in most acute care settings [11]. Even approximation of GFR with a 24 h urinary creatinine clearance is challenging due to urine collection errors, extended intervals of time needed for the collection, and delayed turnaround for results [12]. Therefore, the current recommended tool to estimate drug elimination at the bedside is serum creatinine [13]. However, there are many nonrenal factors that contribute to altered serum creatinine production and elimination, particularly in patients with malignancy, which can lead to a greater risk for an inaccurate renal estimate [8]. Cystatin C is an endogenous low-molecular weight protein produced at a constant rate by all nucleated cells. Unlike creatinine which undergoes proximal tubular secretion in addition to filtration thus overestimating GFR, cystatin C is freely filtered in the glomerulus and >99% is reabsorbed and catabolized in proximal tubular cells [14]. Non-GFR determinants of cystatin C and creatinine differ, with the former being less influenced by body composition and nutritional status, but more affected by inflammation and cell turnover [15–17]. Cystatin C distribution is confined to the extracellular space rather than the more broadly distributed serum creatinine. This volume of distribution difference confers a kinetic advantage to cystatin C and suggests that it could more rapidly respond to changes in underlying kidney function than creatinine [18]. As cystatin C is recommended for use in many settings including in the confirmatory diagnosis of chronic kidney disease, it is widely accessible, reasonably priced, has a standardized and validated assay and internet-based publicly available calculators exist to derive a GFR estimate.

Some studies have suggested that cystatin C could serve as a marker for disease activity and prognosis in lymphoma, independent of renal function [19, 20]. However, recent data indicated that cystatin was not associated with overall survival in patients with DLBCL [21]. Furthermore, cystatin C was found to be a useful marker of renal function in pediatric patients receiving methotrexate [22].

Single plasma MTX concentrations which exceed 0.99 μmol/L between 42 and 48 hours after drug administration have been associated with a higher incidence of MTX toxicity [23]. Additionally, the total duration of exposure to MTX concentrations greater 0.1 μmol/L is a primary determinant of consequent bone marrow suppression [5]. Delayed recognition of toxicity is a missed opportunity to institute supportive measures such as increased leucovorin dose to limit the severity of complications [10]. Since the optimal dose of methotrexate remains unknown, it is important to accurately evaluate all pharmacokinetic parameters, including drug clearance, in order to minimize toxicity without compromising efficacy until prospective, randomized trials can compare superiority of one dose to another [2]. In Case 2, the elevated baseline cystatin C, despite a normal creatinine clearance, prompted an MTX dose decrease that was even greater than that originally planned (44% instead of 20%) and a preemptive increase of leucovorin (100 mg every 6 hours instead of 25 mg every 6 hours). Even though the serum MTX concentration was still elevated at 48-hours (1.7 μmol/L, goal < 1.0 μmol/L), this empiric dose adjustment and supportive care strategy were the likely explanation for a more limited degree and duration of exposure in dose 2 relative to dose 1 (5 days versus 8 days, resp.). One could assume that if the dose had only been reduced by 20%, the 48-hour methotrexate concentration would have been much higher than observed, which would have resulted in prolongation of supportive care and an extended hospitalization.

4. Conclusion

Serum creatinine-based estimated GFR may overestimate true renal function in patients with lymphoma due to low-serum creatinine concentrations in the setting of reduced skeletal muscle mass and cachexia. Use of serum cystatin C as a method to more comprehensively characterize a patient's GFR to inform MTX dosing represents a novel approach to improve care delivery. Although our cases show promise with this strategy, given that dosing regimens were originally developed using creatinine-based estimates of GFR, prospective investigations of MTX dosing regimens based on cystatin C inclusive GFR estimates are needed. Further studies should seek to clarify to what degree serial cystatin C concentrations would be of utility in such patients.

Conflicts of Interest

The authors declare that they have no conflicts of interest to disclose.

References

[1] J. L. Rubenstein, N. K. Gupta, G. N. Mannis, A. K. LaMarre, and P. Treseler, "How I treat CNS lymphomas," *Blood*, vol. 122, no. 14, pp. 2318–2330, 2013.

[2] S. Dalia, S. Price, P. Forsyth, L. Sokol, and M. Jaglal, "What is the optimal dose of high-dose methotrexate in the initial treatment of primary central nervous system lymphoma?," *Leukemia & Lymphoma*, vol. 56, no. 2, pp. 500–502, 2015.

[3] M. A. Perazella and G. W. Moeckel, "Nephrotoxicity from chemotherapeutic agents: clinical manifestations, pathobiology, and prevention/therapy," *Seminars in Nephrology*, vol. 30, no. 6, pp. 570–581, 2010.

[4] S. C. Howard, J. McCormick, C. H. Pui, R. K. Buddington, and R. D. Harvey, "Preventing and managing toxicities of high-dose methotrexate," *Oncologist*, vol. 21, no. 12, pp. 1471–1482, 2016.

[5] H. M. Pinedo and B. A. Chabner, "Role of drug concentration, duration of exposure, and endogenous metabolites in determining methotrexate cytotoxicity," *Cancer Treatment Reports*, vol. 61, pp. 709–715, 1977.

[6] D. W. Cockcroft and M. H. Gault, "Prediction of creatinine clearance from serum creatinine," *Nephron*, vol. 16, no. 1, pp. 31–41, 1976.

[7] T. Batchelor, K. Carson, A. O'Neill et al., "Treatment of primary CNS lymphoma with methotrexate and deferred radiotherapy: a report of NABTT 96-07," *Journal of Clinical Oncology*, vol. 21, no. 6, pp. 1044–1049, 2003.

[8] N. Lameire, W. Van Biesen, and R. Vanholder, "Acute renal problems in the critically ill cancer patient," *Current Opinion in Critical Care*, vol. 14, no. 6, pp. 635–646, 2008.

[9] J.-J. Zhu, E. R. Gerstner, D. A. Engler et al., "High-dose methotrexate for elderly patients with primary CNS lymphoma," *Neuro-Oncology*, vol. 11, no. 2, pp. 211–215, 2009.

[10] A. Nirenberg, C. Mosende, B. M. Mehta et al., "High-dose methotrexate with citrovorum factor rescue: predictive value of serum methotrexate concentrations and corrective measures to avert toxicity," *Cancer Treatment Reports*, vol. 61, pp. 779–783, 1977.

[11] E. R. Gerstner, K. A. Carson, S. A. Grossman, and T. T. Batchelor, "Long-term outcome in PCNSL patients treated with high-dose methotrexate and deferred radiation," *Neurology*, vol. 70, no. 5, pp. 401-402, 2008.

[12] D. E. Gerber, S. A. Grossman, T. Batchelor, and X. Ye, "Calculated versus measured creatinine clearance for dosing methotrexate in the treatment of primary central nervous system lymphoma," *Cancer Chemotherapy and Pharmacology*, vol. 59, no. 6, pp. 817–823, 2007.

[13] G. R. Matzke, G. R. Aronoff, A. J. Atkinson et al., "Drug dosing consideration in patients with acute and chronic kidney disease-a clinical update from Kidney Disease: Improving Global Outcomes (KDIGO)," *Kidney International*, vol. 80, no. 11, pp. 1122–1137, 2011.

[14] M. Mussap and M. Plebani, "Biochemistry and clinical role of human cystatin C," *Critical Reviews in Clinical Laboratory Sciences*, vol. 41, no. 5, pp. 467–550, 2004.

[15] L. A. Stevens, C. H. Schmid, T. Greene et al., "Factors other than glomerular filtration rate affect serum cystatin C levels," *Kidney International*, vol. 75, no. 6, pp. 652–660, 2009.

[16] A. Segarra, J. de la Torre, N. Ramos et al., "Assessing glomerular filtration rate in hospitalized patients: a comparison between CKD-EPI and four cystatin C-based equations," *Clinical Journal of the American Society of Nephrology*, vol. 6, no. 10, pp. 2411–2420, 2011.

[17] J. S. Chew-Harris, C. M. Florkowski, P. M. George, J. L. Elmslie, and Z. H. Endre, "The relative effects of fat versus muscle mass on cystatin C and estimates of renal function in healthy young men," *Annals of Clinical Biochemistry*, vol. 50, no. 1, pp. 39–46, 2013.

[18] O. Tenstad, A. B. Roald, A. Grubb, and K. Aukland, "Renal handling of radiolabelled human cystatin C in the rat," *Scandinavian Journal of Clinical and Laboratory Investigation*, vol. 56, no. 5, pp. 409–414, 1996.

[19] A. Mulaomerović, A. Halilbašić, E. Čičkušić, T. Zavašnik-Bergant, L. Begić, and J. Kos, "Cystatin C as a potential marker for relapse in patients with non-Hodgkin B-cell lymphoma," *Cancer Letters*, vol. 248, no. 2, pp. 192–197, 2007.

[20] A. Softic, L. Begic, A. Halilbasic, T. Vižin, and J. Kos, "The predictive value of cystatin C in monitoring of B non-hodgkin lymphomas: relation to biochemical and clinical parameters," *ISRN Oncology*, vol. 2013, Article ID 752792, 6 pages, 2013.

Refractory Abdominal Pain in a Patient with Chronic Lymphocytic Leukemia: Be Wary of Acquired Angioedema due to C1 Esterase Inhibitor Deficiency

Abdullateef Abdulkareem,[1] Ryan S. D'Souza,[2] Joshua Mundorff,[1] Pragya Shrestha,[1] Oluwaseun Shogbesan,[1] and Anthony Donato[1]

[1]*Department of Medicine, Reading Hospital, West Reading, PA, USA*
[2]*Department of Anesthesiology, Mayo Clinic Hospital, Rochester, MN, USA*

Correspondence should be addressed to Abdullateef Abdulkareem; dayo.abdulkareem@readinghealth.org

Academic Editor: Kate Khair

Acquired angioedema due to C1 inhibitor deficiency (C1INH-AAE) is a rare and potentially fatal syndrome of bradykinin-mediated angioedema characterized by episodes of angioedema without urticaria. It typically manifests with nonpitting edema of the skin and edema in the gastrointestinal (GI) tract mucosa or upper airway. Edema of the upper airway and tongue may lead to life-threatening asphyxiation. C1INH-AAE is typically under-diagnosed because of its rarity and its propensity to mimic more common abdominal conditions and allergic reactions. In this article, we present the case of a 62-year-old male with a history of recently diagnosed chronic lymphocytic leukemia (CLL) who presented to our hospital with recurrent abdominal pain, initially suspected to have *Clostridium difficile* colitis and diverticulitis. He received a final diagnosis of acquired angioedema due to C1 esterase inhibitor deficiency due to concomitant symptoms of lip swelling, cutaneous nonpitting edema of his lower extremities, and complement level deficiencies. He received acute treatment with C1 esterase replacement and icatibant and was maintained on C1 esterase infusions. He also underwent chemotherapy for his underlying CLL and did not experience further recurrence of his angioedema.

1. Introduction

Acquired angioedema due to C1 esterase inhibitor deficiency (C1INH-AAE) is a rare and potentially fatal disorder caused by acquired consumption of C1 esterase inhibitor. Studies estimate a prevalence rate between 1 in 100,000 and 1 in 500,000 patients, although it may be higher as the condition is commonly unrecognized [1]. It may manifest with nonpitting edema of the skin, including the skin of the face, lips, limbs, or genitals, abdominal pain secondary to edema of the gastrointestinal mucosa, and severe life-threatening edema of the upper airway and oral mucosa [2].

2. Case Presentation

A 62-year-old male with a two-month history of recurrent hospital admissions for abdominal pain presented to the emergency room with colicky, generalized abdominal pain. He also reported new asymmetric swelling of his upper and lower lips. He denied associated difficulty swallowing or breathing. He had no previous history of angioedema, food allergies, or new medications. He denied any fever, chills, malaise, trauma, nausea, vomiting, diarrhea, constipation, hematochezia or melena, weight loss, sick contacts, neurological deficits, or recent travel history. Of note, he had never taken angiotensin-converting enzyme inhibitors (ACEi) or angiotensin receptor blocker medications. He was a former smoker and quit 14 years ago and reported only occasional alcohol intake. He had no family history of angioedema. This was the third hospital admission for abdominal pain episodes within six weeks, with prior episodes spontaneously resolving within a few days.

Six weeks prior to current presentation, a computed tomography (CT) scan of the abdomen for a prior bout of this illness revealed diffuse small bowel thickening with mild adjacent mesenteric fat stranding and a thickened, nodular terminal ileum and cecum. He also had a positive *Clostridium difficile* stool toxin test. He was treated with metronidazole for *C. difficile* colitis although diarrhea was not a prominent symptom. Two weeks prior to current presentation, he was admitted for recurrent abdominal pain for which another CT was performed, and on this one, he was found to have severe jejunal edema, new proctocolitis, and several enlarged mesenteric and inguinal lymph nodes. The lymph nodes were biopsied and found to have CD5-positive cells consistent with a new diagnosis of chronic lymphocytic leukemia/small lymphocytic lymphoma (CLL/SLL), later confirmed by bone marrow biopsy. The patient was again treated for presumed *C. difficile* colitis, due to another positive stool toxin test, this time with oral vancomycin. He also received a course of amoxicillin-clavulanate as CT abdomen showed extensive diverticulosis and evidence of sigmoid colitis, introducing the possibility of diverticulitis. Evaluation during that admission included esophagogastroduodenoscopy (EGD) and push enteroscopy. Both were unremarkable except for previously known Barrett's esophagus. Interestingly, he also had asymmetric left lower limb cutaneous swelling and pain during that admission that had an unrevealing workup including a negative Doppler ultrasound.

During the current presentation, vital signs were normal with oxygen saturation at 95% on room air. Physical examination revealed lungs that were clear to auscultation without stridor. Symmetric upper and lower lip swelling without hives was noted (Figure 1). The central abdomen was mildly tender to palpation two inches above the umbilicus with no guarding or rebound. No edema was noted in the lower extremities during this current admission. All other systems examined were normal.

3. Investigations

Complete blood count revealed a white blood count of 4900/μL (normal: 4,800–10,800/μL), hemoglobin of 12.4 (normal: 14–17.5 g/dL), and platelets of 149,000 (normal: 130,000–400,000/μL). Lactic acid, sedimentation rate, C-reactive protein, lipase, and liver function tests were normal. Considering the bouts of unexplained bowel edema and swelling lips without hives, a diagnostic workup for angioedema was pursued. Functional C1 esterase inhibitor level was found to be 4% (normal: >40%), along with C1 esterase inhibitor antigen of <3 mg/dl (normal: 21–39 mg/dl), C4 complement < 1.7 mg/dl (normal: 12–38 mg/dl), and low normal C1q level of 113 μg/ml (normal: 109–242 μg/ml). C3 complement level was normal at 88.6 mg/dl (normal: 59–152 mg/dl). *C. difficile* stool toxin test during this admission was negative. Stool samples were also negative for *Salmonella*, *Shigella*, *Escherichia coli*, *Campylobacter*, *Yersinia enterocolitica*, *Giardia*, *Vibrio*, and *Aeromonas*. CT abdomen and pelvis (Figure 2) showed jejunal enteritis with progressive duodenitis and stable abdominopelvic lymphadenopathy. A repeat C1q level performed 6 months later was low at <50 μg/ml (109–242 μg/ml).

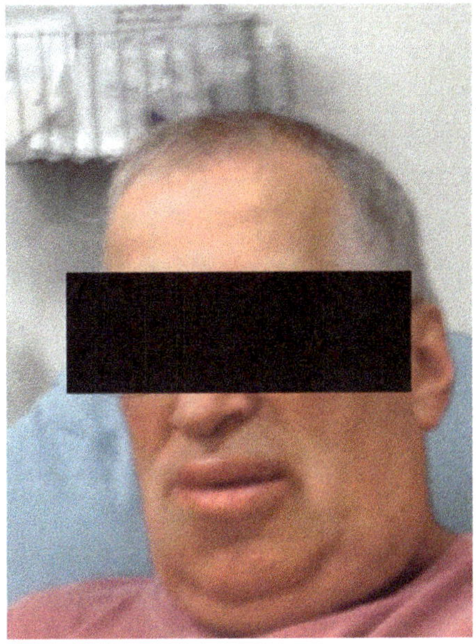

FIGURE 1: Patient with symmetric lip swelling of upper and lower lips.

4. Differential Diagnosis

Given the patient's history of positive *C. difficile* stool tests, a diagnosis of *C. difficile* colitis was initially assigned, although repeat stool toxin assay was negative. Diverticulitis, acute pancreatitis, peptic ulcer disease, acute cholecystitis, and inflammatory bowel syndrome were excluded based on clinical history, negative biochemical and stool tests, EGD, and CT abdomen/pelvis results. Stool studies were negative for bacterial or parasitic infection that could otherwise explain the CT scan findings. Viral gastroenteritis was considered although patient denied any nausea, vomiting, or diarrhea, and symptoms appeared to be recurrent.

Since nonspecific abdominal pain was accompanied with symptoms of lip swelling and recent cutaneous swelling in his lower extremities, a suspicion was formed of angioedema. Allergic angioedema was excluded as the patient denied urticaria and exposure to precipitating agents and had abnormal complement levels in his serum. Similarly, the presence of low C1-INH levels [3] and the absence of ACEi use excluded ACEi-induced angioedema. Hereditary angioedema (HAE) was unlikely because our patient denied a family history of angioedema and experienced onset of symptoms in his 6th decade, as opposed to before the 2nd decade which is more typical of HAE [4].

5. Treatment

Patient was urgently administered intravenous methylprednisolone 125 mg and benadryl. Once a diagnosis of acquired C1 esterase deficiency was made, he received C1 esterase replacement and icatibant (a bradykinin B_2 receptor antagonist). He was subsequently maintained on C1 esterase replacement therapy and given rescue injections of icatibant for acute exacerbations. He also received outpatient chemotherapy for his CLL/SLL with six cycles of rituximab, cyclophosphamide,

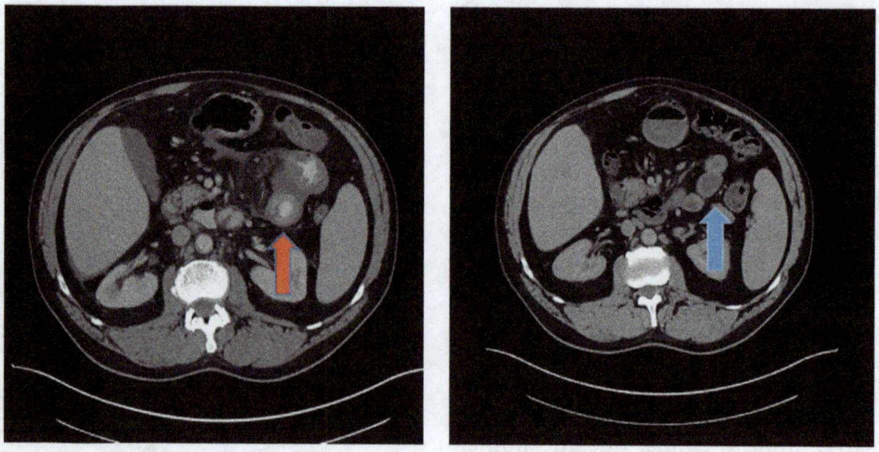

(a) (b)

FIGURE 2: CT abdomen findings before and after treatment. (a) Before treatment, the patient was noted to have jejunal enteritis, which is indicated by the target sign (red arrow). (b) After treatment, the patient had resolution of jejunitis (blue arrow).

vincristine, and prednisone (R-CVP). He had no further episodes of abdominal pain, lip swelling, or lower extremity swelling. Interval imaging with CT abdomen showed resolution of jejunitis and duodenitis (Figure 2).

6. Discussion

Approximately half of patients with C1INH-AAE may have upper airway edema, and consequently death from asphyxiation or anoxic brain injury can occur in up to 30% of patients [3, 5, 6]. However, more benign and nonspecific presentations of GI angioedema and cutaneous edema may be the only manifesting symptoms. GI symptoms of angioedema include nonspecific colicky abdominal pain, vomiting, diarrhea, and abdominal distension [2], which can be mistaken for common abdominal conditions such as gastroenteritis and diverticulitis. Cutaneous edema may manifest as nonpitting edema of the skin, usually affecting the face but may also involve the lower extremities, mimicking allergic reactions and thrombophlebitis.

Because the diagnosis is extremely uncommon and its symptoms are protean, there is frequently a delay in diagnosis. A retrospective nationwide study in France found a median delay in diagnosis of 10 months [3], whereas a national audit in the United Kingdom showed a diagnostic delay of 5 years [7]. Our patient was diagnosed within only 2 months of symptom onset, but after three hospital admissions and incorrect diagnoses of *C. difficile colitis* and diverticulitis.

The key pathologic abnormality in C1INH-AAE is the acquired deficiency of C1-inhibitor enzyme (C1-INH). A major function of C1-INH is the inhibition of kallikrein, which is a protease that cleaves kininogen and releases bradykinin [8]. Consequently, in C1-INH deficiency, the absence of inhibition of kallikrein leads to increased bradykinin levels, which then facilitate vasodilation and increased tissue permeability, resulting in angioedema flares [8]. C1-INH deficiency in acquired angioedema (AAE) may be caused by excessive consumption due to hyperactivation of the classic complement pathways associated with underlying lymphoproliferative diseases or by autoantibodies (autoimmune mediated). Both lymphoproliferative disorders and autoantibodies frequently coexist in the same patients and one may lead to the other [9–11]. Our patient did not have antibodies tested, but he did have CLL (a lymphoproliferative disease).

Laboratory findings include low C1-INH activity, low C3 and C4 levels, and autoantibodies to C1-INH in up to 70% of patients with AAE [12, 13]. C1q level is typically low in up to 70% of patients, although it may be normal in early stages of the disease [14]. Our patient had low C1-INH activity, low C1-INH level, low C4 complement, and an initially low-normal level of C1q but low repeat C1q levels six months after diagnosis.

Most patients afflicted with C1INH-AAE also have concomitant lymphoproliferative and autoimmune disorders [15]. In one review that included 136 cases of acquired C1 inhibitor deficiency, lymphatic malignancies were identified in 35%, MGUS in 32%, autoimmune diseases in 8%, with adenocarcinoma, and other malignancies identified in 6% [15]. Lymphoproliferative disorders and B-cell malignancies are the most commonly associated conditions [10, 16], especially splenic marginal zone lymphomas [17]. Associated autoimmune disorders include systemic lupus erythematosus, cryoglobulinemia, and autoimmune hemolytic anemia [18, 19]. Interestingly, there have also been reports of association with *Helicobacter pylori* [20]. In our case, the patient had been recently diagnosed with CLL, a non-Hodgkin's lymphoma with known association with C1INH-AAE [13, 21–23].

Primary pharmacologic treatment for acute C1INH-AAE includes C1 esterase inhibitor concentrate from human plasma or recombinant C1 inhibitor concentrate, icatibant (a synthetic bradykinin B_2 receptor antagonist), and/or ecallantide (a kallikrein inhibitor). The most widely used therapy is C1 esterase inhibitor concentrate, although resistance to this treatment over time, necessitating higher doses to control symptoms, has been reported [10].

Importantly, unlike more common causes of angioedema including allergic and drug-induced angioedema, acute presentations of C1INH-AAE typically do not respond to corticosteroids, antihistamine, or epinephrine [24]. Prophylactic treatment to prevent recurrent symptoms of C1INH-AAE includes C1 esterase inhibitor concentrate administered every 3-4 days, attenuated androgens (i.e., danazol and stanozolol) and antifibrinolytic agents [17, 25]. Our index patient received C1 esterase inhibitor concentrate and icatibant twice weekly prophylaxis with C1 esterase inhibitor concentrate. He experienced resolution of his symptoms following initiation of that therapy and treatment of his lymphoma with chemotherapy. Other case reports have documented similar improvement in angioedema symptoms following treatment of lymphoma [26].

Physicians caring for patients with unexplained abdominal pain especially with concomitant skin, lip, or airway swelling should consider angioedema as a possibility and should check laboratory testing for confirmation.

7. Teaching Points

(1) Wider appreciation of the possibility of C1INH-AAE in refractory recurrent abdominal pain, particularly in patients with lymphoproliferative disorders, could lead to proper and timely medical therapy and avert fatal respiratory complications from laryngeal and upper airway edema.

(2) Abdominal symptoms in C1INH-AAE may mimic gastroenteritis and diverticulitis, whereas nonpitting cutaneous edema may be mistaken for allergic reactions and thrombophlebitis.

(3) Unlike more common causes of angioedema including allergic and drug-induced angioedema, acute presentations of angioedema secondary to C1 esterase deficiency typically do not respond to corticosteroids, antihistamine, or epinephrine and necessitate treatment with C1 inhibitor replacement therapy, icatibant, ecallantide, or fresh frozen plasma.

(4) If an underlying associated disease is identified in a patient with C1INH-AAE, including lymphoproliferative malignancy or autoimmune disease, treatment of the underlying disease may lead to symptomatic improvement of C1INH-AAE.

Conflicts of Interest

The authors declare that there are no conflicts of interest regarding the publication of this paper.

References

[1] E. Pappalardo, M. Cicardi, C. Duponchel et al., "Frequent de novo mutations and exon deletions in the C1 inhibitor gene of patients with angioedema," *Journal of Allergy and Clinical Immunology*, vol. 106, no. 6, pp. 1147–1154, 2000.

[2] M. Cicardi and A. Zanichelli, "Acquired angioedema," *Allergy, Asthma and Clinical Immunology*, vol. 6, no. 1, p. 14, 2010.

[3] D. Gobert, R. Paule, D. Ponard et al., "A nationwide study of acquired C1-inhibitor deficiency in France: characteristics and treatment responses in 92 patients," *Medicine*, vol. 95, no. 33, p. e4363, 2016.

[4] M. P. Henao, T. Craig, J. Kraschnewski, and T. Kelbel, "Diagnosis and screening of patients with hereditary angioedema in primary care," *Therapeutics and Clinical Risk Management*, vol. 12, pp. 701–711, 2016.

[5] G. Dobson, D. Edgar, and J. Trinder, "Angioedema of the tongue due to acquired C1 esterase inhibitor deficiency," *Anaesthesia And Intensive Care*, vol. 31, no. 1, pp. 99–102, 2003.

[6] K. Bork, K. Siedlecki, S. Bosch, R. E. Schopf, and W. Kreuz, "Asphyxiation by laryngeal edema in patients with hereditary angioedema," *Mayo Clinic Proceedings*, vol. 75, no. 4, pp. 349–354, 2000.

[7] S. Jolles, P. Williams, and E. Carne, "A UK national audit of hereditary and acquired angioedema," *Clinical and Experimental Immunology*, vol. 175, no. 1, pp. 59–67, 2014.

[8] T. Caballero, M. L. Baeza, R. Cabañas et al., "Consensus statement on the diagnosis, management, and treatment of angioedema mediated by bradykinin. Part I. Classification, epidemiology, pathophysiology, genetics, clinical symptoms, and diagnosis," *Journal of Investigational Allergology and Clinical Immunology*, vol. 21, no. 5, pp. 333–347, 2011.

[9] M. Cugno, R. Castelli, and M. Cicardi, "Angioedema due to acquired C1-inhibitor deficiency: a bridging condition between autoimmunity and lymphoproliferation," *Autoimmunity Reviews*, vol. 8, no. 2, pp. 156–159, 2008.

[10] M. Cicardi, L. C. Zingale, E. Pappalardo, A. Folcioni, and A. Agostoni, "Autoantibodies and lymphoproliferative diseases in acquired C1-inhibitor deficiencies," *Medicine*, vol. 82, no. 4, pp. 274–281, 2003.

[11] M. A. Wu and R. Castelli, "The Janus faces of acquired angioedema: C1-inhibitor deficiency, lymphoproliferation and autoimmunity," *Clinical Chemistry and Laboratory Medicine*, vol. 54, no. 2, pp. 207–214, 2016.

[12] M. Cicardi and A. Zanichelli, "Angioedema due to C1 inhibitor deficiency in 2010," *Internal and Emergency Medicine*, vol. 5, no. 6, pp. 481–486, 2010.

[13] M. Jung and L. Rice, ""Surgical" abdomen in a patient with chronic lymphocytic leukemia: a case of acquired angioedema," *Journal of Gastrointestinal Surgery*, vol. 15, no. 12, pp. 2262–2266, 2011.

[14] M. Cicardi, "Acquired C1 Inhibitor Deficiency: Clinical Manifestations, Epidemiology, Pathogenesis, and Diagnosis," *UptoDate*, 2016.

[15] L. C. Zingale, R. Castelli, A. Zanichelli, and M. Cicardi, "Acquired deficiency of the inhibitor of the first complement component: presentation, diagnosis, course, and conventional management," *Immunology and Allergy Clinics of North America*, vol. 26, no. 4, pp. 669–690, 2006.

[16] M. Cicardi, D. Lambertenghi Deliliers, A. Zanichelli, L. C. Zingale, and R. Castelli, "Lymphoproliferative disease and acquired C1 inhibitor (C1-INH) deficiency," *Journal of Allergy and Clinical Immunology*, vol. 119, no. 1, p. S279, 2007.

[17] R. Castelli, M. A. Wu, M. Arquati et al., "High prevalence of splenic marginal zone lymphoma among patients with acquired C1 inhibitor deficiency," *British Journal of Haematology*, vol. 172, no. 6, pp. 902–908, 2016.

[18] P. Cacoub, V. Frémeaux-Bacchi, I. De Lacroix et al., "A new type of acquired C1 inhibitor deficiency associated with systemic lupus erythematosus," *Arthritis and Rheumatism*, vol. 44, no. 8, pp. 1836–1840, 2001.

[19] J. Gelfand, G. R. Boss, C. L. Conley, R. Reinhart, and M. M. Frank, "Acquired C1 esterase inhibitor deficiency and angioedema: a review," *Medicine*, vol. 58, no. 4, pp. 321–328, 1979.

[20] D. Mukeba, K. Chandrikakumari, J. B. Giot et al., "Autoimmune angioneurotic edema in a patient with *Helicobacter pylori* infection," *Helicobacter*, vol. 14, no. 1, pp. 9–11, 2009.

[21] G. Mohyuddin and I. Rabinowitz, "A patient with chronic lymphocytic leukemia and acquired angioedema: correlation of clinical and biochemical response to CLL therapy," *Ecancermedicalscience*, vol. 7, p. 292, 2013.

[22] N. Klossowski, S. A. Braun, V. von Gruben et al., "Acquired angioedema with C1-INH deficiency and accompanying chronic spontaneous urticaria in a patient with chronic lymphatic B cell leukemia," *Der Hautarzt*, vol. 66, no. 10, pp. 723–725, 2015.

[23] R. Castelli, A. Zanichelli, M. Cicardi, and M. Cugno, "Acquired C1-inhibitor deficiency and lymphoproliferative disorders: a tight relationship," *Critical Reviews in Oncology/Hematology*, vol. 87, no. 3, pp. 323–332, 2013.

[24] A. Agostoni, E. Aygören-Pürsün, K. E. Binkley et al., "Hereditary and acquired angioedema: problems and progress: proceedings of the third C1 esterase inhibitor deficiency workshop and beyond," *Journal of Allergy and Clinical Immunology*, vol. 114, no. 3, pp. S51–S131, 2004.

[25] M. Cicardi, C. Suffritti, F. Perego, and S. Caccia, "Novelties in the diagnosis and treatment of angioedema," *Journal of Investigational Allergology and Clinical Immunology*, vol. 26, no. 4, pp. 212–221, 2016.

[26] A. Branellec, L. Bouillet, N. Javaud et al., "Acquired C1-inhibitor deficiency: 7 patients treated with rituximab," *Journal of Clinical Immunology*, vol. 32, no. 5, pp. 936–941, 2012.

Permissions

All chapters in this book were first published in CRH, by Hindawi Publishing Corporation; hereby published with permission under the Creative Commons Attribution License or equivalent. Every chapter published in this book has been scrutinized by our experts. Their significance has been extensively debated. The topics covered herein carry significant findings which will fuel the growth of the discipline. They may even be implemented as practical applications or may be referred to as a beginning point for another development.

The contributors of this book come from diverse backgrounds, making this book a truly international effort. This book will bring forth new frontiers with its revolutionizing research information and detailed analysis of the nascent developments around the world.

We would like to thank all the contributing authors for lending their expertise to make the book truly unique. They have played a crucial role in the development of this book. Without their invaluable contributions this book wouldn't have been possible. They have made vital efforts to compile up to date information on the varied aspects of this subject to make this book a valuable addition to the collection of many professionals and students.

This book was conceptualized with the vision of imparting up-to-date information and advanced data in this field. To ensure the same, a matchless editorial board was set up. Every individual on the board went through rigorous rounds of assessment to prove their worth. After which they invested a large part of their time researching and compiling the most relevant data for our readers.

The editorial board has been involved in producing this book since its inception. They have spent rigorous hours researching and exploring the diverse topics which have resulted in the successful publishing of this book. They have passed on their knowledge of decades through this book. To expedite this challenging task, the publisher supported the team at every step. A small team of assistant editors was also appointed to further simplify the editing procedure and attain best results for the readers.

Apart from the editorial board, the designing team has also invested a significant amount of their time in understanding the subject and creating the most relevant covers. They scrutinized every image to scout for the most suitable representation of the subject and create an appropriate cover for the book.

The publishing team has been an ardent support to the editorial, designing and production team. Their endless efforts to recruit the best for this project, has resulted in the accomplishment of this book. They are a veteran in the field of academics and their pool of knowledge is as vast as their experience in printing. Their expertise and guidance has proved useful at every step. Their uncompromising quality standards have made this book an exceptional effort. Their encouragement from time to time has been an inspiration for everyone.

The publisher and the editorial board hope that this book will prove to be a valuable piece of knowledge for researchers, students, practitioners and scholars across the globe.

List of Contributors

Vadim R. Gorodetskiy
Department of Intensive Methods of Therapy, V.A. Nasonova Research Institute of Rheumatology, Russian Academy of Medical Sciences, Kashirskoye shosse 34A, Moscow 115522, Russia

Natalya A. Probatova and Tatiana T. Kondratieva
Department of Pathology, N.N. Blokhin Russian Cancer Research Center, Russian Academy of Medical Sciences, Kashirskoye shosse 24, Moscow 115478, Russia

M. Guerreiro, A. H. Santos, P. Gomes and C. Marques
Department of Clinical Hematology, Centro Hospitalar São João, Alameda Professor Hernâni Monteiro, 4200-319 Porto, Portugal

F. Príncipe, M. J. Teles and M. Guerreiro
Department of Clinical Pathology, Centro Hospitalar São João, Alameda Professor Hernâni Monteiro, 4200-319 Porto, Portugal

S. Fonseca, A. H. Santos, M. Lima and M. Guerreiro
Department of Hematology, Laboratory of Cytometry, Hospital de Santo António, Centro Hospitalar do Porto, Rua D. Manuel II,s/n, 4099-001 Porto, Portugal

E. Fonseca
Department of Pathology, Centro Hospitalar São João, Alameda Professor Hernâni Monteiro, 4200-319 Porto, Portugal

M. A. Sobas, M. Podolak-Dawidziak, J. Rybka, M. Biedro N, M. Sawicki, J. Dybko and K. Kuliczkowski
Department of Haematology, Blood Neoplasms and Bone Marrow Transplantation,Medical University of Wrocław, Wrocław, Poland

K. Zduniak
Department of Pathology, Medical University Wrocław, Wrocław, Poland

Naoko Kudo and Shinsaku Imashuku
Division of Hematology, Takasago-seibu Hospital, Takasago 676-0812, Japan

Masakatsu Usui and Kenji Miki
Department of Internal Medicine, Uji-Tokushukai Medical Center, Uji 611-0042, Japan

Yukiharu Nakabo
e Center for Hematological Diseases, Takeda General Hospital, Kyoto 601-1495, Japan

Ken-ichi Yoshida
Division of Ophthalmology, Takasago-seibu Hospital, Takasago 676-0812, Japan

Takashi Osafune
Department of Urology, Uji-Tokushukai Medical Center, Uji 611-0042, Japan

Keisuke Nishimura
Department of Pathology, Uji-Tokushukai Medical Center, Uji 611-0042, Japan

Shinsaku Imashuku
Department of Laboratory Medicine, Uji-Tokushukai Medical Center, Uji 611-0042, Japan

Mohamed Hassanein, Lilit Karapetyan, Afshan Khan and Supratik Rayamajhi
Michigan State University, Clinical Center, 788 Service Road, East Lansing, MI 48824, USA

Suyash Dahal
KIST Medical College and Teaching Hospital, Lalitpur, Nepal

Sumit Dahal, Dipesh K. C. Ghimire and Ebad Ur Rahman
Interfaith Medical Center, Brooklyn, NY, USA

Eliza Sharma
Maimonides Medical Center, Brooklyn, NY, USA

Hind Salama and Ayman Alhejazi
Division of Hematology and HSCT, Department of Oncology, King Abdulaziz Medical City, Riyadh, Saudi Arabia

Suleiman Kojan
Department of Neurology, King Abdulaziz Medical City, Riyadh, Saudi Arabia

Suleiman Kojan, Fahad Azzumeea and Ayman Alhejazi
College of Medicine, King Saud bin Abdulaziz University for Health Science, Riyadh, Saudi Arabia

Shaima Abdulrahman and Fahad Azzumeea
Department of Medical Imaging, King Abdulaziz Medical City, Riyadh, Saudi Arabia

Marta Lopes, Maria dos Anjos Teixeira and Cláudia Casais
Serviço de Hematologia Clínica, Hospital de Santo António (HSA), Centro Hospitalar do Porto (CHP), Porto, Portugal

Maria dos Anjos Teixeira
Laboratório de Citometria, Serviço de Hematologia Clínica, Hospital de Santo António (HSA), Centro Hospitalar do Porto (CHP), Porto, Portugal
Unidade Multidisciplinar de Investigação Biomédicas, Instituto de Ciências Biomédicas Abel Salazar da Universidade do Porto (UMIB/ICBAS/UP), Porto, Portugal

Maria Jara-Acevedo
Sequencing Service (NUCLEUS), University of Salamanca, Salamanca, Spain
Institute of Biomedical Research of Salamanca (IBSAL), Salamanca, Spain
Biomedical Research Networking Centre Consortium (CIBER-CIBERONC), Madrid, Spain

Alberto Orfao
Institute of Biomedical Research of Salamanca (IBSAL), Salamanca, Spain
Biomedical Research Networking Centre Consortium (CIBER-CIBERONC), Madrid, Spain
Cytometry Service (NUCLEUS), University of Salamanca, Salamanca, Spain
Cancer Research Centre (IBMCC, USAL-CSIC), University of Salamanca, Salamanca, Spain
Department of Medicine, University of Salamanca, Salamanca, Spain

Mitsutaka Nishimoto, Hirohisa Nakamae and Masayuki Hino
Hematology, Graduate School of Medicine, Osaka City University, 1-4-3 Asahi-machi, Abeno, Osaka, Japan

Kana Matsumoto, Kunihiko Morita and Hirohisa Nakamae
Department of Clinical Pharmaceutics, Faculty of Pharmaceutical Sciences, DoshishaWomen's College of Liberal Arts, Kodo, Kyotanabe, Kyoto, Japan

Yuki Koga and Hirohisa Nakamae
Department of Cardiovascular Medicine, Graduate School of Medicine, Osaka City University, 1-4-3 Asahi-machi, Abeno, Osaka, Japan

Dai Momose
Department of Hematology, Osaka General Hospital,West Japan Railway Company, 1-2-22 Matsuzaki-cho, Abeno, Osaka, Japan

John Patrick O'Neill, Fiona Quinn, Anita Dowling, Jan Walker and Richard Flavin
1St. James's Hospital, Dublin, Ireland

Triona Hayes and Brian Bird
Bons Secours Hospital, Cork, Ireland

Stephen E. Langabeer
Cancer Molecular Diagnostics, St. James's Hospital, Dublin 8, Ireland

Eibhlin Conneally and Catherine M. Flynn
Department of Haematology, St. James's Hospital, Dublin 8, Ireland

Joselle Cook and Steven Song
Department of Medicine, SUNY Downstate Medical Center, Brooklyn, NY 11203, USA

Anthony Ventimiglia
College of Medicine, SUNY Downstate Medical Center, Brooklyn, NY 11203, USA

Carol Luhrs
Division of Hematology and Oncology, SUNY Downstate Medical Center, Brooklyn, NY 11203, USA

Weerapat Owattanapanich and Theera Ruchutrakool
Division of Hematology, Department of Medicine, Faculty of Medicine, Siriraj Hospital, Mahidol University, Bangkok, Thailand

I. Ramasamy
Department of Biochemistry, Worcester Royal Hospital, Worcester, UK

Z. Rudzki
Heart of England NHS Trust, Birmingham, UK

Pin-Zi Chen, Yee-Jen Wu, Chien-Chih Wu and Yu-Wen Wang
Department of Pharmacy, National Taiwan University Hospital, College of Medicine, National Taiwan University, 7 Chung Shan S. Rd., Taipei, Taiwan

Akihito Fujimi, Yasuhiro Nagamachi and Naofumi Yamauchi
Department of Hematology, Sapporo Kiyota Hospital, Sapporo, Japan

Yuji Kanisawa
Department of Hematology and Oncology, Oji General Hospital, Tomakomai, Japan

Eric X. Wei, Menchu G. Ong, Diana M. Veillon, James D. Cotelingam and Rodney E. Shackelford
Department of Pathology and Translational Pathobiology, LSU Health Shreveport, Shreveport, LA, USA

Vasiliki Leventaki, John K. Choi, Susana C. Raimondi, Elizabeth M. Azzato and Sheila A. Shurtleff
Department of Pathology, St. Jude Children's Research Hospital, Memphis, TN, USA

Feng Li, Xiaomei Zhang, Yanting Guo, Yuandong Zhu, Yicun Wu and Yun Ling
Department of Hematology, The First People's Hospital of Changzhou, The Third Affiliated Hospital of Soochow University, Changzhou, Jiangsu, China

Karan Seegobin and Satish Maharaj
Department of Internal Medicine, University of Florida College of Medicine, Jacksonville, FL 32209, USA

Bharatsinh Gharia and Lara Zuberi
Department of Hematology and Oncology, University of Florida College of Medicine, Jacksonville, FL 32209, USA

John Jacob Kinross-Wright, Kalyan Chakravarthy Potu and Randall Lamfers
Department of Internal Medicine, Sanford USD School of Medicine, Sioux Falls, SD, USA

Brandy Pownell and Kalyan Chakravarthy Potu
Department of Pathology, Sanford USD School of Medicine, Sioux Falls, SD, USA

Jonathan S. Bleeker
Division of Hematology and Oncology, Sanford USD School of Medicine, Sioux Falls, SD, USA

Robert Stuver
Beth Israel Deaconess Medical Center, Department of Internal Medicine, 330 Brookline Avenue, Boston, MA 02215, USA

Alec Petersen
Brigham and Women's Hospital, Department of Internal Medicine, 45 Francis Street, Boston, MA 02115, USA

Thomas A. Guerrero-Garcia, Ursula Matulonis, Paul Richardson and Prabhsimranjot Singh
Dana Farber Cancer Institute, 450 Brookline Avenue, Boston, MA 02215, USA

Masaaki Tsuji, Tatsuki Uchiyama, Chisaki Mizumoto, Tomoharu Takeoka, Kenjiro Tomo and Tatsuharu Ohno
Department of Hematology and Immunology, Otsu Red Cross Hospital, 1-1-35 Nagara, Otsu-shi, Shiga, Japan

Alexandros Makis, Zoi Kanta, Dimitrios Kalogeropoulos and Nikoloaos Chaliasos
Department of Pediatrics, University Hospital of Ioannina, Ioannina, Greece

Zhou Yu, Daniel E. Ezekwudo, Foluso Ogunleye, Susanna S. Gaikazian and Ishmael Jaiyesimi
Department of Hematology and Oncology,William Beaumont Hospital, Royal Oak, MI, USA

Zhou Yu, Yifan Pang, Linda Wang, Daniel E. Ezekwudo, Foluso Ogunleye, Susanna S. Gaikazian, Mark Micale, James Huang, Ann Marie Blenc and Ishmael Jaiyesimi
Oakland UniversityWilliam Beaumont School of Medicine, Rochester, MI, USA

Yifan Pang and Linda Wang
Department of Internal Medicine,William Beaumont Hospital, Royal Oak, MI, USA

Mark Micale, James Huang and Ann Marie Blenc
Department of Pathology and Laboratory Medicine,William Beaumont Hospital, Royal Oak, MI, USA

Fares Darawshy and Arieh Ben-Yehuda
Internal Medicine Division, Internal Medicine C Department, Hebrew University-Hadassah Medical Organization,Jerusalem, Israel

Karine Atlan
The Pathology Institute, Hebrew University-Hadassah Medical Organization, Jerusalem, Israel

Deborah Rund
Hematology Department, Hebrew University-Hadassah Medical Organization, Jerusalem, Israel

Manuel R. Espinoza-Gutarra
Department of Internal Medicine, UT Health San Antonio, 7703 Floyd Curl Drive, San Antonio, TX 78229, USA

Sherri L. Cervantez
Department of Hematology-Oncology, Mays Cancer Center, UT Health San Antonio, 7979 Wurzbach Rd., San Antonio, TX 78229, USA

Zohra Nooruddin
Department of Hematology-Oncology, South Texas VA, 7400 Merton Minter, San Antonio, TX 78229, USA

Filipa Mousinho, Tatiana Mendes, Paula Sousa e Santos and Fernando Lima
1Clinical Hematology Department, Hospital de São Francisco Xavier, Centro Hospitalar de Lisboa Ocidental, Lisbon, Portugal

Maria João Acosta, José Pereira and Maria Arroz
Clinical Pathology Department, Flow Cytometry Laboratory, Hospital de São Francisco Xavier, Centro Hospitalar de Lisboa Ocidental, Lisbon, Portugal

Cândido Silva and Ana Paula Azevedo
Clinical Pathology Department, Hematology Laboratory, Hospital de São Francisco Xavier, Centro Hospitalar de Lisboa Ocidental, Lisbon, Portugal

Rita Oliveira and Martinha Chorão
Pathology Department, Hospital de Egas Moniz, Centro Hospitalar de Lisboa Ocidental, Lisbon, Portugal

Kosuke Miki
School of Medicine, University of Tsukuba, Tsukuba, Japan

Naoshi Obara, Kenichi Makishima, Tatsuhiro Sakamoto, Manabu Kusakabe, Takayasu Kato, Naoki Kurita, Hidekazu Nishikii, Yasuhisa Yokoyama, Mamiko Sakata-Yanagimoto, Yuichi Hasegawa and Shigeru Chiba
Department of Hematology, Faculty of Medicine, University of Tsukuba, Tsukuba, Japan

Madiha Iqbal, Salman Ahmed, Prachi Jani, Salvador Alvarez and Han W. Tun
Department of Hematology and Oncology, Mayo Clinic, Jacksonville, FL, USA

Rabia Saleem
University of Oklahoma, Oklahoma City, OK, USA

Daniel S. O'Neil
Herbert Irving Comprehensive Cancer Center, Columbia University Medical Center-College of Physicians and Surgeons, New York, NY, USA

Mark A. Francescone
Department of Radiology, Columbia University Medical Center-College of Physicians and Surgeons, New York, NY, USA

Karen Khan, Owen A. O'Connor and Ahmed Sawas
Center for Lymphoid Malignancies, Columbia University Medical Center-College of Physicians and Surgeons, New York, NY, USA

Alobeid Bachir
Department of Pathology and Cell Biology, Columbia University Medical Center-College of Physicians and Surgeons, New York, NY, USA

Sebastiano Cicco, Antonio G. Solimando, Patrizia Leone, Stefano Battaglia, Roberto Ria, Angelo Vacca and Vito Racanelli
Department of Biomedical Sciences and Human Oncology, Section of Internal Medicine "G. Baccelli", University of Bari Aldo Moro Medical School, Bari, Italy

Abdullah M. Khan, Jameel Muzaffar, Hermant Murthy, John R. Wingard and Jan S. Moreb
Division of Hematology and Oncology, Department of Medicine, University of Florida, Gainesville, FL, USA

Hamza Hashmi and Drew Murray
Division of Hematology and Oncology, University of Louisville, Louisville, KY, USA

Samer Al-Quran
Department of Pathology and Laboratory Medicine, University of Louisville, Louisville, KY, USA

William Tse
Division of Blood and Marrow Transplant, University of Louisville, Louisville, KY, USA

Maria Sunseri and Tanya Wilcox
Department of Medicine, New York University Langone Health, 550 First Avenue, New York, NY 10016, USA

Tania Ahuja
Department of Pharmacy, New York University Langone Health, 550 First Avenue, New York, NY, USA

David Green
Department of Medicine, New York University Langone Health, Division of Hematology, 550 First Avenue, New York, NY, USA

Samuel Adediran and Nicole Agostino
Lehigh Valley Health Network, Departments of Hematology and Oncology and Medicine, Allentown, PA, USA

Fabrizio Accardi, Laura Notarfranchi, Benedetta Dalla Palma, Franco Aversa and Nicola Giuliani
UO di Ematologia e CTMO, Azienda Ospedaliero-Universitaria di Parma and Department of Medicine and Surgery, University of Parma, Parma, Italy

Valentina Papa, Roberta Costa and Giovanna Cenacchi
Department of Biomedical and Neuromotor Sciences, Alma Mater University of Bologna, Bologna, Italy

Anna Rita Capozzi and Vladimiro Pietrini
Muscle and Nerve Histopathology Laboratory, Neurology Unit, Azienda Ospedaliero-Universitaria di Parma, University of Parma, Parma, Italy

Gian Luca Capello and Laura Verga
Department of Diagnostic Medicine, Electron Microscopy Laboratory, IRCCS Fondazione Policlinico San Matteo and University of Pavia, Pavia, Italy

Cristina Mancini and Eugenia Martella
Pathology Unit, Azienda Ospedaliero-Universitaria di Parma, Parma, Italy

Jacob D. Kjelland
Department of Internal Medicine, University of California Davis Medical Center, Sacramento, CA 98517, USA

Denis M. Dwyre
Department of Pathology, University of California Davis Medical Center, Sacramento, CA 98517, USA

Brian A. Jonas
Department of Internal Medicine, Division of Hematology and Oncology, University of California Davis Medical Center, Sacramento, CA 98517, USA
VA Northern California Health Care System, Mather, CA 95655, USA

Leena T. Rahmat, Aaron C. Logan and Gabriel N. Mannis
Department of Hematologic Malignancies and Blood and Marrow Transplant, University of California, San Francisco, CA, USA

Anna Nguyen and Sonam Prakash
Department of Pathology, University of California, San Francisco, CA, USA

Haifaa Abdulhaq
Department of Hematology and Oncology, University of California, San Francisco, CA, USA

Heather Katz and Mohamed Alsharedi
Department of Hematology/Oncology, Joan C. Edwards School of Medicine Marshall University, 1600 Medical Center Dr, Huntington, WV 25701, USA

Steven Sagun
Joan C. Edwards School of Medicine Marshall University, 1600 Medical Center Dr, Huntington, WV 25701, USA

Doreen Griswold
Department of Pathology, Joan C. Edwards School of Medicine Marshall University, 1600 Medical Center Dr, Huntington, WV 25701, USA

Jason N. Barreto and Erin Frazees
Department of Pharmacy, Mayo Clinic, Rochester, MN, USA

Allison L. McClanahan and Carrie A. Thompson
Division of Hematology, Department of Internal Medicine, Mayo Clinic, Rochester, MN, USA

Andrew D. Rule
Division of Nephrology and Hypertension, Department of Internal Medicine, Mayo Clinic, Rochester, MN, USA
Division of Epidemiology, Department of Health Sciences Research, Mayo Clinic, Rochester, MN, USA

Erin Frazee
Robert D. and Patricia E. Kern Center for the Science of Health Care Delivery, Mayo Clinic, Rochester, MN, USA

Abdullateef Abdulkareem, Joshua Mundorff, Pragya Shrestha, Oluwaseun Shogbesan and Anthony Donato
Department of Medicine, Reading Hospital, West Reading, PA, USA

Ryan S. D'Souza
Department of Anesthesiology, Mayo Clinic Hospital, Rochester, MN, USA

Index

www.ingramcontent.com/pod-product-compliance
Lightning Source LLC
LaVergne TN
LVHW060548210926
848485LV00005B/1276